UNIFORM ANATOMICAL GIFT ACT:

A State-by-State Guide

ISBN 0-922802-07-6

Published by:

Kessinger Publishing Company
P.O. Box 160
Kila, MT 59920

ISBN 0-922802-07-6

Printed in U.S.A.

Disclaimer

This publication is designed to provide accurate and authoritative information in regard to the subject matter covered. It is sold with the understanding that the publisher and author are not engaged in rendering legal, accounting or other professional service. If legal advice or other expert assistance is required, the services of a competent professional person should be sought.—From a Declaration of Principles jointly adopted by a Committee of the American Bar Association and a Committee of Publishers and Associations.

The author has used his best efforts in collecting and preparing material for inclusion in this book, but does not warrant that the information herein is complete or accurate, and does not assume, and hereby disclaims, any liability to any person for any loss or damage caused by errors or omissions in this book whether such errors or omissions result from negligence, accident or any other cause.

This publication contains certain selected statutes only and is not intended to be complete or all inclusive in the subject matter presented. Although every effort has been made to ensure the accuracy of this information, it is not intended as a substitute for the law or for opinions and decisions of the courts.

The publisher and author will not be held responsible for typographical errors, misprints, and misinformation which may be found herein.

This publication is intended purely for educational purposes. Because the United States currently functions under an evolutionary legal system, the reader bears the burden of assuring that the principles of law stated in this work are current and binding at the time of any intended use or application. Caution: The law in this country is subject to change arbitrarily and without prior notice.

TABLE OF CONTENTS

ALABAMA

UNIFORM ANATOMICAL GIFT ACT

§ 22-19-40. Short title.

This article may be cited as the Alabama Uniform Anatomical Gift Act.

§ 22-19-41. Definitions.

For the purposes of this article, the following terms shall have the meanings respectively ascribed to them by this section:

(1) BANK OR STORAGE FACILITY. A facility licensed, accredited or approved under the laws of any state for the storage of human bodies, or parts thereof.

(2) DECEDENT. A deceased individual and includes a stillborn infant or fetus.

(3) DONOR. An individual who makes a gift of all, or part of, his body.

(4) HOSPITAL. A hospital licensed under the laws of the state of Alabama, or any subdivision thereof, or under the laws and regulations of the United States government, or any agency thereof.

(5) PART. Organs, tissues, eyes, bones, arteries, blood or other fluids and any other portions of a human body.

(6) PERSON. An individual, corporation, government or governmental subdivision or agency, business trust, estate trust, partnership or association or any other legal entity.

(7) PHYSICIAN OR SURGEON. A physician or surgeon licensed or authorized to practice under the laws of any state.

§ 22-19-42. Who may donate all, or part of, body; rights of donees.

(a) Any individual of sound mind and 18 years of age or older may give all, or any part of, his body for any purposes specified in section 22-19-43, the gift to take effect upon death.

(b) Any of the following persons, in order of priority stated, when persons in prior classes are not available at the time of death, and in the absence of actual notice of contrary indications by the decedent or actual notice of opposition by a member of the same or a prior class, may give all, or any part of, the decedent's body for any purpose specified in section 22-19-43:

(1) The spouse;

(2) An adult son or daughter;

(3) Either parent;

(4) An adult brother or sister;

(5) A guardian of the person of the deceased at the time of his death; or

(6) Any other person authorized or under obligation to dispose of the body.

(c) If the donee has actual notice of contrary indications by the decedent or that a gift by a member of a class is opposed by a member of the same or of a prior class, the donee shall not accept the gift. The persons authorized by subsection (b) of this section may make the gift after or immediately before death.

(d) A gift of all, or part of, a body authorizes any examination necessary to assure medical acceptability of the gift for the purposes intended.

(e) The rights of the donee created by the gift are paramount to the rights of others, except as provided by subsection (d) of section 22-19-47.

§ 22-19-43. Institutions or persons who may become donees; purposes for which anatomical gifts may be made.

The following persons may become donees of gifts of bodies, or parts thereof, for the purposes stated:

(1) Any hospital, surgeon or physician for medical or dental education, research, advancement or medical or dental science, therapy or transplantation;

(2) Any accredited medical or dental school or college or university for education, research, advancement of medical or dental science or therapy;

(3) Any bank or storage facility for medical or dental education, research, advancement of medical or dental science, therapy or transplantation; or

(4) Any specified individual for therapy or transplantation needed by him.

§ 22-19-44. Modes of executing gift.

(a) A gift of all or part of the body under subsection (a) of section 22-19-42 may be made by will. The gift becomes effective upon the death of the testator without waiting for probate. If the will is not probated, or if it is declared invalid for testamentary purposes, the gift, to the extent that it has been acted upon in good faith, is nevertheless valid and effective.

(b) A gift of all or part of the body under subsection (a) of section 22-19-42 may also be made by document other than a will. The gift becomes effective upon the death of the donor. The document, which may be a card designed to be carried on the person, must be signed by the donor in the presence of two witnesses, who must sign the document in his presence. If the donor cannot sign, the document may be signed for him at his direction and in his presence and in the presence of two witnesses, who must sign the document in his presence. Delivery of the document of gift during the donor's lifetime is not necessary to make the gift valid.

(c) The gift may be made either to a specified donee or without naming a donee. If the donee is not named, the attending physician may accept as donee upon or following death. If the gift is made to a specified donee who is not available at the time and place of death, the attending physician may, in the absence of any expressed indication that the donor desired otherwise, accept the gift as donee. The physician who becomes a donee under this subsection shall not participate in the procedures for removing or transplanting a part.

(d) The donor may designate in his will, card or other document of gift the surgeon or physician to carry out the appropriate procedures. In the absence of a designation, or if the designee is not available, the donee or other person authorized to accept the gift may comply or authorize any surgeon or physician for the purpose.

(e) Any gift by a person designated in subsection (b) of section 22-19-42 shall be made by a document signed by him or made by his telegraphic, recorded telephonic or other recorded message.

§ 22-19-45. Delivery or deposit of gift document.

If the gift is made by the donor to a specified donee, the will, card or other document, or an executed copy thereof, may be delivered to the donee to expedite the appropriate procedures immediately after death. Delivery is not necessary to the validity of the gift. The will, card or other document, or an executed copy thereof, may be deposited in any hospital, bank or storage facility or registry office that accepts it for safekeeping or for facilitation of procedures after death. On request of any interested party upon, or after, the donor's death, the person in possession shall produce the document for examination.

§ 22-19-46. Amendment or revocation of gift.

(a) If the will, card or other document, or executed copy thereof, has been delivered to a specified donee, the donor may amend or revoke the gift by:

(1) The execution and delivery to the donee of a signed statement;

(2) An oral statement made in the presence of two persons and communicated to the donee;

(3) A statement during a terminal illness or injury addressed to an attending physician and communicated to the donee; or

(4) A signed card or document found on his person or in his effects.

(b) Any document of gift which has not been delivered to the donee may be revoked by the donor in the manner set out in subsection (a) of this section or by destruction, cancellation or mutilation of the document and all executed copies thereof.

(c) Any gift made by a will may also be amended or revoked in the manner provided for amendment or revocation of wills or as provided in subsection (a) of this section.

§ 22-19-47. Powers, duties and liabilities upon death.

(a) The donee may accept or reject the gift. If the donee accepts a gift of the entire body, he may, subject to the terms of the gift, authorize embalming and the use of the body in funeral services. If the gift is of a part of the body, the donee, upon the death of the donor and prior to embalming, shall cause the part to be removed without unnecessary mutilation. After removal of the part, custody or the remainder of the body vests in the surviving spouse, next of kin or other persons under obligations to dispose of the body.

(b) The time of death shall be determined by a physician who attends the donor at his death or, if none, the physician who certifies the death. The physician shall not participate in the procedures for removing or transplanting a part.

(c) A person who acts in good faith in accord with the terms of this article or with the anatomical gift laws of another state or a foreign country is not liable for damages in any civil action or subject to prosecution in any criminal proceeding for his act.

(d) The provisions of this article are subject to the laws of this state prescribing powers and duties with respect to autopsies.

ANATOMICAL GIFTS BY HOLDERS OF DRIVERS' LICENSES OR NONDRIVER IDENTIFICATION CARDS

§ 22-19-60. Gift made by execution of affidavit to be filed with department of public safety; notice of intent and specific gift to be noted on driver's license or nondriver identification card; when gift effective; execution and acknowledgment of affidavit; effect of expiration, revocation, renewal, etc., of license or card.

(a) A gift of all or part of the body may be made by the holder of a valid Alabama driver's license or nondriver identification card by the execution of a sworn affidavit to be filed with the department of public safety.

(b) Notice of intent to make a gift shall be noted on the driver's license or nondriver identification card of the donor in a manner to be determined by the department of public safety and there shall also be noted thereon the specific gift of the donor in accordance with the following legend:

E — Eye
K — Kidney
H — Heart
Li — Liver

L — Lungs

A — All (everything)

(c) The gift shall become effective on the death of the donor without any formal requirements of delivery.

(d) The affidavit shall be signed by the holder of the driver's license or nondriver identification card in the presence of two witnesses who shall acknowledge the affidavit in the presence of the donor.

(e) The gift shall become invalidated upon the expiration, cancellation, revocation or suspension of a driver's license or nondriver identification card.

(f) The gift shall not become invalidated if the driver's license or nondriver identification card is properly renewed before the expiration date.

(g) The amendatory provisions of subsection (b) of this section shall commence on the date of renewal of the driver's license or nondriver identification card of the donor.

ALASKA

UNIFORM ANATOMICAL GIFT ACT

Sec. 13.50.010. Persons who may execute an anatomical gift.

(a) A person of sound mind who is 18 or more years of age may make a gift to take effect upon death, of all or a part of the person's body for a purpose specified in AS 13.50.020.

(b) When persons in prior classes are not available at the time of death, and in the absence of actual notice of contrary indications by the decedent or actual notice of opposition by a member of the same or a prior class, any of the following persons, in order of priority listed, may give all or a part of the decedent's body for a purpose specified in AS 13.50.020:

(1) the spouse;

(2) an adult son or daughter;

(3) either parent;

(4) an adult brother or sister;

(5) a guardian of the decedent at the time of death;

(6) any other person authorized or under obligation to dispose of the body.

(c) The persons authorized by (b) of this section may make the gift after or immediately before death.

(d) If the donee has actual notice of contrary indications by the decedent or that a gift by a member of a class is opposed by a member of the same or a prior class, the donee may not accept the gift.

(e) A gift of all or a part of a body authorizes any examination necessary to assure medical acceptability of the gift for the purpose intended.

(f) The rights of the donee created by the gift are superior to the rights of others except as provided in AS 13.50.060(d).

Sec. 13.50.014. Requests by hospitals for anatomical gifts.

(a) When a person dies in a hospital or is pronounced dead after arriving at a hospital, the administrator or a designated employee shall request a gift under AS 13.50.010(b), unless the administrator or employee knows that the person has executed a gift.

(b) Each hospital in the state shall develop procedures for identifying potential donors of gifts, notifying and coordinating with eye banks, tissue banks, and organ procurement agencies, and assisting in the procurement, removal, storage, and transportation of gifts. The procedures must specify the circumstances under which it is inappropriate to request a gift, such as if the gift is unsuitable, if the request is likely to offend the donor's religious beliefs, or if asked to make the request is likely to cause undue emotional distress to the person who would be making the gift. The procedures must encourage reasonable discretion and sensitivity.

(c) The commissioner of health and social services shall exempt from the requirements of this section a hospital that lacks the means to properly remove, store, or transport gifts.

Sec. 13.50.016. Investigations by law enforcement and medical personnel.

Law enforcement or medical personnel who respond to the scene of an accident or emergency involving the death of a person and who know that the person executed a gift shall inform appropriate hospital personnel of the gift.

Sec. 13.50.020. Potential donees and purposes for which anatomical gifts may be made.

The following persons may become donees of gifts of a decedent's body or a part of a decedent's body for the purposes stated:

(1) a hospital, surgeon, or physician, for medical or dental education, research, advancement of medical or dental science, therapy, or transplantation;

(2) an accredited medical or dental school, college or university for education, research, advancement of medical or dental science, or therapy;

(3) a bank or storage facility, for medical or dental education, research, advancement of medical or dental science, therapy, or transplantation; or

(4) a specified individual for therapy or transplantation needed by the individual.

Sec. 13.50.030. Manner of executing anatomical gifts.

(a) A gift of all or a part of the body under AS 13.50.010(a) may be made by will. The gift takes effect upon the death of the testator before probate. If the will is not probated, or is declared invalid for testamentary purposes, the gift, to the extent that it has been acted upon in good faith, is valid and effective.

(b) A gift of all or a part of the body under AS 13.50.010(a) may be made by a document other than a will. The gift takes effect upon the death of the donor. The document, which may be a card designed to be carried on the person, shall be signed by the donor in the presence of two witnesses who shall sign the document in the donor's presence. If the donor cannot sign, the document may be signed for the donor at the donor's direction and in the donor's presence in the presence of two witnesses who must sign the document in the donor's presence. Delivery of the document of gift during the donor's lifetime is not necessary to make the gift valid.

(c) A gift may be made to a specified donee or without specifying a donee. If a donee is not specified, the gift may be accepted by the attending physician as donee upon or after death. If the gift is made to a specified donee who is not available at the time and place of death, the attending physician upon or following death, in the absence of any express indication that the donor desired otherwise, may accept the gift as donee.

(d) The donor may designate in a will, card, or other document of gift the surgeon or physician to carry out the appropriate procedure for removing or transplanting a part of the decedent's body. In the absence of a designation or if the designee is not available, the donee or other person authorized to accept the gift may employ or authorize any surgeon or physician for the purpose of removing or transplanting a part of the decedent's body.

(e) A gift by a person designated in AS 13.50.010(b) shall be made by a document signed by the person or made by the person's telegraphic, recorded telephonic, or other recorded message.

Sec. 13.50.040. Delivery of document of gift.

If the gift is made by the donor to a specified donee, the will, card, or other document, or an executed copy of it, may be delivered to the donee to expedite the appropriate procedure for removing or transplanting a part of the decedent's body immediately after death. Delivery is not necessary for a valid gift. The will, card, or other document, or an executed copy of it, may be deposited in a hospital, bank or storage facility, or registry office to facilitate the procedure for removing or transplanting a part of the decedent's body after death. On the request of any interested person upon or after the donor's death, the person in possession of the document shall produce the document for examination.

Sec. 13.50.050. Amendment or revocation of the gift.

(a) If the will, card, or other document or executed copy of it is delivered to a specified donee, the donor may amend or revoke the gift by
    (1) the execution and delivery to the donee of a signed statement;
    (2) an oral statement made in the presence of two persons and communicated to the donee;
    (3) a statement during a terminal illness or injury addressed to an attending physician and communicated to the donee; or
    (4) a signed card or document found on the donor's person or in the donor's effects.

(b) A document of gift which is not delivered to the donee may be revoked by the donor as provided in (a) of this section or by destruction, cancellation, or mutilation of the document and all executed copies of it.

(c) A gift made by a will may be amended or revoked in the manner provided for amendment or revocation of wills or as provided in (a) of this section.

Sec. 13.50.060. Rights and duties at death.

(a) The donee may accept or reject the gift. If the donee accepts a gift of the entire body, the donee may, subject to the terms of the gift, authorize embalming and the use of the body in funeral services. If the gift is of a part of the body, the donee, upon the death of the donor and before embalming shall have the part removed without unnecessary mutilation. After removal of the part of the body, custody of the remainder of the body vests in the surviving spouse, next of kin, or a person other than the spouse or next of kin who is authorized to dispose of the body. A person described in AS 13.50.010(b) and the estate of the donor may not be held liable for the cost of an examination under AS 13.50.010(e) or any costs related to the removal, storage, or transportation of a gift.

(b) The time of death shall be determined by a physician who attends the donor at death, or, if no physician attends, by the physician who certifies the death. The physician may not participate in the procedures for removing or transplanting a part of the body, except as provided in AS 13.50.030(d).

(c) A person who acts in good faith in accordance with the terms of this chapter or the anatomical gift laws of another state or country is not liable for damages for the act in a civil action or subject to prosecution in a criminal proceeding for the act.

(d) The provisions of this chapter are subject to the state autopsy laws under AS 12.65.

Sec. 13.50.065. Regulations.

The commissioner of health and social services shall adopt regulations for the appropriate training of hospital employees who are designated under AS 13.50.014 to request gifts and for the implementation of this chapter.

Sec. 13.50.070. Definitions.

In this chapter
    (1) "bank or storage facility" means a facility licensed, accredited, or approved under the laws of any state for storage of human bodies or parts of them;
    (2) "decedent" means a deceased individual, stillborn infant, or fetus;
    (3) "donor" means an individual who makes a gift of all or a part of the individual's body;

(4) "gift" means an anatomical gift of all or part of a person's body;

(5) "hospital" means a hospital licensed, accredited, or approved under the laws of any state; or a hospital operated by the United States government, or a subdivision thereof, although not required to be licensed under state laws;

(6) "part" means organs, tissues, eyes, bones, arteries, blood, other fluids and any other portions of a human body;

(7) "physician" or "surgeon" means a physician or surgeon licensed or authorized to practice under the laws of any state;

(8) "state" includes any state, district, commonwealth, territory, insular possession, and any other area subject to the legislative authority of the United States.

Sec. 13.50.080. Uniformity of interpretation.

This chapter shall be construed and interpreted so as to carry out its general purpose to make uniform the laws in those states which enact it.

Sec. 13.50.090. Short title.

This chapter may be cited as the Uniform Anatomical Gift Act.

ARIZONA

UNIFORM ANATOMICAL GIFT ACT

§ 36-841. Definitions.

In this article, unless the context otherwise requires:

1. "Bank or storage facility" means a facility licensed, accredited, or approved under the laws of any state for storage of human bodies or parts thereof.

2. "Decedent" means a deceased individual and includes a stillborn infant or fetus.

3. "Donor" means an individual who makes a gift of all or part of his body.

4. "Hospital" means a hospital licensed, accredited, or approved under the laws of any state and includes a hospital operated by the United States government, a state, or a subdivision thereof, although not required to be licensed under state laws.

5. "Part" means organs, tissues, eyes, bones, arteries, blood, other fluids and any other portions of a human body.

6. "Person" means an individual, corporation, government or governmental subdivision or agency, business trust, estate, trust, partnership or association, or any other legal entity.

7. "Physician" or "surgeon" means a physician or surgeon licensed or authorized to practice under the laws of any state.

8. "State" includes any state, district, commonwealth, territory, insular possession, and any other area subject to the legislative authority of the United States of America.

§ 36-842. Persons who may execute an anatomical gift.

A. Any individual of sound mind and eighteen years of age or more may give all or any part of his body for any purpose specified in § 36-843, the gift to take effect upon death.

B. Any of the following persons, in order of priority stated, when persons in prior classes are not available at the time of death, and in the absence of actual notice of contrary indications by the decedent or actual notice of opposition by a member of the same or a prior class, may give all or any part of the decedent's body for any purpose specified in § 36-843:

1. The spouse.
2. An adult son or daughter.
3. Either parent.
4. An adult brother or sister.
5. A guardian of the person of the decedent at the time of his death.
6. Any other person authorized or under obligation to dispose of the body.

C. If the donee has actual notice of contrary indications by the decedent or that a gift by a member of a class is opposed by a member of the same or a prior class, the donee shall not accept the gift. The persons authorized by subsection B, of this section may make the gift after or immediately before death.

D. A gift of all or part of a body authorizes any examination necessary to assure medical acceptability of the gift for the purposes intended.

E. The rights of the donee created by the gift are paramount to the rights of others except as provided by § 36-847, subsection D.

§ 36-843. Persons who may become donees; purpose for which anatomical gifts may be made.

The following persons may become donees of gifts of bodies or parts thereof for the purposes stated:

1. Any hospital, surgeon or physician, for medical or dental education, research, advancement of medical or dental science, therapy or transplantation.

2. Any accredited medical or dental school, college or university for education, research, advancement of medical or dental science, or therapy.

3. Any bank or storage facility, for medical or dental education, research, advancement of medical or dental science, therapy or transplantation.

4. Any specified individual for therapy or transplantation needed by him.

5. The department of health services, for delivery to any of the institutions or persons listed in paragraphs 1 through 4 which have registered with the department and have requested in writing to be notified by the department of the availability of such gifts of bodies or parts thereof. All expenses of delivery of bodies or parts thereof to such person or institution pursuant to this paragraph shall be paid by the person or institution receiving the body or parts thereof.

§ 36-844. Manner of executing anatomical gifts.

A. A gift of all or part of the body under § 36-842, subsection A may be made by any of the following:

1. A will. The gift becomes effective upon the death of the testator without waiting for probate. If the will is not probated, or if it is declared invalid for testamentary purposes, the gift, to the extent that it has been acted upon in good faith, is nevertheless valid and effective.

2. A sworn affidavit provided by and filed with the motor vehicle division of the department of transportation at the time of application for an operator's or chauffeur's license. Such affidavit shall be in a form prescribed by the director of the department of transportation. The gift becomes effective upon the death of the donor. A gift made under this paragraph shall become invalid upon surrender of the license or execution of the gift revocation signed by the licensee on the reverse of the license. A new affidavit shall be filed upon application for renewal or duplicate issuance of a license. The affidavit shall not be construed to be a last will and testament.

3. A document other than a will or a license. The gift becomes effective upon the death of the donor. The document, which may be a card designed to be carried on the person, must be signed by the donor in the presence of two witnesses who must sign the document in his presence. If the donor cannot sign, the document may be signed for him at his direction and in his presence in the presence of two witnesses who must sign the document in his presence. Delivery of the document of gift during the donor's lifetime is not necessary to make the gift valid.

B. The gift may be made to a specified donee or without specifying a donee. If the latter, the gift may be accepted by the attending physician as donee upon or following death. If the gift is made to a specified donee who is not available at the time and place of death, the attending physician upon or following death, in the absence of any expressed indication that the donor desired otherwise, may accept the gift as donee. The physician who becomes a donee under this subsection shall not participate in the procedures for removing or transplanting a part.

C. Notwithstanding § 36-847, subsection B, the donor may designate in his will, card or other document of gift the surgeon or physician to carry out the appropriate procedures. In the absence of a designation or if the designee is not available, the donee or other person authorized to accept the gift may employ or authorize any surgeon or physician for the purpose.

D. Any gift by a person designated in § 36-842, subsection B, shall be made by a document signed by him or made by his telegraphic, recorded telephonic, or other recorded message.

§ 36-845. Delivery of document of gift.

If the gift is made by the donor to a specified donee, the will, card, license or other document, or an executed copy thereof, may be delivered to the donee to expedite the appropriate procedures immediately after death. Delivery is not necessary to the validity of the gift. The will, card, license or other document, or an executed copy thereof, may be deposited in any hospital, bank or storage facility or registry office that accepts it for safekeeping or for facilitation of procedures after death. On request of any interested party upon or after the donor's death, the person in possession shall produce the document for examination.

§ 36-846. Amendment or revocation of the gift.

A. If the will, card, license or other document or executed copy thereof, has been delivered to a specified donee, the donor may amend or revoke the gift by any of the following methods:

1. The execution and delivery to the donee of a signed statement.
2. An oral statement made in the presence of two persons and communicated to the donee.
3. A statement during a terminal illness or injury addressed to an attending physician and communicated to the donee.
4. A signed card or document found on his person or in his effects.

B. Any document of gift which has not been delivered to the donee may be revoked by the donor in the manner set out in subsection A of this section or by destruction, cancellation or mutilation of the document and all executed copies thereof.

C. Any gift made by a will may also be amended or revoked in the manner provided for amendment or revocation of wills, or as provided in subsection A of this section.

§ 36-847. Rights and duties at death.

A. The donee may accept or reject the gift. If the donee accepts a gift of the entire body, he may, subject to the terms of the gift, authorize embalming and the use of the body in funeral services. If the gift is a part of the body, the donee, upon the death of the donor and prior to embalming, shall cause the part to be removed without unnecessary mutilation. After removal of the part, custody of the remainder of the body vests in the surviving spouse, next of kin, or other persons under obligation to dispose of the body.

B. The time of death shall be determined by a physician who tends the donor at his death, or, if none, the physician who certifies the death. The physician shall not participate in the procedures for removing or transplanting a part.

C. A person who acts in good faith in accord with the terms of this article or with the anatomical gift laws of another state or a foreign country is not liable for damages in any civil action or subject to prosecution in any criminal proceeding for his act.

D. The provisions of this article are subject to the laws of this state prescribing powers and duties with respect to inquests and autopsies.

E. Any person who does not have actual notice of an anatomical gift made under this article or the anatomical gift laws of another state or a foreign country and acts in good faith shall not be liable for damages in any civil action or subject to prosecution in any criminal proceeding for an otherwise lawful act which may render a body or parts thereof unusable to a donee.

§ 36-848. Short title.

This article may be cited as the uniform anatomical gift act.

§ 36-849. Organ and tissue procurement protocol; notification of death to organ or tissue procurement agency; consent to donate; waiver of confidentiality; definition.

A. The person in charge of a hospital, or his designated representative, shall establish an organ and tissue procurement for transplant protocol which includes the notification of an appropriate organ or tissue procurement agency pursuant to subsection B of this section, defining who may obtain any and all consents pursuant to subsection C of this section and requiring specified training for the person who requests such consent in proper and appropriate procedures.

B. At or near the occurrence of death in a hospital, the person in charge of the hospital or his designated representative, other than the physician connected with the determination of death, shall notify an appropriate organ or tissue procurement agency within a period of time to permit a viable donation.

C. At or near the occurrence of death in a hospital, a person who is authorized to obtain consent by the protocol required by subsection A of this section shall, in conformity with the protocol established pursuant to subsection A of this section, attempt to obtain consent to donate pursuant to § 36-842, subsection B the gift of all or any part of the decedent's body for any purpose specified in § 36-843.

D. If, pursuant to § 11-594, subsection A, the county medical examiner must conduct an investigation of the facts surrounding death, the organ or tissue procurement agency shall obtain the consent of the county medical examiner before seeking consent to donate pursuant to § 36-842, subsection B. This section does not relieve a hospital of its duty to report certain deaths to the county medical examiner pursuant to § 11-593.

E. A person authorized pursuant to this section may obtain the consent to donate from a patient or from a minor patient's parent on admission to the hospital as part of its standard admitting procedure.

F. No hospital, person or entity is subject to civil damages or legal action as a consequence of good faith acts or omissions related to procurement of organs or tissue in compliance with this article. All acts and omissions are presumed to be in good faith unless the acts or omissions are done with intent to maliciously cause injury.

G. A consent to donate constitutes a limited waiver of a patient's confidentiality provided by § 12-2235 to the extent that the appropriate organ or tissue procurement agency has access to and may obtain a copy of all or any portion of a medical record necessary to determine whether a person is a suitable organ or tissue donor. A hospital shall release copies of records on request if the agency agrees to pay reasonable copying charges. An organ or tissue procurement agency shall keep the records as confidential and privileged to the same extent as required of the hospital from which they are released.

H. For purposes of this section, "attempt to obtain consent" means reasonable efforts to contact the appropriate person pursuant to § 36-842, subsection B.

ARKANSAS

UNIFORM ANATOMICAL GIFT ACT

20-17-601. Definitions.

As used in this subchapter:

(1) "Anatomical gift" means a donation of all or part of a human body to take effect upon or after death;

(2) "Decedent" means a deceased individual and includes a stillborn infant or fetus;

(3) "Document of a gift" means a card, a statement attached to or imprinted on a motor vehicle operator's or chauffeur's license, a will, or other writing used to make an anatomical gift;

(4) "Donor" means an individual who makes an anatomical gift of all or part of the individual's body;

(5) "Enucleator" means an individual who is certified by the Department of Ophthalmology of the University of Arkansas College of Medicine to remove or process eyes or parts of eyes;

(6) "Hospital" means a facility licensed, accredited, or approved as a hospital under the law of any state or a facility operated as a hospital by the United States government, a state, or a subdivision of a state; by the United states government, a state, or a subdivision of a state;

(7) "Part" means an organ, tissue, eye, bone, artery, blood, fluid, or other portion of a human body;

(8) "Person" means an individual, corporation, business trust, estate, trust, partnership, joint venture, association, government, governmental subdivision or agency, or any other legal or commercial entity;

(9) "Physician" or "surgeon" means an individual licensed or otherwise authorized to practice medicine and surgery or osteopathy and surgery under the laws of any state;

(10) "Procurement organization" means a person licensed, accredited, or approved under the laws of any state for procurement, distribution, or storage of human bodies or parts;

(11) "State" means a state, territory, or possession of the United States, the District of Columbia, or the Commonwealth of Puerto Rico;

(12) "Technician" means any person, who is not a physician or surgeon, who is acting under the direction or supervision of a physician, surgeon, or hospital to remove or process a part.

20-17-602. Making, amending, revoking, and refusing to make anatomical gifts by individual.

(a) An individual who is at least eighteen (18) years of age may:

(i) Make an anatomical gift to one or more of those purposes stated in 20-17-606(a);

(ii) Limit an anatomical gift to one or more of those purposes; or

(iii) Refuse to make an anatomical gift.

(b) An anatomical gift may be made only by a document of gift signed by the donor. If the donor cannot sign, the document of gift must be signed by another individual and by two (2) witnesses, all of whom have signed at the direction and in the presence of the donor and of each other, and state that it has been so signed.

(c) If a document of gift is attached to or imprinted on a donor's motor vehicle operator's or chauffeur's license, the document of gift must comply with subsection (b) of this section. Revocation, suspension, expiration, or cancellation of the license does not invalidate the anatomical gift.

(d) A document of gift may designate a particular physician or surgeon to carry out the appropriate procedures. In the absence of a designation or if the designee is not available, the donee or other person authorized to accept the anatomical gift may employ or authorize any physician, surgeon, technician, or enucleator to carry out the appropriate procedures.

(e) An anatomical gift by will takes effect upon death of the testator, whether or not the will is probated. If, after death, the will is declared invalid for testamentary purposes, the validity of the anatomical gift is unaffected.

(f) A donor may amend or revoke an anatomical gift, not made by will, only by:

(1) A signed statement;

(2) An oral statement made in the presence of two (2) individuals;

(3) Any form of communication during a terminal illness or injury addressed to a physician or surgeon; or

(4) The delivery of a signed statement to a specified donee to whom a document of gift had been delivered.

(g) The donor of an anatomical gift made by will may amend or revoke the gift in the manner provided for amendment or revocation of wills, or as provided in subsection (f) of this section.

(h) An anatomical gift that is not revoked by the donor before death is irrevocable and does not require the consent or concurrence of any person after the donor's death.

(i) An individual may refuse to make an anatomical gift of the individual's body or part by:

(i) Writing signed in the same manner as a document of gift;

(ii) A statement attached to or imprinted on a donor's motor vehicle operator's or chauffeur's license; or

(iii) Any other writing used to identify the individual as refusing to make an anatomical gift. During a terminal illness or injury, the refusal may be an oral statement or other form of communication.

(j) In the absence of contrary indications by the donor, an anatomical gift of a part is neither a refusal to give other parts nor a limitation on an anatomical gift under § 20-17-603 or on a removal or release of other parts under 20-17-604.

(k) In the absence of contrary indications by the donor, a revocation or amendment of an anatomical gift is not a refusal to make another anatomical gift. If the donor intends a revocation to be a refusal to make an anatomical gift, the donor shall make the refusal pursuant to subsection (i) of this section.

(l) The Office of Driver Services of the Department of Finance and Administration shall provide on the reverse side of each operator's or chauffeur's license issued a statement whereby the owner of the license may certify his willingness to make an anatomical gift under this subchapter.

(m) A document of gift may, but is not required to be, in the following form:

ANATOMICAL GIFT BY A LIVING DONOR

Pursuant to the Anatomical Gift Act, § 20-17-601 et seq., upon my death, I hereby give (check boxes applicable):

1. { } Any needed organs, tissues, or parts;
2. { } The following organs, tissues, or parts only_____:
3. { } For the following purposes only

_____
(transplant-therapy-research-education)

_____   _____
Date of Birth   Signature of Donor

_____   _____
Date Signed   Address of Donor

20-17-603. Making, revoking, and objecting to anatomical gifts, by others.

(a) Any member of the following classes of persons, in the order or priority listed, may make an anatomical gift of all or a part of the decedent's body for an authorized purpose, unless the decedent, at the time of death, has made an unrevoked refusal to make that anatomical gift:

(1) The spouse of the decedent;
(2) An adult son or daughter of the decedent;
(3) Either parent of the decedent;
(4) An adult brother or sister of the decedent;
(5) A grandparent of the decedent; and
(6) A guardian of the person of the decedent at the time of death.

(b) An anatomical gift may not be made by a person listed in subsection (a) of this section if:

(1) A person in a prior class is available at the time of death to make an anatomical gift;
(2) The person proposing to make an anatomical gift knows of a refusal or contrary indications by the decedent; or
(3) The person proposing to make an anatomical gift knows of an objection to making an anatomical gift by a member of the person's class or a prior class.

(c) An anatomical gift by a person authorized under subsection (a) of this section must be made by: (i) a document of gift signed by the person or: (ii) the person's telegraphic, recorded telephonic, or other recorded message, or other form of communication from the person that is contemporaneously reduced to writing and signed by the recipient.

(d) An anatomical gift by a person authorized under subsection (a) of this section may be revoked by any member of the same or a prior class if, before procedures have begun for the removal of a part from the body of the decedent, the physician, surgeon, technician, or enucleator removing the part knows of the revocation.

(e) A failure to make anatomical gift under subsection (a) of this section is not an objection to the making of an anatomical gift.

20-17-604. Authorization by coroner or hospital administrator.

(a) The coroner or hospital administrator may release and permit the removal of a part from a body within that coroner's or administrator's custody, for transplantation or therapy, if:

(1) The official or administrator has received a request for the part from a hospital, physician, surgeon, or procurement organization;
(2) The official or administrator has made a reasonable effort, taking into account the useful life of the part, to locate and examine the decedent's medical records and inform persons listed in § 20-17-603(a) of their option to make, or object to making, an anatomical gift;
(3) The official administrator does not know of a refusal or contrary indication by the decedent or objection by a person having priority to act as listed in § 20-17-603(a);
(4) The removal will be by a physician, surgeon, or technician; but in the case of eyes, by one of them or by an enucleator;
(5) The removal will not interfere with any autopsy or investigation;

(6) The removal will be in accordance with accepted medical standards; and

(7) Cosmetic restoration will be done, if appropriate.

(b) A coroner or hospital administrator releasing and permitting the removal of a part shall maintain a permanent record of the name of the decedent, the person making the request, the date and purpose of the request, the part requested, and the person to whom it was released.

20-17-605. Required request — Search and notification.

(a) If, at or near the time of death of a patient, there is no medical record that the patient has made or refused to make an anatomical gift, the hospital administrator or a representative designated by the administrator or a representative designated by the administrator or the attending physician shall discuss the option to make or refuse to make an anatomical gift and request the making of an anatomical gift pursuant to § 20-17-603(a). The request must be made with reasonable discretion and sensitivity to the circumstances of the family. A request is not required if the gift is not suitable, based upon accepted medical standards, for a purpose specified in § 20-17-606. An entry must be made in the medical record of the patient, stating the name and affiliation of the individual making the request, and of the name, response, and relationship to the patient of the person to whom the request was made.

(b) The following persons shall make a reasonable search for a document of gift or other information identifying the bearer as a donor or as an individual who has refused to make an anatomical gift:

(1) A law enforcement officer, fireman, paramedic, or other emergency rescuer finding an individual who the searcher believes is dead or near death; and

(2) A hospital, upon the admission of an individual at or near the time of death, if there is not immediately available any other source of that information.

(c) If a document of gift or evidence of refusal to make an anatomical gift is located by the search required by subsection (b)(1) of this section, and the individual or body to whom it relates is taken to a hospital, the hospital must be notified of the contents and the document or other evidence must be sent to the hospital.

(d) If, at or near the time of death of a patient, a hospital knows that an anatomical gift has been made pursuant to § 20-17-603(a) or a release and removal of a part has been permitted pursuant to § 20-17-604, or that a patient or an individual identified as in transit to the hospital is a donor, the hospital shall notify the donee if one is named and known to the hospital; if not, it shall notify an appropriate procurement organization. The hospital shall cooperate in the implementation of the anatomical gift or release and removal of a part.

(e) A person who fails to discharge the duties imposed by this section is not subject to criminal or civil liability but is subject to appropriate administrative sanctions.

20-17-606. Persons who may become donees — Purposes for which anatomical gifts may be made.

(a) The following persons may become donees of anatomical gifts for the purposes stated:

(1) A hospital, physician, surgeon, or procurement organization, for transplantation, therapy, medical or dental education, research, or advancement of medical or dental science;

(2) An accredited medical or dental school, college, or university for education, research, advancement of medical or dental science; or

(3) A designated individual for transplantation or therapy needed by that individual.

(b) An anatomical gift may be made to a designated donee or without designating a donee. If a donee is not designated or if the donee is not available or rejects the anatomical gift, the anatomical gift may be accepted by any hospital.

(c) If the donee knows of the decedent's refusal or contrary indications to make an anatomical gift or that an anatomical gift by a member of a class having priority to act is opposed by a member of the same class or a prior class under § 20-17-603(a), the donee may not accept the anatomical gift.

20-17-607. Delivery of document of gift.

(a) Delivery of a document of gift during the donor's lifetime is not required for the validity of an anatomical gift.

(b) If an anatomical gift is made to a designated donee, the document of gift, or a copy, may be delivered to the donee to expedite the appropriate procedures after death. The document of gift, or a copy, may be deposited in any hospital, procurement organization, or registry office that accepts it for safekeeping or for facilitation of procedures after death. On request of an interested person, upon or after the donor's death, the person in possession shall allow the interested person to examine or copy the document of gift.

20-17-608. Rights and duties at death.

(a) Rights of a donee created by an anatomical gift are superior to rights of others except with respect to autopsies under § 20-17-611(b). A donee may accept or reject an anatomical gift. If a donee accepts an anatomical gift of an entire body, the donee, subject to the terms of the gift, may allow embalming and use of the body in funeral services. If the gift is a part of a body, the donee, upon the death of the donor and before embalming, shall cause the part to be removed without unnecessary mutilation. After removal of the part, custody of the remainder of the body vests in the person under obligation to dispose of the body.

(b) The time of death must be determined by a physician or surgeon who attends the donor at death or, if none, the physician or surgeon who certifies the death. Neither the physician or surgeon who determines the time of death may participate in the procedures for removing or transplanting a part unless the document of gift designates a particular physician or surgeon pursuant to 20-17-602(d).

(c) If there has been an anatomical gift, a physician, surgeon, or technician may remove any donated parts and an enucleator may remove any donated eyes or parts of eyes, after determination of death by a physician or surgeon.

20-17-609. Coordination of procurement and use.

Each hospital in this state, after consultation with other hospitals and procurement organizations, shall establish agreements or affiliations for coordination of procurement and use of human bodies and parts.

20-17-610. Sales or purchase of parts prohibited.

(a) A person may not knowingly, for valuable consideration, purchase or sell a part for transplantation or therapy, if removal of the part is intended to occur after the death of the decedent.

(b) Valuable consideration does not include reasonable payment for the removal, processing, disposal, preservation, quality control, storage, transportation, or implantation of a part.

(c) A person who violates this section is guilty of a Class C felony.

20-17-611. Examination — Autopsy — Liability.

(a) An anatomical gift authorizes any reasonable examination necessary to assure medical acceptability of the gift for the purposes intended.

(b) The provisions of this subchapter are subject to the laws of this state governing autopsies.

(c) A hospital, physician, surgeon, coroner, hospital administrator, enucleator, technician, or the person, who acts in accordance with this subchapter or with the applicable anatomical gift law of another state or attempts in good faith to do so, is not liable for that act in a civil action or criminal proceeding.

(d) An individual who makes an anatomical gift pursuant to §§ 20-17-602 or 20-17-603 and the individual's estate are not liable for any injury or damage that may result from the making or the use of anatomical gift.

20-17-612. Transitional provisions.

This subchapter applies to a document of gift, revocation, or refusal to make an anatomical gift signed by the donor or person authorized to make or object to making an anatomical gift before, on, or after March 9, 1989.

20-17-613. Uniformity of application and construction.

This subchapter shall be applied and construed to effectuate its general purpose to make uniform the law with respect to the subject of this subchapter among states enacting it.

20-17-614. [Reserved.]

20-17-615. Short title.

This subchapter may be cited as the "Arkansas Anatomical Gift Act".

20-17-616. [Reserved.]

CALIFORNIA

CHAPTER 3.5.
UNIFORM ANATOMICAL GIFT ACT

§7150. Citation.
This chapter may be cited as the "Uniform Anatomical Gift Act."

§7150.01. Definitions.
As used in this chapter:

(a) "Anatomical gift" means a donation of all or part of a human body or a pacemaker to take effect upon or after death.

(b) "Decedent" means a deceased individual and includes a stillborn infant or fetus.

(c) "Document of gift" means a card, a statement attached to or imprinted on a motor vehicle operator's or chauffeur's license, a will, or other writing used to make an anatomical gift.

(d) "Donor" means an individual who makes an anatomical gift of all or part of the individual's body or a pacemaker.

(e) "Enucleator" means an individual who removes or processes eyes or parts of eyes.

(f) "Hospital" means a facility licensed, accredited, or approved as a hospital under the law of any state or a facility operated as a hospital by the United States government, a state, or a subdivision of a state.

(g) "Part" means an organ, tissue, eye, bone, artery, blood, fluid, or other portion of a human body or a pacemaker.

(h) "Person" means an individual, corporation, business trust, estate, trust, partnership, joint venture, association, government, governmental subdivision or agency, or any other legal or commercial entity.

(i) "Physician" or "surgeon" means an individual licensed or otherwise authorized to practice medicine and surgery or osteopathy and surgery under the laws of any state.

(j) "Procurement organization" means a person licensed, accredited, or approved under the laws of any state or by the State Department of Health Services for procurement, distribution, or storage of human bodies or parts.

(k) "State" means a state, territory, or possession of the United States, the District of Columbia, or the Commonwealth of Puerto Rico.

(l) "Technician" means an individual who has completed training in removal of parts for transplant, therapeutic, or scientific purposes, which the donee determines to be adequate for the purpose.

§7150.5. Making, amending, revoking and refusing to make anatomical gifts by individual.

(a) An individual who is at least 18 years of age may make anatomical gift for any of the purposes stated in subdivision (a) of Section 1753, limit an anatomical gift to one or more of those purposes, or refuse to make an anatomical gift.

(b) An anatomical gift may be made only by a document of gift signed by the donor. If the donor cannot sign, the document of gift must be signed by another individual and by two witnesses, all of whom have signed at the direction and in the presence of the donor and of each other, and state that it has been so signed.

(c) If a document of gift is attached to or imprinted on a donor's motor vehicle operator's or chauffeur's license, the document of gift must comply with subdivision (b). Revocation, suspension, expiration, or cancellation of the license does not invalidate the anatomical gift.

(d) A document of gift may designate a particular physician or surgeon to carry out the appropriate procedures. In the absence of a designation or if the designee is not available, the donee or other person authorized to accept the anatomical gift may employ or authorize any physician, surgeon, technician, or enucleator to carry out the appropriate procedures.

(e) An anatomical gift by will takes effect upon death of the testator, whether or not the will is probated. If, after death, the will is declared invalid for testamentary purposes, the validity of the anatomical gift is unaffected.

(f) A donor may amend or revoke an anatomical gift, not made by will, only by one or more of the following:

(1) A signed statement.

(2) An oral statement made in the presence of two individuals.

(3) Any form of communication during a terminal illness or injury addressed to a physician or surgeon.

(4) The delivery of a signed statement to a specified donee to whom a document of gift in the manner provided for amendment or revocation of wills, or as provided in subdivision (f).

(h) An anatomical gift that is not revoked by the donor before death is irrevocable and does not require the consent or concurrence of any person after the donor's death.

(i) An individual may refuse to make an anatomical gift of the individual's body or part by a writing signed in the same manner as a document of gift, a statement attached to or imprinted on a donor's motor vehicle operator's or chauffeur's license, or any other writing used to identify the individual as refusing to make an anatomical gift. During a terminal illness or injury, the refusal may be an oral statement or other form of communication.

(j) In the absence of contrary indications by the donor, an anatomical gift of a part is neither a refusal to give other parts nor a limitation on an anatomical gift under Section 7151.5.

(k) In the absence of contrary indications by the donor, a revocation or amendment of an anatomical gift is not a refusal to make another anatomical gift. If the donor intends a revocation to be a refusal to make an anatomical gift, the donor shall make the refusal pursuant to subdivision (i).

§7151. Making, revoking, and objecting to anatomical gifts, by others.

(a) Except as provided in Section 7152, any member of the following classes of persons, in the order of priority listed, may make an anatomical gift of all or part of the decedent's body or a pacemaker for an authorized purpose, unless the decedent, at the time of death, has made an unrevoked refusal to make that anatomical gift:

(1) The attorney-in-fact under a valid durable power of attorney that expressly authorizes the attorney-in-fact to make an anatomical gift of all or part of the principal's body or a pacemaker.

(2) The spouse of the decedent.

(3) An adult son or daughter of the decedent.

(4) Either parent of the decedent.

(5) An adult brother or sister of the decedent.

(6) A grandparent of the decedent.

(7) A guardian or conservator of the person of the decedent at the time of death.

(b) An anatomical gift may not be made by a person listed in subdivision (a) if any of the following occur:

(1) A person in a prior class is available at the time of death to make an anatomical gift.

(2) The person proposing to make an anatomical gift knows of a refusal or contrary indications by the decedent.

(3) The person proposing to make an anatomical gift knows of an objection to making an anatomical gift by a member of the person's class or a prior class.

(c) An anatomical gift by a person authorized under subdivision (a) shall be made by a document of gift signed by the person or the person's telegraphic, recorded telephonic, or other recorded message, or other form of communication from the person that is contemporaneously reduced to writing and signed by the recipient.

(d) An anatomical gift by a person authorized under subdivision (a) may be revoked by any member of the same or a prior class if, before procedures have begun for the removal of a part from the body of the decedent, the physician, surgeon, technician, or enucleator removing the part knows of the revocation.

(e) A failure to make anatomical gift under subdivision (a) is not an objection to the making of an anatomical gift.

§7151.5. Authorization by coroner or medical examiner, hospital, or local public health officer; records.

(a) Except as provided in Section 7152, the coroner or medical examiner may release and permit the removal of a part from a body within that official's custody, for transplantation, therapy, or reconditioning, if all of the following occur:

(1) The official has received a request for the part from a hospital, physician, surgeon, or procurement organization or, in the case of a pacemaker, from a person who reconditions pacemakers.

(2) A reasonable effort has been made to locate and inform persons listed in subdivision (a) of Section 7151 of their option to make, or object to making, an anatomical gift. Except in the case of corneal material to be used for the purpose of transplantation or where the useful life of the part does not permit, a reasonable effort shall be deemed to have been made when a search for the persons has been underway for at least 24 hours.

(3) The official does not know of a refusal or contrary indication by the decedent or objection by a person having priority to act as listed in subdivision (a) of Section 7151.

(4) The removal will be by a physician, surgeon, or technician; but in the case of eyes, by one of them or by an enucleator.

(5) The removal will not interfere with any autopsy or investigation.

(6) The removal will be in accordance with accepted medical standards.

(7) Cosmetic restoration will be done, if appropriate.

(b) Except as provided in Section 7152, if the body is not within the custody of the coroner or medical examiner, a hospital may release and permit the removal of a part from a body if the hospital, after a reasonable effort has been made to locate and inform persons listed in subdivision (a) of Section 7151 of their option to make, or object to the making, an anatomical gift, determines and certifies that the persons are not available. A search for the persons listed in subdivision (a) of Section 7151 may be initiated in anticipation of death, but, except in the case of corneal material to be used for the purpose of transplantation or where the useful life of the part does not permit, the determination may not be made until the search has been underway for at least 24 hours. The search shall include a check of local police missing persons records, examination of personal effects, and the questioning of any persons visiting the decedent before his or her death or in the hospital, accompanying the decedent's body, or reporting the death, in order to obtain information that might lead to the location of any persons listed in subdivision (a) of Section 7151.

(c) Except as provided in Section 7152, if the body is not within the custody of the coroner or medical examiner or a hospital, the local public health officer may release and permit the removal of any part from a body in the local public health officer's custody for transplantation, therapy, or reconditioning if the requirements of subdivision (a) are met.

(d) An official or hospital releasing and permitting the removal of a part shall maintain a permanent record of the name of the decedent, the person making the request, the date and purpose of the request, the part requested, and the person to whom it was released.

§7151.6. Repealed by Stats. 1988, c. 1095, § 1

§7151.7. Repealed by Stats. 1988, c. 1095, § 1

§7152. Members of faith healing sect or religions with tenets in opposition to anatomical gifts; donations only by decedent.

Only an individual may make an anatomical gift of all or part of the individual's body or a pacemaker, if it is made known that the individual at the time of death was a member of a religion, church, sect, or denomination which relies solely upon prayer for the healing of disease or which has religious tenets that would be violated by the disposition of the human body or parts thereof or a pacemaker for any of the purposes stated in subdivision (a) of Section 7153.

§7152.5 Protocol by hospitals to identify potential donors; search for document and notification.

(a) If, at or near the time of death of a patient, there is no medical record that the patient has made or refused to make an anatomical gift, the hospital shall comply with the protocol developed pursuant to Section 7184.

(b) The following persons shall make a reasonable search for a document of gift or other information identifying the bearer as a donor or as an individual who has refused to make an anatomical gift:

(1) A law enforcement officer finding an individual who the officer believes is dead or near death.

(2) A hospital, upon the admission of an individual at or near the time of death, if there is not immediately available any other source of that information.

(c) If a document of gift or evidence of refusal to make an anatomical gift is located by the search required by paragraph (1) of subdivision (b), and the individual or body to whom it relates is taken to a hospital, the hospital shall be notified of the contents and the document or other evidence shall be sent to the hospital.

(d) If, at or near the time of death of a patient, a hospital knows that an anatomical gift has been made pursuant to subdivision (a) of Section 7151 or a release and removal of a part has been permitted pursuant to Section 7151.5, or that a patient or an individual identified as in transit to the hospital is a donor, the hospital shall notify the donee if one is named and known to the hospital; if not, it shall notify an appropriate procurement organization. The hospital shall cooperate in the implementation of the anatomical gift or release and removal of a part.

(e) A person who fails to discharge the duties imposed by this section is not subject to criminal or civil liability but is subject to appropriate administrative sanctions.

§7153. Person who may become donees; purposes for which anatomical gifts may be made.

(a) The following persons may become donees of anatomical gifts for the purposes stated:

(1) A hospital, physician, surgeon, or procurement organization, for transplantation, therapy, medical or dental education, research, or advancement of medical or dental science.

(2) An accredited medical or dental school, college, or university for education, research, or advancement of medical or dental science.

(3) A designated individual for transplantation or therapy needed by that individual.

(4) In the case of a pacemaker, a person who reconditions pacemakers.

(b) An anatomical gift may be made to a designated donee or without designating a donee. If a donee is not designated or if the donee is not available or rejects the anatomical gift, the anatomical gift may be accepted by any hospital or, in the case of a pacemaker, the pacemaker may be accepted by any person who reconditions pacemakers.

(c) If the donee knows of the decedent's refusal or contrary indications to make an anatomical gift or that an anatomical gift by a member of a class having priority to act is opposed by a member of the same class or a prior class under subdivision (a) of Section 7151, the donee may not accept the anatomical gift.

§7153.5. Delivery of document of gift; examination by interested person.

(a) Delivery of a document of gift during the donor's lifetime is not required for the validity of an anatomical gift.

(b) If an anatomical gift is made to a designated donee, the document of gift, or a copy, may be delivered to the donee to expedite the appropriate procedures after death. The document of gift, or a copy, may be deposited in any hospital, procurement organization, or registry office that accepts it for safekeeping or for facilitation of procedures after death. On request of an interested person, upon or after the donor's death, the person in possession shall allow the interested person to examine or copy the document of gift.

§7154. Rights and duties at death.

(a) Rights of a donee created by an anatomical gift are superior to rights of others except with respect to autopsies under subdivision (b) of Section 7155.5. A donee may accept or reject an anatomical gift. If a donee accepts an anatomical gift of an entire body, the donee, subject to the terms of the gift, may allow embalming and use of the body in funeral services. If the gift is of a part of a body or a pacemaker, the donee, upon the death of the donor and before embalming, shall cause the part or pacemaker to be removed without unnecessary mutilation. After removal of the part or pacemaker, custody of the remainder of the body vests in the person specified in Section 7100.

(b) The time of death must be determined by a physician or surgeon who attends the donor at death, or, if none, the physician or surgeon who certifies the death. Neither the physician or surgeon who attends the donor at death nor the physician or surgeon who determines the time of death may participate in the procedures for removing or transplanting a part unless the document of gift designates a particular physician or surgeon pursuant to subdivision (d) of Section 7150.5.

(c) If there has been an anatomical gift, a technician may remove any donated parts and an enucleator may remove any donated eyes or parts of eyes, after determination of death by a physician or surgeon.

§7154.5 Coordination of procurement and use.

Each hospital in this state, after consultation with other hospitals and procurement organizations, shall establish agreements or affiliations for coordination of procurement and use of human bodies and parts.

§7155. Sale or purchase of parts; prohibition; penalties.

(a) A person may not knowingly, for valuable consideration, purchase or sell a part for transplantation, therapy, or reconditioning, if removal of the part is intended to occur after the death of the decedent.

(b) Valuable consideration does not include reasonable payment for the removal, processing, disposal, preservation, quality control, storage, transplantation, or implantation of a part.

(c) A person who violates this section is guilty of a felony and upon conviction shall be punished by imprisonment in the state prison for three, five, or seven years, a fine not exceeding fifty thousand dollars ($50,000), or both.

§7155.5. Examination; autopsy; immunity from liability.

(a) An anatomical gift authorizes any reasonable examination necessary to assure medical acceptability of the gift for the purposes intended. All donors shall be screened for infectious diseases, including human immunodeficiency virus (HIV) antibody testing, pursuant to regulations adopted by the State Department of Health Services.

(b) The provisions of this chapter are subject to the laws of this state governing autopsies.

(c) A hospital, physician, surgeon, coroner, medical examiner, local public health officer, enucleator, technician, or other person, who acts in accordance with this chapter or with the applicable anatomical gift law of another state or a foreign country or attempts in good faith to do so is not liable for that act in a civil action or criminal proceeding.

(d) An individual who makes an anatomical gift pursuant to Section 7150.5 or 7151 and the individual's estate are not liable for any injury or damage that may result from the making or the use of the anatomical gift.

§7155.6. Repealed by Stats. 1988, c. 1095, § 1

§7156. Date of application.

This chapter applies to a document of gift, revocation, or refusal to make an anatomical gift signed by the donor or a person authorized to make or object to making an anatomical gift before, on, or after January 1, 1989.

§7156.5. Uniformity of application and construction.

This chapter shall be applied and construed to effectuate its general purpose to make uniform the law with respect to the subject of this chapter among states enacting it.

§7157. Repealed by Sats. 1988, c. 1095, § 1.

COLORADO

UNIFORM ANATOMICAL GIFT ACT

§ 12-34-101. Short title.

This part 1 shall be known and may be cited as the "Uniform Anatomical Gift Act".

§ 12-34-101.5. Legislative declaration.

The general assembly hereby finds and declares that the use of anatomical gifts, including the donation of organs or tissue, for the purpose of transplantation is of great interest to the well-being of the citizens of this state and may save or prolong the life or improve the health of extremely ill and dying persons. The general assembly therefore finds that it is in the best interests of the state to encourage such donations for transplants and to encourage the use of the authorization for anatomical gifts required to be printed on the back of drivers' licenses and identification cards indicating that the signer has consented to the donation of organs or tissue and indicating, if known, the results of HLA typing for the purpose of matching such anatomical gifts for transplants. The general assembly further finds that it is beneficial to the state for employers to encourage such donations by allowing employees time off for the purpose of making such donations and, to that end, that it is necessary to direct that the state personnel board, consistent with section 24-50-104 (9)(c), C.R.S., adopt a rule that provides for two days per year of paid leave for employees in the state personnel system for the purpose of donating organs, tissue, or bone marrow for a transplant.

§ 12-34-102. Definitions.

As used in this part 1, unless the context otherwise requires:

(1) "Bank or storage facility" means a facility licensed, accredited, or approved under the laws of any state for storage of human bodies or parts thereof.

(2) "Decedent" means a deceased individual and includes a stillborn infant or fetus.

(3) "Donor" means an individual who makes a gift of all or part of his body.

(4) "Hospital" means a hospital licensed, accredited, or approved under the laws of any state and includes a hospital operated by the United States government, a state, or a political subdivision thereof, although not required to be licensed under state laws.

(5) "Part" includes organs, tissues, eyes, bones, arteries, blood, other fluids, and other portions of a human body.

(6) "Person" means an individual, corporation, government or political subdivision or agency thereof, business trust, estate, trust, partnership, association, or any other legal entity.

(7) "Physician" or "surgeon" means a physician or surgeon licensed or authorized to practice under the laws of any state.

(7.5) "Procurement agency" means any agency that has been certified or recertified by the secretary of the United States department of health and human services or any agency certified by the executive director of the Colorado department of health as a qualified organ or tissue agency.

(8) "State" includes any state, district, commonwealth, territory, insular possession, and any other area subject to the legislative authority of the United States of America.

§ 12-34-103. Persons who may execute an anatomical gift.

(1) Any individual of sound mind and eighteen years of age or more may give all or any part of his body, the gift to take effect upon death, for any purpose specified in section 12-34-104.

(2) Any of the following persons, in the order of priority stated, when persons in prior classes are not available at the time of death, and in the absence of actual notice of a contrary indication as defined in section 12-34-107, or actual notice of opposition by a member of the same or a prior class, may give all or any part of the decedent's body for any purposes specified in section 12-34-104:

(a) The spouse;

(b) An adult son or daughter;

(c) Either parent;

(d) An adult brother or sister;

(e) A guardian of the person of the decedent at the time of his death;

(f) Any other person authorized or under obligation to dispose of the body.

(3) If the donee has actual notice of a contrary indication as defined in section 12-34-107, or that a gift by a member of a class is opposed by a member of the same or a prior class, the donee shall not accept the gift. The persons authorized by subsection (2) of this section may make the gift after death or immediately before death.

(4) A gift of all or part of a human body authorizes any examination necessary to assure medical acceptability of the gift for the purposes intended.

(5) The rights of the donee created by the gift are paramount to the rights of others except as provided by section 12-34-108 (4).

§ 12-34-104. Persons who may become donees, and purposes for which anatomical gifts may be made.

(1) The following persons may become donees of gifts of bodies or parts thereof for the purposes stated:

(a) Any hospital, surgeon, or physician for medical or dental education, research, advancement of medical or dental science, therapy, or transplantation; or

(b) Any accredited medical or dental school, college, or university for education, research, advancement of medical or dental science, or therapy; or

(c) Any bank or storage facility, for medical or dental education, research, advancement of medical or dental science, therapy, or transplantation; or

(d) Any specified individual for therapy or transplantation needed by him.

§ 12-34-105. Manner of executing anatomical gifts.

(1) A gift of all or part of a human body under section 12-34-103 (1) may be made by any of the following:

(a) By will. The gift becomes effective upon the death of the testator without waiting for probate. If the will is not probated or if it is declared invalid for testamentary purposes, the gift, to the extent that it has been acted upon in good faith, is nevertheless valid and effective.

(b) Repealed, L. 85, p. 513, § 4, effective January 1, 1986.

(c) By document other than a will or license. The gift becomes effective upon the death of the donor. The document, which may be a card designed to be carried on the person, shall be signed by the donor in the presence of two witnesses who must then sign the document in his presence. If the donor cannot sign, the document may be signed for him at his direction and in his presence and in the presence of two witnesses who must then sign the document in his presence. Delivery of the document of gift during the donor's lifetime is not necessary to make the gift valid.

(2) The gift of all or part of a human body may be made either to a specified donee or without specifying a donee. If the latter, the gift may be accepted by the attending physician as donee upon or following death if he is not the physician determining the time and probable cause of death pursuant to section 12-34-108 (2). If the gift is made to a specified donee who is not available at the time and place of death, the attending physician upon or following death, in the absence of any expressed indication that the donor desired otherwise, may accept the gift as donee. The physician who becomes a donee under this subsection (2) shall not participate in the procedures for removing or transplanting a part.

(3) Notwithstanding the provisions of section 12-34-108 (2), the donor may designate in his will, license, card, or other document of gift the surgeon or physician to carry out the appropriate procedures. In the absence of a designation, or if the designee is not available, the donee or other person authorized to accept the gift may employ or authorize any surgeon or physician for the purpose.

(4) Any gift by a person designated in section 12-34-103 (2) shall be made by a document signed by him or by his telegraphic, recorded telephonic, or other recorded message.

(5) (a) The department of revenue shall place on the back of each driver's license, provisional driver's license, and identification card issued pursuant to article 2 of title 42, C.R.S., a card, as provided in paragraph (c) of subsection (1) of this section, in the form as follows:

I hereby give, at the time of my death, any of my organs and tissues designated below that may be needed for transplantation, therapy, research, or education. I give:

A. ___ Any needed organ or tissue   Date:_____

B. ___ Organs or tissue listed:_____

Signature

of Donor:_____HLA typing (if known):_____

Witness:_____Witness:_____

(b) A gift made by a card as provided in this subsection (5) shall be deemed revoked on the expiration date of the license to which it is attached. The gift shall also be deemed revoked at any time the license is revoked or suspended.

(c) At the time the driver's license, provisional driver's license, or identification card is issued, the department of revenue, or any private organization approved by the department of revenue, may provide literature which explains the "Uniform Anatomical Gift Act" and which contains information about transplantable organs and tissues.

§ 12-34-106. Delivery of document of gift.

If the gift is made by the donor to a specified donee, the will, card, or other document, or an executed copy thereof, may be delivered to the donee to expedite the appropriate procedures immediately after death, but delivery is not necessary to the validity of the gift. The will, card, or other document, or an executed copy thereof, may be deposited in any hospital, bank or storage facility, or registry office that accepts the same for safekeeping or for facilitation of procedures after death. On request of any interested party upon or after the donor's death, the person in possession shall produce the document for examination.

§ 12-34-107. Amendment or revocation of the gift.

(1) If the will, card, or other document, or an executed copy thereof, has been delivered to a specified donee, the donor may amend or revoke the gift by:

(a) The execution and delivery to the donee of a signed statement; or

(b) An oral statement made in the presence of two persons and communicated to the donee; or

(c) A statement during a terminal illness or injury addressed to an attending physician and communicated to the donee; or

(d) A signed card or document found on his person or in his effects.

(2) Any document of gift which has not been delivered to the donee may be revoked by the donor in the manner set out in subsection (1) of this section or by destruction, cancellation, or mutilation of the document and all executed copies thereof.

(3) Any gift made by a will may also be amended or revoked in the manner provided for amendment or revocation of wills, or as provided in subsection (1) of this section.

(4) The donor of an anatomical gift made pursuant to section 12-34-105 (5) (a) may revoke the gift by crossing off his signature on the card.

§ 12-34-108. Rights and duties at death.

(1) The donee may accept or reject the gift. If the donee accepts a gift of the entire body, he may, subject to the terms of the gift, authorize embalming and the use of the body in funeral services. If the gift is of a part of the body, the donee, upon the death of the donor and prior to embalming, shall cause the part to be removed without unnecessary mutilation. After removal of the part, custody of the remainder of the body vests in the surviving spouse, next of kin, or any other person authorized or under obligation to dispose of the body.

(2) Prior to the time the donee accepts the body, or a part thereof, the attending physician or, if none, the physician certifying death shall determine, record, and attest by his signature the time and probable cause of death in a permanent written record kept by such physician or hospital or the institution in which the death occurred, which record shall be open to the public. Such physician shall not be a donee. This physician shall not participate in the procedures for removing or transplanting a part.

(3) A person who acts in good faith in accordance with the terms of this part 1, or under the anatomical gift laws of another state or a foreign country, is not liable for damages in any civil action or subject to prosecution in any criminal proceeding for his act.

(4) The provisions of this part 1 are subject to the laws of this state prescribing powers and duties with respect to autopsies.

(5) In the case of a gift of an eye as provided for in this part 1, a mortuary science practitioner, as defined in part 1 of article 54 of this title, who has successfully completed a course in eye enucleation and has received a certificate of competence from the department of ophthalmology of the university of Colorado school of medicine or who has successfully completed a similar course elsewhere may enucleate eyes for such gift, without charge to the estate or family of the donor, after the proper certification of death by a physician and compliance with any other requirements of this part 1 in relation to such gift.

§ 12-34-108.5. Anatomical gift protocol required.

(1) In order to ensure that donors or families of donors be informed of the option to make an anatomical gift, every hospital licensed or certified pursuant to section 25-1-107 (1) (I) or (1) (I) (II), C.R.S., shall develop and implement, by October 1, 1987, an organ and tissue procurement protocol for the purpose of identifying potential donors.

(2) The protocol developed pursuant to this section shall encourage discretion and sensitivity to family circumstances in all discussions regarding the making of an anatomical gift.

(3) Each hospital protocol shall:

(a) Designate individuals who shall make requests for anatomical gifts. Such individuals may be physicians, employees of the hospital, or any other persons designated by the hospital administrator.

(b) Describe the circumstances under which the request for an anatomical gift may be made.

(4) Each person designated by a hospital protocol to make requests for anatomical gifts shall be trained to make such requests by the hospital or by a procurement agency.

(5) Requests for anatomical gifts shall be of the persons listed in section 12-34-103 (2) in the order of priority stated therein.

(6) The attending physician or his designee physician shall be responsible for:

(a) The identification of all potential donors;

(b) The notification of the individuals designated in the protocol as to when the request for the anatomical gift should be made;

(c) The notification of the appropriate hospital personnel as to when the anatomical gift should be obtained from the donor; and

(d) Making the appropriate entry in the medical record of the donor as to the fact that an anatomical gift was made.

(7) Each hospital, in conjunction with procurement agencies, shall establish medical criteria for determining the suitability of potential donors.

(8) No request for an anatomical gift shall be made when:

(a) The hospital or the attending physician, or his designee physician, has actual notice of a contrary indication by the decedent or by a member of a class listed in section 12-34-103 (2); or

(b) The attending physician has notified the hospital that a donation is not suitable for medical reasons; or

(c) Circumstances surrounding the death are such that a report to the county coroner is required pursuant to section 30-10-606, C.R.S. In such cases, however, the coroner may direct the anatomical gift protocol of the hospital to be implemented or inform a member of a class listed in section 12-34-103 (2) of the option to make an anatomical gift, so long as the coroner is still able to fulfill his statutory duties. Each individual designated in the hospital protocol as the person responsible for making the request for an anatomical gift may request the coroner to implement the protocol.

(9) The individual designated in the protocol to make the request for an anatomical gift shall, after being notified by the attending physician pursuant to paragraph (b) of subsection (6) of this section, make the request for an anatomical gift. Such request shall be noted in the medical record of the donor and shall indicate who made the request, the person of whom the request was made and his relationship to the donor, whether the request was granted, and, if the request was granted, the organs or tissue donated.

(10) Any hospital which determines that its resources or geographical location makes it impractical to implement a protocol covering all types of organs and tissues for anatomical gifts in a particular situation may request an exemption from the requirements of this section. When such a determination is made, the governing body of the hospital shall notify the executive director of the department of health in writing as to the reasons for such determination. The executive director of the department of health, upon receipt of a request from a hospital seeking an exemption, may grant or deny such request or, prior to denying or granting the request, may request additional information.

(11) All costs associated with the administration of this section shall be paid by the procurement agency requesting the anatomical gift. Payment for such costs shall be made by the procurement agency within sixty days from the date on which the agency receives the bill.

(12) It is the responsibility of all procurement agencies to:

(a) Inform hospitals and coroners of the needs for organs and tissue;

(b) Assist hospitals and other providers in the training of personnel and the development of the protocols required by this section;

(c) Coordinate with all other procurement agencies a central clearinghouse which is available twenty-four hours per day for the purpose of allowing hospitals and coroners to contact one source so that the procurement process is expedited.

(13) In the event there is more than one procurement agency seeking the same anatomical gift, the hospital obtaining the anatomical gift may designate which agency will receive the gift.

(14) Any person who in good faith participates in any activity required or authorized by this section, including the development or implementation of any protocol, shall be immune from any civil or criminal liability.

§ 12-34-109. Uniformity of interpretation.

This part 1 shall be so construed to effectuate its general purpose to make uniform the law of those states which enact it.

CONNECTICUT

CHAPTER 368I
ANATOMICAL DONATIONS

Sec. 19A-279a. Anatomical gifts: Definitions.

As used in sections 19a-279 to 19a-2791, inclusive:

(1) "Anatomical gift" means a donation of all or part of a human body to take effect upon or after death.

(2) "Decedent" means a deceased person and includes a stillborn infant or fetus.

(3) "Document of gift" means a card, a statement attached to or imprinted on a motor vehicle operator's or chauffeur's license, a will or other writing used to make an anatomical gift.

(4) "Donor" means a person who makes an anatomical gift of all or part of his body.

(5) "Hospital" means a hospital licensed under chapter 368v or licensed, accredited or approved as a hospital under the law of any state or a facility operated as a hospital by the United States government, a state or a subdivision of a state.

(6) "Part" means an organ, tissue, eye, bone, artery, blood, fluid or other portion of a human body.

(7) "Person" means an individual, corporation, business trust, estate, trust, partnership, joint venture, association, government, governmental subdivision or agency or any other legal or commercial entity.

(8) "Physician" or "surgeon" means a person licensed to practice medicine and surgery or osteopathy and surgery under chapter 370 or 371 or the law of any other state.

(9) "Procurement organization" means a person licensed, accredited or approved under the laws of any state for procurement, distribution or storage of human bodies or parts.

(10) "State" means a state, territory or possession of the United States, the District of Columbia or the Commonwealth of Puerto Rico.

(11) "Technician" means a technician of an organ or tissue procurement organization which meets the requirements of the American Association of Tissue Banks or the Eyebank Association of America.

Sec. 19a-279b. Making, amending, revoking and refusing to make an anatomical gift by an individual.

(a) A person who is at least eighteen years of age may (1) make an anatomical gift for any of the purposes stated in subsection (a) of section 19a-279f, (2) limit an anatomical gift to one or more of such purposes, or (3) refuse to make an anatomical gift.

(b) An anatomical gift may be made by a document of gift signed by the donor. If the donor cannot sign, the document of gift shall be signed by another person and by two witnesses, all of whom have signed at the direction and in the presence of the donor and of each other, and state that it has been so signed.

(c) If a document of gift is attached to or imprinted on a donor's motor vehicle operator's license, the document of gift shall comply with subsection (b) of this section. Revocation, suspension, expiration or cancellation of the license shall not invalidate the anatomical gift.

(d) A document of gift may designate a particular physician or surgeon to carry out the appropriate procedures. In the absence of a designation or if the designee is not available, the donee or other person authorized to accept the anatomical gift may employ or authorize any physician or surgeon to carry out the appropriate procedure.

(e) An anatomical gift by will shall take effect upon the death of the testator, whether or not the will is probated. If, after death, the will is declared invalid for testamentary purposes, the validity of the anatomical gift is unaffected.

(f) A donor may amend or revoke an anatomical gift, not made by will, only by: (1) A signed statement; (2) an oral statement made in the presence of two persons; (3) any form of communication during a terminal illness or injury addressed to a physician or surgeon; or (4) the delivery of a signed statement to a specified donee to whom a document of gift had been delivered.

(g) The donor of an anatomical gift made by will may amend or revoke the gift in the manner provided for amendment or revocation of wills, or as provided in subsection (f) of this section.

(h) An anatomical gift that is not revoked by the donor before death is irrevocable and shall not require the consent or concurrence of any person after the death of the donor.

(i) A person may refuse to make an anatomical gift of his body or part by (1) a writing signed in the same manner as a document of gift, (2) a statement attached to or imprinted on a donor's motor vehicle operator's or chauffeur's license or (3) any other writing used to identify the person as refusing to make an anatomical gift. During a terminal illness or injury, the refusal may be an oral statement or other form of communication.

(j) In the absence of contrary indications by the donor, an anatomical gift of a part is neither a refusal to give other parts nor a limitation on an anatomical gift under section 19a-279c or on a removal or release of other parts under section 19a-279d.

(k) In the absence of contrary indications by the donor, a revocation or amendment of an anatomical gift is not a refusal to make another anatomical gift, the donor shall make the refusal pursuant to subsection (i) of this section.

Sec. 19a-279c. Classes of persons who may make an anatomical gift of all or a part of decedent's body.

(a) Any member of the following classes of persons, in the order of priority listed, may make an anatomical gift of all or a part of the decedent's body for an authorized purpose, unless the decedent, before or at the time of death, has made an unrevoked refusal to make that anatomical gift: (1) The spouse of the decedent; (2) an adult son or daughter of the decedent; (3) either parent of the decedent; (4) an adult brother or sister of the decedent; (5) a grandparent of the decedent; and (6) a guardian of the person of the decedent at the time of death.

(b) An anatomical gift may not be made by a person listed in subsection (a) of this section if: (1) A person in a prior class is available at the time of death to make an anatomical gift; (2) the person proposing to make an anatomical gift knows of a refusal or contrary indications by the decedent; or (3) the person proposing to make an anatomical gift knows of an objection to making an anatomical gift by a member of the person's class or prior class.

(c) An anatomical gift by a person authorized under subsection (a) of this section shall be made by (1) a document of gift signed by the person or (2) the person's telegraphic, recorded telephonic or other recorded message, or other form of communication from the person that is contemporaneously reduced to writing and signed by the recipient.

(d) An anatomical gift by a person authorized under subsection (a) of this section revoked by any member of the same or a prior class if, before procedures have begun for the removal of a part from the body of the decedent, the physician, surgeon or technician removing the part knows of the revocation.

(e) A failure to make an anatomical gift under subsection (a) of this section is not an objection to the making of an anatomical gift.

Sec. 19a-279d. Role of chief medical examiner.

The chief medical examiner shall serve as a facilitator for tissue harvesting and organ procurement within the constraints imposed by his official investigative responsibilities.

Sec. 19a-279e. Routine inquiry and required request; search and notification.

(a) On or before admission to a hospital, or as soon as possible thereafter, a person designated by the hospital shall ask each patient who is at least eighteen years of age: "Are you an organ or tissue donor?" If the answer is affirmative the person shall request a copy of the document of gift. If the answer is negative or there is no answer and the attending physician consents, the person designated shall discuss with the option to make or refuse to make an anatomical gift. The answer to the question, an available copy of any document of gift or refusal to make an anatomical gift, and any other relevant information, shall be placed in the patient's medical record.

(b) If, at or near the time of death of a patient, there is no medical record that the patient has made or refused to make an anatomical gift, the hospital administrator or a representative designated by the administrator shall discuss the option to make or refuse to make an anatomical gift and request the making of an anatomical gift pursuant to subsection (a) of section 19a-279c. The request shall be made with reasonable discretion and sensitivity to the circumstances of the family. A request is not required if the gift is not suitable, based upon accepted medical standards, for a purpose specified in section 19a-279f. An entry shall be made in the medical record of the patient stating the name and affiliation of the person making the request, and the name, response and relationship to the patient of the person to whom the request was made.

(c) The following persons shall make a reasonable search for a document of gift or other information identifying the bearer as a donor or as a person who has refused to make an anatomical gift: (1) A law enforcement officer, fireman, paramedic or other emergency rescuer finding a person who the searcher believes is dead or near death; and (2) a hospital, upon the admission of a person at or near the time of death, if there is not immediately available any other source of that information.

(d) If a document of gift or evidence of refusal to make an anatomical gift is located by the search required by subdivision (1) of subsection (c) of this section, and the person or body to whom it relates is taken to a hospital, the hospital shall be notified of the contents and the document or other evidence shall be sent to the hospital.

(e) If, at or near the time of death of a patient, a hospital knows that an anatomical gift has been made pursuant to subsection (a) of section 19a-279c or a release and removal of a part has been permitted pursuant to section 19a-279d, or that a patient or a person identified as in transit to the hospital is a donor, the hospital shall notify the donee if one is named and known to the hospital; if not, it shall notify an appropriate procurement organization. The hospital shall cooperate in the implementation of the anatomical gift or release and removal of a part.

(f) A person who fails to discharge the duties imposed by this section shall not be subject to criminal or civil liability but shall be subject to appropriate administrative sanctions.

Sec. 19a-279f. Persons who may become donees; purposes for which anatomical gifts may be made.

(a) The following persons may become donees of anatomical gifts for the purposes stated: (1) A hospital, physician, surgeon or procurement organization, for transplantation, therapy, medial or dental education, research, or advancement of medical or dental science; (2) an accredited medical or dental school, college or university for education, research advancement of medical or dental science; or (3) a designated person for transplantation or therapy needed by that individual.

(b) An anatomical gift may be made to a designated donee or without designating a donee. If a donee is not designated or if the donee is not available or rejects the anatomical gift, the anatomical gift may be accepted by any hospital.

(c) If the donee knows of the decedent's refusal or contrary indications to make an anatomical gift or that an anatomical gift by a member of a class having priority to act is opposed by a member of the same class or a prior class under subsection (a) of section 19a-279c, the donee may not accept the anatomical gift.

Sec. 19a-279g. Delivery of document of gift.

(a) Delivery of a document of gift during the donor's lifetime is not required for the validity of an anatomical gift.

(b) If an anatomical gift is made to a designated donee, the document of gift, or a copy, may be delivered to the donee to expedite the appropriate procedures after death. The document of gift, or a copy, may be deposited in any hospital, procurement organization or registry office that accepts it for safekeeping or for facilitation of procedures after death. On request of an interested person, upon or after the donor's death, the person in possession shall allow the interested person to examine or copy the document of gift.

Sec. 19a-279h. Rights and duties at death.

(a) Rights of a donee created by an anatomical gift are superior to rights of others except with respect to autopsies under subsection (b) of section 19a-279j. A donee may accept or reject an anatomical gift. If a donee accepts an anatomical gift of an entire body, the donee, subject to the terms of the gift, may allow embalming and use of the body in funeral services. If the gift is of a part of a body, the donee, upon the death of the donor and before embalming, shall cause the part to be removed without unnecessary mutilation. After removal of the part, custody of the remainder of the body shall vest in the person under obligation to dispose of the body.

(b) The time of death shall be determined by two physicians who attend the donor at death or, if none, the physicians who certify the death. Without limiting any other method of determining death, a donor may be pronounced dead if two physicians determine, in accordance with the usual and customary standards of medical practice, that the donor has suffered a total and irreversible cessation of all brain function. A total and irreversible cessation of all brain function shall mean that the heart and lungs of the donor cannot function, and are not functioning, without artificial supportive measures. Neither the physicians who attend the donor at death nor the physicians who determine the time of death may participate in the procedures for removing or transplanting a part unless the document of gift designates a particular physician or surgeon pursuant to subsection (d) of section 19a-279b.

Sec. 19a-279i. Coordination of procurement and use.

Each hospital in this state, after consultation with other hospitals and procurement organizations, shall establish agreements or affiliations for coordination of procurement and use of human bodies and parts.

Sec. 19a-279j. Examination, autopsy, liability.

(a) An anatomical gift shall authorize any reasonable examination necessary to assure medical acceptability of the gift for the purposes intended.

(b) The provisions of sections 19a-279a to 19a-279l, inclusive, shall be subject to the laws of this state governing autopsies.

(c) A hospital, physician, surgeon, medical examiner or other person, who acts in accordance with sections 19a-279a to 19a-279l, inclusive, or with the applicable anatomical gift law of another state or attempts in good faith to do so shall not be liable for that act in a civil action or criminal proceeding.

(d) A person who makes an anatomical gift pursuant to section 19a-279b or 19a-279c and the person's estate shall not be liable for any injury or damage that may result from the making or the use of the anatomical gift.

Sec. 19a-279k. Transitional provision.

Sections 19a-279a to 19a-279l, inclusive, shall apply to a document of gift, revocation or refusal to make an anatomical gift signed by the donor or a person authorized to make or object to making an anatomical gift before, on or after July 1, 1988.

Sec. 19a-279l. Regulations.

The commissioner of health services shall adopt regulations, in accordance with the provisions of chapter 54, for purposes of sections 19a-279a to 19a-279k, inclusive.

Sec. 19a-280. (Formerly Sec. 19-139l). Sale of blood, tissue and organs.

The implied warranties of merchantability and fitness shall not be applicable to a contract for the sale of human blood plasma, or other human tissue or organs from a blood bank or reservoir of such other tissues or organs. Such blood, blood plasma, and the components, derivatives or fractions thereof, or tissue or organs shall not be considered commodities subject to sale or barter, but shall be considered as medical services.

Sec. 19a-280a. Prohibition against transfer for valuable consideration of any human organ for use in human transplantation. Penalty.

(a) For the purposes of this section:

(1) "Human organ" means human kidney, liver, heart, lung, pancreas, eye, bone, skin, fetal tissue or any other human organ

or tissue, but does not include hair or blood, blood components including plasma, blood derivatives, or blood reagents.

(2) "Valuable consideration" does not include (A) a fee paid to a physician or to other medical personnel for services rendered in the usual course of medical practice or a fee paid for hospital or the clinical services; (B) reimbursement of legal or medical expenses incurred for the benefit of the ultimate receiver of the organ; or (C) reimbursement of expenses of travel, housing and lost wages incurred by the donor of a human organ in connection with the donation of the organ.

(b) No person shall knowingly acquire, receive or otherwise transfer for valuable consideration any human organ for use in human transplantation.

(c) Any person who violates the provisions of this section shall be guilty of a class A misdemeanor.

DELAWARE

ANATOMICAL GIFTS AND STUDIES

§ 2710. Definitions.

As used in this subchapter:

(1) "Bank or storage facility" means a facility licensed, accredited or approved under the laws of any state for storage of human bodies or parts thereof.

(2) "Decedent" means a deceased individual and includes a stillborn infant or fetus.

(3) "Donor" means an individual who makes a gift of all or part of his body.

(4) "Hospital" means a hospital licensed, accredited or approved under the laws of any state and includes a hospital operated by the United States government, a state or a subdivision thereof, although not required to be licensed under state laws.

(5) "Part" includes organs, tissues, eyes, bones, arteries, blood, other fluids and other portions of a human body, and "part" includes "parts."

(6) "Person" means an individual, corporation, government or governmental subdivision or agency, business trust, estate, trust, partnership or association or any other legal entity.

(7) "Physician" or "surgeon" means a physician or surgeon licensed or authorized to practice under the laws of any state.

(8) "State" includes any state, district, commonwealth, territory, insular possession and any other area subject to the legislative authority of the United States of America.

§ 2711. Persons who may execute an anatomical gift.

(a) Any individual of sound mind and 18 years of age or more or an individual not of such age who has parental consent may give all or any part of his or her body for any purposes specified in § 2712 of this title, the gift to take effect upon the donor's death. However, a married minor may make such a donation without parental consent.

(b) "Parental consent" as used in this section shall be defined as the written permission by any of the following persons in order of priority stated below when persons of prior classes are no longer living or no longer have contractual capacity and when there is no notice to a donee of an objection, written or otherwise, by a person of the same class:

(1) Either parent;

(2) A legal guardian;

(3) Any individual having legal custody.

(c) Any of the following persons in order of priority stated, when persons in prior classes are not available at the time of death and in the absence of actual notice of contrary indications by the decedent or actual notice of opposition by a member of the same or a prior class, may give all or any part of the decedent's body for any purpose specified in § 2712 of this title:

(1) The spouse;

(2) An adult son or daughter, 18 years of age or older;

(3) Either parent;

(4) An adult brother or sister;

(5) A guardian of the person of the decedent at the time of his death;

(6) Any other person authorized or under obligation to dispose of the body.

(d) If the donee has actual notice of contrary indications by the decedent or that a gift by a member of a class is opposed by a member of the same or a prior class, the donee shall not accept the gift. The persons authorized by subsection (b) of this section may make the gift after death or immediately before death.

(e) A gift of all or part of a body authorizes any examination necessary to assure medical acceptability of the gift for the purposes intended.

(f) The rights of the donee created by the gift are paramount to the rights of others except as provided by § 2716(e) of this title.

§ 2712. Persons who may become donees, and purposes for which anatomical gifts may be made.

The following persons may become donees of gifts of bodies or parts thereof for the purposes stated:

(1) Any hospital, surgeon or physician, for medical or dental education, research, advancement of medical or dental science, therapy or transplantation; or

(2) Any accredited medical or dental school, college or university for education, research, advancement of medical or dental science or therapy; or

(3) Any bank or storage facility, for medical or dental education, research, advancement of medical or dental science, therapy or transplantation; or

(4) Any specified individual for therapy or transplantation needed by him.

§ 2713. Manner of executing anatomical gifts.

(a) A gift of all or part of the body under § 2711(a) of this title may be made by will. The gift becomes effective upon the death of the testator without waiting for probate. If the will is not probated, or if it is declared invalid for testamentary purposes, the gift, to the extent that it has been acted upon in good faith, is nevertheless valid and effective.

(b) A gift of all or part of the body under § 2711(a) of this title may also be made by document other than a will. The gift becomes effective upon the death of the donor. The document, which may be a card designed to be carried on the person, must be signed by the donor in the presence of 2 witnesses who need not be in the presence of each other but who must sign the document in his presence. If the donor cannot sign, the document may be signed for him at his discretion and in his presence and in the presence of 2 witnesses who must sign the document in his presence. Delivery of the document of gift during the donor's lifetime is not necessary to make the gift valid.

(c) The gift may be made to a specified donee or without specifying a donee. If the latter, the gift may be accepted by the attending physician as donee upon or following death. If the gift is made to a specified donee who is not available at the time and place of death, the attending physician upon or following death, in the absence of any expressed indication that the donor desired otherwise, may accept the gift as donee. The physician who becomes a donee under this subsection shall not participate in the procedures for removing or transplanting a part.

(d) Notwithstanding § 2716(b) of this title, the donor may designate in his will, card or other document of gift the surgeon or physician to carry out the appropriate procedures. In the absence of a designation or if the designee is not available, the donee or other person authorized to accept the gift may employ or authorize any surgeon or physician for the purpose or, in the case of a gift of eyes, he may employ or authorize an undertaker licensed by the State who has successfully completed a course in eye enucleation approved by the Medical Examiner of the State to enucleate eyes for the gift after certification of death by a physician. A qualified undertaker acting in accordance with this subsection shall be free from civil and criminal liability with respect to the eye enucleation.

(e) Any gift by a person designated in § 2711(b) of this title shall be made by a document signed by him or made by his telegraphic, recorded, telephonic or other recorded message.

(f) A person who so directs the manner in which his body or any part of his body shall be disposed of shall receive no remuneration or other thing of value for such disposition.

§ 2714. Delivery of document of gift.

If the gift is made by the donor to a specified donee, the will, card or other document, or an executed copy thereof, may be delivered to the donee to expedite the appropriate procedures immediately after death, but delivery is not necessary to the validity of the gift. The will, card or other document, or an executed copy thereof, may be deposited in any hospital, bank or storage facility or registry office that accepts them for safekeeping or for facilitation of procedures after death. On request of any interested party upon or after the donor's death, the person in possession shall produce the document for examination.

§ 2715. Amendment or revocation of the gift.

(a) If the will, card or other document or executed copy thereof has been delivered to a specified donee, the donor may amend or revoke the gift by:

(1) The execution and delivery to the donee of a signed statement; or

(2) An oral statement made in the presence of 2 persons and communicated to the donee; or

(3) A statement during a terminal illness or injury addressed to an attending physician and communicated to the donee; or

(4) A signed card or document found on his person or in his effects.

(b) Any document of gift which has not been delivered to the donee may be revoked by the donor in the manner set in subsection (a) of this section or by destruction, cancellation or mutilation of the document and all executed copies thereof.

(c) Any gift made by a will may also be amended or revoked in the manner provided for amendment or revocation of wills or as provided in subsection (a) of this section.

§ 2716. Rights and duties at death.

(a) The donee may accept or reject the gift. If the donee accepts a gift of the entire body, he may, subject to the terms of the gift, authorize embalming and the use of the body in funeral services. If the gift is of a part of the body, the donee, upon the death of the donor and prior to embalming, shall cause the part to be removed without unnecessary mutilation. After removal of the part, custody of the remainder of the body vests in the surviving spouse, next of kin or other persons under obligation to dispose of the body. The heir of any donor, at the time the disposition of the body takes place, may submit a request in writing to the donee that the body be returned to the heir at such time as the donee either refuses the disposition of the entire body or the parts thereof or determines that he no longer has use of the remains.

(b) A surgeon, physician, funeral director or eye bank technician who is authorized to remove any part in accordance with this subchapter is also authorized to draw or secure a blood sample from the donor, in order to screen the tissue received for medical purposes.

(c) The time of death shall be determined by a physician who attends the donor at his death or, if none, the physician who certifies the death. This physician shall not participate in the procedures for removing or transplanting a part.

(d) A person who acts in good faith in accord with the terms of this subchapter or under the anatomical gift laws of another state (or a foreign county) is not liable for damages in any civil action or subject to prosecution in any criminal proceeding for his act.

(e) Where no other provision for the same exists, a body, or the remains thereof, after it is no longer needed for the purpose indicated by the donor, may be buried at public expense on order of the Medical Council of Delaware, but in no case shall the expense of the burial exceed $100.

(f) This subchapter is subject to the laws of this State prescribing powers and duties with respect to autopsies.

§ 2717. Uniformity of interpretation.

This subchapter shall be so construed as to effectuate its general purpose to make uniform the law of those states which enact it.

§ 2718. Short title.

This subchapter may be cited as the Uniform Anatomical Gift Act.

§ 2719. Forms.

The following forms may be used to accomplish the purposes of this subchapter:

Anatomical Gift by Next of Kin or Other Authorized Person

I, _____, hereby make this anatomical gift of or from to the body of _____ who died on _____ at the _____ in _____. The marks in the appropriate squares and the words filled into the blanks below indicate my relationship to the deceased and my desires respecting the gift.

I am the surviving: ❏ spouse; ❏ adult son or daughter; ❏ parent; ❏ adult brother or sister; ❏ guardian; ❏ _____, authorized to dispose of the body:

I give ❏ the body of deceased; ❏ any needed organs or parts; ❏ the following organs or parts _____;

To the following person (or institution) _____ (insert the name of a physician, hospital, research or educational institution, storage bank or individual), for the following purposes: ❏ any purpose authorized by law; ❏ transplantation; ❏ therapy; ❏ research; ❏ medical education.

Dated _____ City and State _____.

_____
Signature of Survivor

_____
Address of Survivor

Anatomical Gift by a Living Donor

I am of sound mind and 18 years or more of age.

I hereby make this anatomical gift to take effect upon by death. The marks in the appropriate squares and words filled into the blanks below indicate my desires.

I give: ❏ my body; ❏ any needed organs or parts; ❏ the following organs or parts

_____;

To the following person or institutions ❏ the physician in attendance at my death; ❏ the hospital in which I die; ❏ the following named physician, hospital, storage bank or other medical institution _____; ❏ the following individual for treatment _____; for the purposes: ❏ any purpose authorized by law; ❏ transplantation; ❏ therapy; ❏ research; ❏ medical education.

Dated _____ City and State _____

Signed by the Donor in the presence of the following who sign as witnesses.

_____
Witness

_____
Signature of Donor

_____
Witness

_____
Address of Donor

Anatomical Gift by a Living Minor Donor

I am of sound mind and under 18 years of age.

I hereby make this anatomical gift to take effect upon my death with the parental consent of the undersigned. The marks in the appropriate squares and the words filled into the blanks below indicate my desires.

I give: ❏ my body; ❏ any needed organs or parts; ❏ the following organs or parts

_____ ;

To the following person or institutions ❏ the physician in attendance at my death; ❏ the hospital in which I die; ❏ the following named physician, hospital, storage bank or other medical institution _____; ❏ the following individual for treatment _____; for the following purposes; ❏ any purpose authorized by law; ❏ transplantation; ❏ therapy; ❏ research; ❏ medical education.

Dated _____ City and State _____

The undersigned parent or other person authorized by law grants permission for the above anatomical gift.

Signed by the Donor and the person giving parental consent in the presence of the following who sign as witnesses.

_____
Signature of Donor

_____
Witness

_____
Address of Donor

_____
Signature of Parent or other
Person Authorized by Law

_____
Witness

_____
Address of Consenting Party

§ 2721. Requests for anatomical gifts.

(a) It must be determined that the death of the patient in an acute care general hospital is imminent. On or before the occurrence of death, the hospital shall make a request of the first person or persons available in a class set forth in § 2722 of this title, in the order of the priority stated. Where no person is available in a prior class at the time of the request, and in the absence of actual notice of consent or denial by the patient or a person in a prior class, the hospital shall make the request for an anatomical gift from the person or persons in the next class. Any consent or refusal relating to the donation of specific parts, organs or tissues need only be obtained from the person or persons in the highest priority class in which there is a person or persons available.

(b) The hospital medical staff shall develop a protocol for identifying potential organ and tissue donors. The hospital shall require that, when the death of the patient is imminent, the persons designated in § 2722 of this title be asked whether the patient has previously agreed to donate any tissues or organs. If not, the appropriate person or persons under § 2722 of this title shall be informed of the option to donate organs and tissues or organs from the patient, the hospital shall then notify an organ and tissue procurement organization, and cooperate in the procurement of the anatomical gift or gifts.

(c) The protocols developed by the hospitals shall include a mechanism for appropriate training of the personnel making the request for anatomical donation.

(d) Where the hospital has received actual notice that either the patient, or the first person or persons available in a class set forth in § 2722 of this title, does not wish to make an anatomical gift, the hospital shall not request consent to an anatomical gift.

(e) "Acute care general hospital" shall mean a hospital that provides diagnostic and therapeutic services to patients for a variety of medical conditions both surgical and nonsurgical and in which the average length of stay for all patients is less than 30 days.

§ 2722. Persons qualified to consent.

The following persons may, in the order set forth herein, consent to or deny a request for an anatomical gift of any specific parts, organs or tissues of the body of a patient in a terminal condition and incompetent or a deceased person who has not made an anatomical gift. Such consent or denial shall be in writing. If there is a conflict among members of a class, the denial will control:

(1) The spouse of the patient or decedent;

(2) A son or daughter of the patient or decedent, if such son or daughter is 18 years of age or older;

(3) Either parent of the patient or decedent;

(4) A brother or sister of the patient or decedent, if such brother or sister is 18 years of age or older; and

(5) The guardian of the patient or decedent at the time of the decedent's death.

§ 2723. Certification of donation.

Where an anatomical gift is requested in accordance with this subchapter, the hospital shall complete a "Certificate of Request of an Anatomical Gift," on a form promulgated by the Bureau of Vital Statistics. Said certificate shall include a statement to the effect that a request for consent to an anatomical gift has been made; a statement whether or not such consent was granted; the name of the person granting or refusing such request, and the relationship of such person to the patient. Where a request is made pursuant to this subchapter, such request and its disposition shall be noted in the patient's medical record, and on the death certificate.

§ 2724. Exceptions.

Where, in the opinion of the attending physician, based on medical criteria, a request under this subchapter would not yield a donation which would be suitable, a request for an anatomical donation is not required. The hospital shall, however, keep a record of each instance in which a request under this subchapter was not made, and the reason such request was not made.

§ 2725. Declaration concerning medical treatment.

Consent to an anatomical gift under this statute shall not override an individual's declaration regarding medical treatment under Chapter 25 of this title.

§ 2726. Liability.

A hospital or physician who acts in good faith in accord with the terms of this subchapter is not liable for damages in any civil action or subject to prosecution in any criminal proceeding for his act.

DISTRICT OF COLUMBIA

ANATOMICAL GIFTS

§2-1501. Definitions; short title.

(a) As used in this chapter, the term:

(1) "Bank or storage facility" means a facility licensed, accredited, or approved under the laws of any state for storage of human bodies or parts thereof.

(2) "Decedent" means a deceased individual and includes a stillborn infant or fetus.

(3) "Donor" means an individual who makes a gift of all or part of his body.

(4) "Hospital" means a hospital licensed, accredited, or approved under the laws of any state and includes a hospital operated by the United States government, a state, or a subdivision thereof, although not required to be licensed under state laws.

(5) "Part" includes organs, tissues, eyes, bones, arteries, blood, other fluids, and other portions of a human body, and "part" includes "parts."

(6) "Person" means an individual, corporation, government, or governmental subdivision or agency, business trust, estate, trust, partnership, or association or any other legal entity.

(7) "Physician" or "surgeon" means a physician or surgeon licensed or authorized to practice under the laws of any state.

(8) "State" includes any state, district, commonwealth, territory, insular possession, the District of Columbia, and any other area subject to the legislative authority of the United States of America.

(b) This chapter shall be known as the "District of Columbia Anatomical Gift Act."

§2-1502. Persons eligible to execute gifts; nonacceptance by donee; rights of donee created by gift.

(a) Any individual of sound mind and 18 years of age or more may give all or any part of his body for any purposes specified in §2-1503, the gift to take effect upon death.

(b) Any of the following persons, in order of priority stated, when persons in prior classes are not available at the time of death, and in the absence of actual notice of contrary indications by the decedent, or actual notice of opposition by a member of the same or a prior class, may give all or any part of the decedent's body for any purposes specified in §2-1503:

(1) The spouse:

(2) An adult son or daughter;

(3) Either parent;

(4) An adult brother or sister;

(5) A guardian of the person of the decedent at the time of his death; or

(6) Any other person authorized or under obligation to dispose of the body.

(c) If the donee has actual notice of contrary indications by the decedent, or that a gift by a member of a class is opposed by a member of the same or a prior class, the donee shall not accept the gift. The persons authorized by subsection (b) of this section may make the gift after death or immediately before death.

(d) A gift of all or part of a body authorizes any examination necessary to assure medical acceptability of the gift for the purposes intended.

(e) The rights of the donee created by the gift are paramount to the rights of others except as provided by §2-1507 (d).

§2-1503. Persons who may become donees; purposes for which gifts may be made.

The following persons may become donees of gifts of bodies or parts thereof for the purposes stated:

(1) Any hospital, surgeon, or physician, for medical or dental education, research, advancement of medical or dental science, therapy, or transplantation; or

(2) Any accredited medical or dental school, college, or university, for education, research, advancement of medical or dental science, or therapy; or

(3) Any bank or storage facility, for medical or dental education, research, advancement of medical or dental science, therapy, or transplantation; or

(4) Any specified individual for therapy or transplantation needed by him.

§2-1504. Manner of executing gifts.

(a) A gift of all or part of the body under §2-1502 (a) may be made by will. The gift becomes effective upon the death of the testator without waiting for probate. If the will is not probated, or if it is declared invalid for testamentary purposes, the gift, to the extent that it has been acted upon in good faith, is nevertheless valid and effective.

(b) (1) A gift of all or part of the body under §2-1502 (a) may also be made by document other than a will. The gift becomes effective upon death of the donor. The document, which may be a card designed to be carried on the person, must be signed by the donor, in the presence of 2 witnesses who must sign the document in his presence. If the donor cannot sign, the document may be signed for him at his direction and in his presence, and in the presence of 2 witnesses who must sign the document in his presence.

Delivery of the document of gift during the donor's lifetime is not necessary to make the gift valid.

(2) Any such document referred to in paragraph (1) of this subsection may be in the following form and contain the following information:

UNIFORM DONOR CARD
of

_____
print or type name of donor

In the hope that I may help others, I hereby make this anatomical gift, if medically acceptable, to take effect upon my death. The words and marks below indicate my desires.

I give: (a)—any needed organs or parts
       (b)—only the following organs or parts

_____
specify the organ(s) or part(s)

for the purposes of transplantation, therapy, medical research, or education;
       (c)—my body for anatomical study if needed.

Limitations or special wishes, if any:_____

(Other side of card)

Signed by the donor and the following 2 witnesses in the presence of each other:

_____   _____
Signature of donor   Date of birth of donor

_____   _____
Date signed   City and State

_____   _____
Witness   Witness

This is a legal document under the District of Columbia Anatomical Gift Act or similar laws.

(c) The gift may be made to a specified donee or without specifying a donee. If the latter, the gift may be accepted by the attending physician as donee upon or following death. If the gift is made to a specified donee who is not available at the time and place of death, the attending physician upon or following death, in the absence of any expressed indication that the donor desired otherwise, may accept the gift as donee. The physician who becomes a donee under this subsection shall not participate in the procedures for removing or transplanting a part.

(d) Notwithstanding §2-1507 (b), the donor may designate in his will, card, or other document of gift the surgeon or physician to carry out the appropriate procedures. In the absence of a designation, or if the designee is not available, the donee or other person authorized to accept the gift may employ or authorize any surgeon or physician for the purpose.

(e) Any gift by a person designated in §2-1502 (b) shall be made by a document signed by him, or made by his telegraphic, recorded telephonic, or other recorded message.

§2-1505. Delivery of documents of gift.

If the gift is made by the donor to a specified donee, the will, card, or other document, or any executed copy thereof, may be delivered to the donee to expedite the appropriate procedures immediately after death, but delivery is not necessary to the validity of the gift. The will, card, or other document, or an executed copy thereof, may be deposited in any hospital, bank or storage facility, or registry office that accepts them for safekeeping or for facilitation of procedures after death. On request of any interested party upon or after the donor's death, the person in possession shall produce the document for examination.

§2-1506. Amendment or revocation of gift.

(a) If the will, card, or other document or executed copy thereof, has been delivered to a specified donee, the donor may amend or revoke the gift by:

(1) The execution and delivery to the donee of a signed statement; or

(2) An oral statement made in the presence of two persons and communicated to the donee; or

(3) A statement during a terminal illness or injury addressed to an attending physician and communicated to the donee; or

(4) A signed card or document found on his person or in his effects.

(b) Any document of gift which has not been delivered to the donee may be revoked by the donor in the manner set out in subsection (a) of this section or by destruction, cancellation, or mutilation of the document and all executed copies thereof.

(c) Any gift made by a will may also be amended or revoked in the manner provided for amendment or revocation of wills, or as provided in subsection (a) of this section.

§2-1507. Duties of donee, determination of time of death; immunity.

(a) The donee may accept or reject the gift. If the donee accepts a gift of the entire body, he may, subject to the terms of the gift, authorize embalming and the use of the body in funeral services. If the gift is of a part of the body, the donee, upon the death of the donor and prior to embalming, shall cause part to be removed without unnecessary mutilation. After removal of the part, the custody of the remainder of the body vests in the surviving spouse, next of kin or other persons under obligation to dispose of the body.

(b) The time of death shall be determined by a physician who attends the donor at this death, or, if none, the physician who certifies the death. This physician shall not participate in the procedures for removing or transplanting a part.

(c) A person, who acts in good faith, in accord with the terms of this chapter or under the anatomical gift laws of another state, is not liable for damages in any civil action or subject to prosecution in any criminal proceeding for his act.

(d) The provisions of this chapter are subject to the laws of the District of Columbia prescribing powers and duties with respect to autopsies.

§2-1508. Construction.

This chapter shall be so construed as to effectuate its general purpose to make uniform the law of those states which enacted it.

§2-1509. Duties of hospitals and hospices.

(a) As of January 1, 1988, whenever a patient of a hospital or hospice dies, is determined to be a suitable candidate for organ or tissue donation, and has not made an anatomical gift by will or uniform donor card, a representative of the hospital or hospice shall, in accordance with §2-1502 (b) and (c), request a person authorized by § 2-1502 (b) to consent to an anatomical gift of all or part of the decedent's body.

(b) The request required by subsection (a) of this section shall be made only if a nonprofit organ or tissue bank or retrieval organization has notified the hospital that a donation can be properly obtained and used in a manner consistent with accepted medical standards.

(c) Upon the discovery of a properly executed uniform donor card or the receipt of a consent under subsection (a) of this section, a hospital or hospice shall immediately notify a nonprofit organ or tissue bank or retrieval organization and shall cooperate in procuring the anatomical gift.

§2-1510. Certificate requirement.

(a) Whenever a request for consent is made pursuant to §2-1509, the hospital or hospice representative making the request shall complete a certificate of request for an anatomical gift on a form to be supplied by the Mayor. The certificate shall include the following:

(1) A statement indicating that a request for an anatomical gift was made;

(2) The name and affiliation of the person making the request;

(3) An indication of whether consent was granted and, if so, what organs and tissues were donated; and

(4) The name of the person granting or refusing the request, and his or her relationship to the decedent.

(b) A copy of the certificate described in subsection (a) of this section shall be included in the decedent's medical record.

§2-1511. Rules.

The Mayor shall, no later than August 1, 1987, and pursuant to subchapter I of Chapter 15 of Title, 1, issued all rules necessary to carry out the purposes of §§ 2-1509 and 2-1510. These rules shall at a minimum include:

(1) Standards for the training and qualification of those hospital and hospice representatives who have been designated to make consent requests pursuant to §2-1509;

(2) Procedures to be used when making consent requests under §2-1509; and

(3) Procedures to facilitate effective coordination among hospitals, hospices, other health-care facilities and agencies, organ and tissue banks, and retrieval organizations.

FLORIDA

ANATOMICAL GIFTS

732.910 Legislative declaration.

Because of the rapid medical progress in the fields of tissue and organ preservation, transplantation of tissue, and tissue culture, and because it is in the public interest to aide the medical developments in these fields, the Legislature in enacting this part intends to encourage and aid the development of reconstructive medicine and surgery and the development of medical research by facilitating premortem and postmortem authorizations for donations of tissue and organs. It is the purpose of this part to regulate the gift of a body or parts of a body, the gift to be made after the death of a donor.

732.911 Definitions.

For the purpose of this part:

(1) "Bank" or "storage facility" means a facility licensed, accredited, or approved under the laws of any state for storage of human bodies or parts thereof.

(2) "Donor" means an individual who makes a gift of all or part of his body.

(3) "Hospital" means a hospital licensed, accredited, or approved under the laws of any state and includes a hospital operated by the United States Government or a state, or a subdivision thereof, although not required to be licensed under state laws.

(4) "Physician" or "surgeon" means a physician or surgeon licensed to practice under chapter 458 or chapter 459 or similar laws of any state. "Surgeon" includes dental or oral surgeon.

732.912 Person who may make an anatomical gift.

(1) Any person who may make a will may give all or part of his body for any purpose specified in s. 732.910, the gift to take effect upon death.

(2) In the order of priority stated and in the absence of actual notice of contrary indications by the decedent of actual notice of opposition by a member of the same or a prior class, any of the following persons may give all or any part of the decedent's body for any purpose specified in s. 732.910:

(a) The spouse of the decedent;

(b) An adult son or daughter of the decedent;

(c) Either parent of the decedent;

(d) An adult brother or sister of the decedent;

(e) A guardian of the person of the decedent at the time of his death; or

(f) A representative ad litem who shall be appointed by a court of competent jurisdiction forthwith upon a petition heard ex parte filed by any person, which representative ad litem shall ascertain that no person of higher priority exists who objects to the gift of all or any part of the decedent's body and that no evidence exists of the decedent's having made a communication expressing a desire that his body or body parts not be donated upon death;

but no gift shall be made by the spouse if any adult son or daughter objects, and provided that those of higher priority, if they are reasonably available, have been contacted and made aware of the proposed gift, and further provided that a reasonable search is made to show that there would have been no objection on religious grounds by the decedent.

(3) If the donee has actual notice of contrary indications by the decedent or objection of an adult son or daughter or actual notice that a gift by a member of a class is opposed by a member of the same or a prior class, the donee shall not accept the gift.

(4) The person authorized by subsection (2) may make the gift after the decedent's death or immediately before the decedent's death.

(5) A gift of all or part of a body authorizes any examination necessary to assure medical acceptability of the gift for the purposes intended.

(6) The rights of the donee created by the gift are paramount to the rights of others, except as provided by s. 732.917.

732.913 Person who may become donees; purposes for which anatomical gifts may be made.

The following persons may become donees of gifts of bodies or parts of them for the purposes stated:

(1) Any hospital, surgeon, or physician for medical or dental education or research, advancement of medical or dental science, therapy, or transplantation.

(2) Any accredited medical or dental school, college, or university for education, research, advancement of medical or dental science, or therapy.

(3) Any bank or storage facility for medical or dental education, research, advancement of medical or dental science, therapy, or transplantation.

(4) Any specified individual for therapy or transplantation needed by him.

732.914 Manner of executing anatomical gifts.

(1) A gift of all or part of the body under s. 732.912(1) may be made by will. The gift becomes effective upon the death of the testator without waiting for probate. If the will is not probated or if it is declared invalid for testamentary purposes, the gift is nevertheless valid to the extent that it has been acted upon in good faith.

(2)(a) A gift of all or part of the body under s. 732.912(1) may also be made by a document other than a will. The gift becomes effective upon the death of the donor. The document must be signed by the donor in the presence of two witnesses who shall sign the document in his presence. If the donor cannot sign, the document may be signed for him at his direction and in his presence and the presence of two witnesses who must sign the document in his presence. Delivery of the document of gift during the donor's lifetime is not necessary to make the gift valid.

(b) The following form of written instrument shall be sufficient for any person to give all or part of his body for the purposes of this part:

UNIFORM DONOR CARD

The undersigned hereby makes this anatomical gift, if medically acceptable, to take effect on death. The words and marks below indicate my desires:

I give:

(a)____any needed organs or parts;

(b)____only the following organs or parts specify the organ(s) or part(s)
for the purpose of transplantation, therapy, medical research, or education;

(c)____my body for anatomical study if needed. Limitations or special wishes, if any:
(If applicable, list specific donee)
Signed by the donor and the following witnesses in the presence of each other:

(Signature of donor)   (Date of birth of donor)
(Date signed)   (City and State)
(Witness)   (Witness)
(Address)   (Address)

(3) The gift may be made to a specified donee or without specifying a donee. In the latter case, the gift may be accepted by the attending physician as donee upon or following the donor's death. If the gift is made to a specified donee who is not available at the time and place of death, the attending physician may accept the gift as donee upon or following death in the absence of any expressed indication that the donor desired otherwise. The physician who becomes a donee under this subsection shall not participate in the procedures for removing or transplanting a part.

(4) Notwithstanding s. 732.917(2), the donor may designate in his will or other document of gift the surgeon or physician to carry out the appropriate procedures. In the absence of a designation or if the designee is not available, the donee or other person authorized to accept the gift may employ or authorize any surgeon or physician for the purpose.

(5) Any gift by a person designated in s. 732.912(2) shall be made by a document signed by him or made by his telegraphic, recorded telephonic, or other recorded message.

732.915 Delivery of document.

(1) If a gift is made through the program established by the Department of Health and Rehabilitative Services and the Department of Highway Safety and Motor Vehicles under the authority of s. 732.921, the completed donor registration card shall be delivered to the Department of Highway Safety and Motor Vehicles and recorded on microfilm, but delivery is not necessary to the validity of the gift. If the donor withdraws the gift, the records of the Department of Highway Safety and Motor Vehicles shall be updated to reflect such withdrawal.

(2) If a gift is not made through the program established by the Department of Health and Rehabilitative Services and the Department of Highway Safety and Motor Vehicles under the authority of s. 732.921 and is made by the donor to a specified donee, the document, other than a will, may be delivered to the donee to expedite the appropriate procedures immediately after death, but delivery is not necessary to the validity of the gift. Such document may be deposited in any hospital, bank, storage facility, or registry office that accepts such documents for safekeeping or for facilitation of procedures after death.

(3) On the request of any interested party upon or after the donor's death, the person in possession shall produce the document for examination.

732.916 Amendment or revocation of the gift.

(1) If the will or other document authorized under the provisions of s. 732.915(2) has been delivered to a specified donee, the donor may amend or revoke the gift by:

(a) The execution and delivery to the donee of a signed statement.

(b) An oral statement made in the presence of two persons and communicated to the donee.

(c) A statement during a terminal illness or injury addressed to an attending physician and communicated to the donee.

(d) A signed document found on his person or in his effects.

(2) A document of gift that has not been delivered to the donee may be revoked by the donor in the manner set out in subsection (1) or by destruction, cancellation, or mutilation of the document.

(3) Any gift made by a will may also be amended or revoked in the manner provided for amendment or revocation of wills or as provided in subsection (1).

732.917 Rights and duties at death.

(1) The donee, as specified under the provisions of s. 732.915(2), may accept or reject the gift. If the donee accepts a gift of the entire body or a part of the body to be used for scientific purposes other than a transplant, he may authorize embalming and the use of the body in funeral services, subject to the terms of the gift. If the gift is of a part of the body, the donee shall cause the part to be removed without unnecessary mutilation upon the death of the donor and before or after embalming. After removal of the part, custody of the remainder of the body vests in the surviving spouse, next of kin, or other persons under obligation to dispose of the body.

(2) The time of death shall be determined by a physician who attends the donor at his death or, if there is no such physician, the physician who certifies the death. This physician shall not participate in the procedures for removing or transplanting a part.

(3) A person who acts in good faith and without negligence in accord with the terms of this part or under the anatomical gift laws of another state or a foreign country is not liable for damages in any civil action or subject to prosecution for his acts in any criminal proceeding.

(4) The provisions of this part are subject to the laws of this state prescribing powers and duties with respect to autopsies.

732.918 Eye banks.

(1) Any state, county, district, or other public hospital may purchase and provide the necessary facilities and equipment to establish and maintain an eye bank for restoration of sight purposes.

(2) The Department of Education may have prepared, printed, and distributed:

(a) A form document of gift for a gift of the eyes.

(b) An eye bank register consisting of the names of persons who have executed documents for the gift of their eyes.

(c) Wallet cards reciting the document of gift.

732.9185 Corneal removal by medical examiners.

(1) In any case in which a patient is in need of corneal tissue for a transplant, a district medical examiner or an appropriately qualified designee with training in ophthalmologic techniques may, upon request of any eye bank authorized under s. 732.918, provide the cornea of a decedent whenever all of the following conditions are met:

(a) A decedent who may provide a suitable cornea for the transplant is under the jurisdiction of the medical examiner and an autopsy is required in accordance with s. 406.11.

(b) No objection by the next of kin of the decedent is known by the medical examiner.

(c) The removal of the cornea will not interfere with the subsequent course of an investigation or autopsy.

(2) Neither the district medical examiner nor his appropriately qualified designee nor any eye bank authorized under s. 732.918 may be held liable in any civil or criminal action for failure to obtain consent of the next of kin.

732.919 Enucleation of eyes by licensed funeral directors.

With respect to a gift of any eye as provided for in this part, a licensed funeral director as defined in chapter 470 who has completed a course in eye enucleation and has received a certificate of competence from the Department of Ophthalmology of the University of Florida School of Medicine, the University of South Florida School of Medicine, or the University of Miami School of Medicine may enucleate eyes for gift after proper certification of death by a physician and in compliance with the intent of the gift as defined in this chapter. No properly certified funeral director acting in accordance with the terms of this part shall have any civil or criminal liability for eye enucleation.

732.921 Donations as part of driver license or identification card process.

(1) The Department of Health and Rehabilitative Services and the Department of Highway Safety and Motor Vehicles shall develop and implement a program encouraging and allowing persons to make anatomical gifts as a part of the process of issuing identification cards and issuing and renewing driver licenses. The donor registration card distributed by the Department of Highway Safety and Motor Vehicles shall include the material specified by s. 732.914(2)(b) and may require such additional information, and include such additional material, as may be deemed necessary by that department. The Department of Highway Safety and Motor Vehicles shall also develop and implement a program to identify donors, which program may include notations on identification cards, driver licenses, and driver records or such other methods as the department may develop. The Department of Health and Rehabilitative Services shall provide the necessary supplies and forms through funds appropriated from general revenue or contributions from interested voluntary, nonprofit organizations. The Department of Highway Safety and Motor Vehicles shall provide the necessary recordkeeping system through funds appropriated from general revenue. The Department of Highway Safety and Motor Vehicles and the Department of Health and Rehabilitative Services shall incur no liability in connection with the performance of any acts authorized herein.

(2) The Department of Highway Safety and Motor Vehicles, after consultation with and concurrence by the Department of

Health and Rehabilitative Services, shall promulgate rules and regulations to implement the provisions of this section according to the provisions of chapter 120.

(3) Funds expended by the Department of Health and Rehabilitative Services to carry out the intent of this section shall not be taken from any funds appropriated for patient care.

32.9215 Education program relating to anatomical gifts.

The Department of Health and Rehabilitative Services, subject to the concurrence of the Department of Highway Safety and Motor Vehicles, shall develop a continuing program to educate and inform medical professionals, law enforcement agencies and officers and the public regarding the laws of this state relating to anatomical gifts and the need for anatomical gifts.

(1) The program shall be implemented by contract with one or more medical schools located in the state.

(2) The Legislature finds that particular difficulties exist in making members of the various minority communities within the state aware of laws relating to anatomical gifts and the need for anatomical gifts. Therefore, the program shall include, as a demonstration project, activities especially targeted at providing such information to the nonwhite, Hispanic, and Caribbean populations of the state.

(3) The Department of Health and Rehabilitative Services shall, no later than March 1 of each year, submit a report to the Legislature containing statistical data on the effectiveness of the program in procuring donor organs and the effect of the program on state spending for health care.

732.922 Duty of certain hospital administrators.

(1) When used in this section, "hospital" means any establishment licensed under chapter 395 except psychiatric and rehabilitation hospitals.

(2) Where, based on accepted medical standards, a hospital patient is a suitable candidate for organ or tissue donation, the hospital administrator or his designee shall at or near the time of death request any of the persons specified in s. 732.912, in the order of priority stated, when persons in prior classes are not available and in the absence of actual notice of contrary intentions by the decedent or actual notice of opposition by a member of any of the classes specified in s. 732.912, to consent to the gift of all or any part of the decedent's body for any purpose specified in this part.

(3) Where the hospital administrator or his designee has actual notice of opposition from any of the persons specified in s. 732.912, such gift of all or any part of the decedent's body shall not be requested. Except as provided in s. 732.912, in the absence of actual notice of opposition, consent or refusal need only be obtained from the person or persons in the highest priority class available.

(4) A gift made pursuant to a request required by this section shall be executed pursuant to s. 732.914.

(5) The Department of Health and Rehabilitative Services shall establish rules and guidelines concerning the education of individuals who may be designated to perform the request and the procedures to be used in making the request. The department is authorized to adopt rules concerning the documentation of the request, where such request is made.

(6) No recovery shall be allowed nor shall civil or criminal proceedings be instituted in any court in this state against the licensed hospital or the hospital administrator or his best judgment, he deems such a request for organ donation to be inappropriate according to the procedures established by the Department of Health and Rehabilitative Services, or he has made every reasonable effort to comply with the provisions of this section.

GEORGIA

ANATOMICAL GIFTS

44-5-140. Short title.

This article may be cited as the "Georgia Anatomical Gift Act."

44-5-141. Intent; legislative purpose.

This article shall be so construed as to effectuate its general purpose to make uniform the law of those states which enact it.

44-5-142. Definitions.

As used in this article, the term:

(1) "Bank or storage facility" means a tissue bank or eye bank licensed or approved by the State of Georgia and also means an organ procurement agency or other facilities for the storage of human bodies or parts thereof in this state.

(2) "Decedent" means a deceased individual and includes a stillborn infant or fetus.

(3) "Donor" means an individual who makes a gift of all or part of his body.

(4) "Hospital" means a hospital licensed, accredited, or approved under the laws of any state, although not required to be licensed under state laws, and includes hospitals operated by the United States government or by the state or a subdivision thereof.

(4.5) "Organ procurement agency" means an organization located in the State of Georgia that is designated by the Health Care Financing Administration of the federal Department of Health and Human Services under the end stage renal disease facility regulations to perform or coordinate the performance of all of the following services:

(A) Procurement of donated kidneys;

(B) Preservation of donated kidneys;

(C) Transportation of donated kidneys; and

(D) Maintenance of a system to locate prospective recipients of procured organs.

An organ procurement agency may also perform these services for extrarenal vital organs and includes any organization certified by the federal Department of Health and Human Services as an organ procurement agency.

(5) "Part" means organs, tissues, eyes, bones, arteries, blood and other fluids, and any other portions of a human body. The term "part" also means a heart pacemaker.

(6) "Person" means an individual, corporation, government or governmental subdivision or agency, business trust, estate, trust, partnership or association, or any other legal entity.

(7) "Physician" or "surgeon" means a physician or surgeon licensed or authorized to practice under the laws of any state.

(8) "State" means any state, district, commonwealth, territory, insular possession, and any other area subject to the legislative authority of the United States of America.

44-5-143. Adult decedents.

(a) Any individual who is 18 years of age or older and of sound mind may give all or part of his body for any purpose specified in Code Section 44-5-144, the gift to take effect upon death.

(b) On or before the occurrence of death in a hospital, when persons in prior classes are not available and in the absence of actual notice of contrary indications by the decedent or actual notice of opposition by a member of the same or a prior class, the person in charge of the hospital or his designated representative shall notify the applicable type of bank or storage facility which shall, if appropriate, request that any of the following persons, in order of priority stated, give all or any part of the decedent's body for any purpose specified in Code Section 44-5-144:

(1) The spouse;

(2) An adult son or daughter;

(3) Either parent;

(4) An adult brother or sister:

(5) A guardian of the person of the decedent at the time of his death other than a guardian ad litem appointed for such purpose; or

(6) Any other person authorized or under obligation to dispose of the body.

(c) (1) The person in charge of the hospital or his designated representative shall record in a book kept for this purpose a statement to the effect that the applicable type of bank or storage facility has been notified and whether, if appropriate, a request for a consent to an anatomical gift has been made and shall further indicate whether or not consent was granted, the name of the person granting the consent, and his or her relationship to the decedent.

(2) A request under subsection (b) of this Code section is appropriate only when consent would yield a donation suitable for use pursuant to medical and other criteria as defined by regulations of the Board of Human Resources.

(d) If the donee has actual notice of contrary indications by the decedent or actual notice that a gift by a member of a class is opposed by a member of the same or a prior class, the donee shall not accept the gift. The persons authorized by subsection (b) of this Code section may make the gift after or immediately before death. Upon admission of a person to any hospital, at his request, the hospital shall record in a book kept for the purpose the expression of intent of such person with regard to the disposition of his body and such expression shall be deemed to be sufficient notice under this Code section not to be contravened by opposition from persons listed in subsection (b) of this Code section.

(e) A gift of all or part of a body authorizes any examination necessary to assure medical acceptability of the gift for the purposes intended.

(f) The rights of the donee created by the gift are paramount to the rights of others except as provided by subsection (d) of Code Section 44-5-148.

(g) The Board of Human Resources shall establish regulations concerning the training of any person or persons who may be designated to perform the request and the procedures to be employed in making it. In addition, the board shall establish such regulations as are necessary to implement appropriate hospital procedures to facilitate the delivery of donations from receiving hospitals to potential recipients.

(h) The Board of Human Resources shall establish such additional rules and regulations as are necessary for the implementation of this Code section.

(i) In promulgating or amending all rules and regulations required for the proper implementation and administration of this Code section, the Board of Human Resources shall consult with and receive input from any and all affected associations, agencies, or entities including but not limited to the Medical Association of Georgia, the Atlanta Regional Organ Procurement Agency, the Atlanta Regional Tissue Bank, the Medical College of Georgia Regional Organ Procurement Program, the Georgia Lions Eye Bank, Inc., and the Georgia Hospital Association.

(j) In the absence of a specification by a decedent or a person authorized to give all or part of the decedent's body, any bank or storage facility that becomes the donee shall give preference to potential recipients of that donation who are residents of this state if:

(1) The donation is medically acceptable to the potential recipients who are residents of this state;

(2) Potential recipients who are residents of other states are not in greater need of the donation than potential recipients who are residents of this state; and

(3) The requisite medical procedure required for the potential recipient to receive the donation will be performed in this state.

44-5-143.1. Minor decedents.

(a) The parents, legal guardian, or other person authorized under subsection (b) of this Code section may, unless otherwise directed by a will, give all or any part of the body of a person who is under 18 years of age for any purpose specified in Code Section 44-5-144, the gift to take effect upon death.

(b) On or before the occurrence of death in a hospital, when persons in prior classes are not available and in the absence of actual notice of contrary indications by the decedent or actual notice of opposition by a member of the same or a prior class, the person in charge of the hospital or his designated representative shall notify the applicable type of bank or storage facility which shall, if appropriate, request that any of the following persons, in order of priority stated, give all or any part of the decedent's body for any purpose specified in Code Section 44-5-144:

(1) Both parents;

(2) If both parents are not readily available and no contrary indications of the absent parent are known, one parent;

(3) If the parents are divorced or legally separated, the custodial parent;

(4) In the absence of the custodial parent, when no contrary indications of the absent parent are known, the noncustodial parent;

(5) If there are no parents, the legal guardian; or

(6) Any other person authorized or obligated to dispose of the body.

(c)(1) The person in charge of the hospital or his designated representative shall record in a book kept for this purpose a statement to the effect that the applicable type of bank or storage facility has been notified and whether, if appropriate, a request for a consent to an anatomical gift has been made and shall further indicate whether or not consent was granted, the name of the person granting the consent, and his or her relationship to the decedent.

(2) A request under subsection (b) of this Code section is appropriate only when consent would yield donation suitable for use pursuant to medical and other criteria as defined by regulations of the Board of Human Resources.

(d) If the donee has actual notice of contrary indications by the decedent or actual notice that a gift by a member of a class is opposed by a member of the same or a prior class, the donee shall not accept the gift. The persons authorized by subsection (b) of this code section may make the gift after or immediately before death. Upon admission of a person to any hospital, at his request, the hospital shall record, in a book kept for the purpose, the expression of intent of such person with regard to the disposition of his body and such expression shall be deemed to be sufficient notice under this code section not to be contravened by opposition from persons listed in subsection (b) of this Code section.

(e) A gift of all or part of a body authorizes any examination necessary to assure medical acceptability of the gift for the purposes intended.

(f) The rights of the donee created by the gift are paramount to the rights of others except as provided by subsection (d) of Code Section 44-5148.

(g) The Board of Human Resources shall establish regulations concerning the training of any person or persons who may be designated to perform the request and the procedures to be employed in making it. In addition, the board shall establish such regulations as are necessary to implement appropriate hospital procedures to facilitate the delivery of donations from receiving hospitals to potential recipients.

(h) The Board of Human Resources shall establish such additional rules and regulations as are necessary for the implementation of this Code section.

(i) In promulgating or amending all rules and regulations required for the proper implementation and administration of this Code section, the Board of Human Resources shall consult with and receive input from any and all affected associates, agencies, or entities including but not limited to the Medical Association of Georgia, the Atlanta Regional Organ Procurement Agency, the Atlanta Regional Tissue Bank, the Medical College of Georgia Regional Organ Procurement Program, the Georgia Lions Eye Bank, Inc., and the Georgia Hospital Association.

(j) In the absence of a specification by a decedent or a person authorized to give all or part of the decedent's body, any bank or storage facility that becomes the donee shall give preference to potential recipients of that donation who are residents of this state if:

(1) The donation is medically acceptable to the potential recipients who are residents of this state;

(2) Potential recipients who are residents of other states are not in greater need of the donation than potential recipients who are residents of this state; and

(3) The requisite medical procedure required for the potential recipient to receive the donation will be performed in this state.

44-5-144. Permissible donees and purposes of anatomical gifts.

The following persons may become donees of gifts of bodies or parts thereof for the purposes stated:

(1) Any hospital, surgeon, or physician, for medical or dental education, research, advancement of medical or dental science, therapy, or transplantation;

(2) Any accredited medical or dental school, college, or university, for education, research, advancement of medical or dental science, or therapy;

(3) Any bank or storage facility, for medical or dental education, research, advancement of medical or dental science, therapy, or transplantation; or

(4) Any specified individual, for therapy or transplantation needed by him.

44-5-145. Gifts made by will, donor card, or other instrument; specification of donee, etc; procedures in absence of specified donee, etc.; certain physicians not to participate in procedures; signatures or recordings.

(a) A gift of all or part of the body under subsection (a) of code Section 44-5-143 may be made by will. The gift becomes effective upon the death of the testator without waiting for probate. If the will is not probated or if it is declared invalid for testamentary purposes, the gift, to the extent that it has been acted upon in good faith, is nevertheless valid and effective.

(b) A gift of all or part of the body under subsection (a) of Code Section 44-5-143 may also be made by a document other than a will.

44-5-146. Delivery of gift document to specific donee or deposit in hospital, bank, etc.; necessity for delivery.

If the gift is made by the donor to a specified donee, the will, card, other document, or an executed copy thereof may be delivered to the donee to expedite the appropriate procedures immediately after death. Delivery is not necessary to the validity of the gift. The will, card, other document, or an executed copy thereof may be deposited in any hospital, bank or storage facility, or registry office that accepts it for safekeeping or for facilitation of procedures after death. Upon the request of any interested party upon or after the donor's death. Upon the request of any interested party upon or after the donor's death, the person in possession shall produce the document for examination.

44-5-147. Amendment or revocation of gift.

(a) If the will, card, other document, or an executed copy thereof has been delivered to a specified donee, the donor may amend or revoke the gift by:

(1) The execution and delivery to the donee of a signed statement;

(2) An oral statement made in the presence of two persons and communicated to the donee;

(3) A statement during a terminal illness or injury, which statement is addressed to an attending physician and communicated to the donee; or

(4) A signed card or document found on his person or in his effects.

(b) Any document of gift which has not been delivered to the donee may be revoked by the donor in the manner set out in subsection (a) of this code section or by the destruction, cancellation, or mutilation of the document and all executed copies thereof.

(c) Any gift made by a will may also be amended or revoked in the manner provided for the amendment or revocation of wills or as provided in subsection (a) of this Code section.

44-5-148. Acceptance by donee; embalming, removal of donated part, etc.; time of death; certain physicians not to participate; civil liability; autopsies.

(a) The donee may accept or reject the gift. If the donee accepts a gift of the entire body, he may, subject to the terms of the gift, authorize embalming and using the body in funeral services. If the gift is of a part of the body, the donee, upon the death of the donor and prior to embalming, shall cause the part to be removed without unnecessary mutilation. After removal of the part, custody of the remainder of the body vests in the surviving spouse, next of kin, or other persons under obligation to dispose of the body.

(b) The time of death shall be determined by a physician who attends the donor at his death or, if there is no attending physician, by the physician who certifies the death. The physician shall not participate in the procedures for removing or transplanting a part.

(c) A person who acts in good faith in accordance with the terms of this article is not liable for damages in any civil action or subject to prosecution in any criminal proceeding for his act.

(d) This article is subject to the laws of this state prescribing powers and duties with respect to autopsies.

44-5-149. Creation of Advisory Board on Anatomical Gift Procurement; membership; terms; officers; meetings; compensation.

(a) There is created an advisory board to be known as the Advisory Board on Anatomical Gift Procurement. The board shall be composed of the following appointed persons:

    (1) The Governor shall appoint:

        (A) One representative of an eye bank;

        (B) One representative of a tissue bank;

        (C) One representative of a bone bank;

        (D) One representative of an organ procurement agency;

        (E) One representative of hospitals in this state;

        (F) One representative of the medical profession in this state;

        (G) One representative of the Department of Human Resources;

        (H) One representative of the Department of Medical Assistance; and

        (I) One representative of the Health Planning Agency;

    (2) The Speaker of the House of Representatives shall appoint three members of the House of Representatives; and

    (3) The President of the Senate shall appoint three members of the Senate.

(b) Each person shall be appointed for a term of two years. Legislative members shall be appointed for a term concurrent with a term of office.

(c) The advisory board shall select a chairman and such other officers as it deems necessary and is empowered to make such rules for governing of the affairs of the board as it deems appropriate. The board shall meet on the call of the chairman.

(d) The members of the board shall receive no compensation. Members appointed under paragraphs (2) and (3) of subsection (a) of this Code section shall receive the allowances authorized for legislative members of interim legislative committees for each day of attendance upon the business of the board.

44-5-150. Duties of Advisory Board on Anatomical Gift Procurement.

The Advisory Board on Anatomical Gift Procurement shall:

    (1) Consult with, advise, and lend expertise to the Department of Human Resources in the implementation and administration of rules and regulations regarding this article;

    (2) Identify areas of need in supply and demand for human organs and tissues in this state and encourage the cooperation of banks and storage facilities under this article in meeting such needs;

    (3) Encourage and recommend the implementation of a formal policy in this state to foster a state-wide network maintained by banks and storage facilities regarding coverage of hospitals and other facilities to assure that anatomical gifts are requested and procured;

    (4) Negotiate and recommend for adoption by the department agreements with other states and with banks and storage facilities of other states, whether through protocols, compacts, or other agreements, and cooperation and reciprocity provisions in the interstate procurement of anatomical gifts;

    (5) Recommend solutions and actions relative to participation in a national network of anatomical gift sharing;

    (6) Encourage improved public education and awareness regarding anatomical gifts; and

    (7) Report biennially to the Governor, the Health and Ecology Committee of the House of Representatives, and the Human Resources Committee of the Senate regarding the progress and actions of the advisory board.

44-5-151. HIV test of body part or donor; disposition if infected; notice to donor or physician; for certain blood testing.

(a) Any term used in this Code section and defined in Code Section 31-22-9.1 shall have the meaning provided for that term in Code Section 31-22-9.1.

(b) Each health care facility, health care provider, blood bank, tissue bank, sperm bank, or other similar legal entity which procedures, processes, distributes, or uses any human body part determined by the Department of Human Resources to have a reasonable probability of transmitting HIV shall subject or have subjected such part, or the donor of such part, to an HIV test prior to making that body part available for use in the body of another human being. Any such body part thus determined to be infected with HIV and any body part the donor of which has thus been determined to be infected with HIV shall not be used in the body of another human being but shall be safely and promptly disposed of or made available for medical research, as provided in the regulations of the Department of Human Resources.

(c) When any body part or the donor thereof has been determined to be infected with HIV pursuant to subsection (b) of this Code section, the person or legal entity which ordered the HIV test of the body part or donor thereof shall:

(1) If the donor is alive and the records of that person or legal entity reflect where the donor can be located, provide personal and confidential notification of such determination to the donor; or

(2) If the donor is deceased, provide confidential notification of such determination to any known physician of the donor, which physician shall have the sole discretion whether the person who executed the gift of the body part or any person at risk of being infected with HIV by the donor should be notified by that physician of such determination.

(d) In a medical emergency constituting a serious threat to the life of a potential recipient of blood, if blood that has been subjected to the HIV test required under subsection (b) of this Code section is not available, the testing otherwise required under subsection (b) shall not be required regarding such blood.

(e) Any person or legal entity which violates subsection (b) of this Code section shall be guilty of a misdemeanor.

HAWAII

CHAPTER 327
UNIFORM ANATOMICAL GIFT ACT

§327.1 Definitions.

As used in this chapter:

"Anatomical gift" means a donation of all or part of a human body to take effect upon or after death.

"Decedent" means a deceased individual and includes a stillborn infant or fetus.

"Document of gift" means a card, a statement attached to or imprinted on a motor vehicle operator's or chauffeur's license, a will, or other writing used to make an anatomical gift.

"Donor" means an individual who makes an anatomical gift of all or part of the individual's body.

"Enucleator" means an individual who has successfully completed a course of training acceptable to the board of medical examiners to remove or process eyes or parts of eyes.

"Hospital" means a facility licensed, accredited, or approved as a hospital under a state law.

"Part" means an organ, tissue, eye, bone, artery, blood, fluid, or other portion of a human body.

"Person" means an individual, corporation, business trust, estate, trust, partnership, joint venture, association, government, governmental subdivision or agency, or any other legal or commercial entity.

"Physician" or "surgeon" means an individual licensed or otherwise authorized to practice medicine and surgery under chapter 453 or osteopathy and surgery under chapter 460.

"Procurement organization" means a person licensed, accredited, or approved under the laws of any state for procurement, distribution, or storage of human bodies or parts.

"State" means a state, territory, or possession of the United States, the District of Columbia, or the Commonwealth of Puerto Rico.

"Technician" means an individual who, under the supervision of a licensed physician, removes or processes a part.

§327-2 Making, amending, revoking, and refusing to make anatomical gifts by individual.

(a) An individual who is at least eighteen years of age may:

(1) Make an anatomical gift for any of the purposes stated in section 327-6;

(2) Limit an anatomical gift to one of those purposes; or

(3) Refuse to make an anatomical gift.

(b) An anatomical gift may be made only by a document of gift signed by the donor. If the donor cannot sign, the document of gift shall be signed by another individual and by two witnesses, all of whom have signed at the direction and in the presence of the donor and of each other, and state that it has been so signed.

(c) If a document of gift is attached to or imprinted on a donor's motor vehicle operator's or chauffeur's license, the document of gift shall comply with subsection (b). Revocation, suspension, expiration, or cancellation of the license shall not invalidate the anatomical gift.

(d) A document of gift may designate a particular physician or surgeon to carry out the appropriate procedures. In the absence of a designation or if the designee is not available, the donee or other person authorized to accept the anatomical gift may employ or authorize any physician, surgeon, technician, or enucleator to carry out the appropriate procedures.

(e) An anatomical gift by will shall take effect upon death of the testator, whether or not the will is probated. If, after death, the will is declared invalid for testamentary purposes, the validity of the anatomical gift is unaffected.

(f) A donor may amend or revoke an anatomical gift, not made by will, only by:

(1) A signed statement;

(2) An oral statement made in the presence of two individuals;

(3) Any form of communication during a terminal illness or injury addressed to a physician or surgeon; or

(4) The delivery of a signed statement to a specified donee to whom a document of gift had been delivered.

(g) The donor of an anatomical gift made by will may amend or revoke the gift in the manner provided for amendment or revocation of wills, or as provided in subsection (f).

(h) An anatomical gift that is not revoked by the donor before death is irrevocable and does not require the consent or concurrence of any person after the donor's death.

(i) An individual may refuse to make an anatomical gift of the individual's body or part by:

(1) A writing signed in the same manner as a document of gift;

(2) A statement attached to or imprinted on a donor's motor vehicle operator's or chauffeur's license; or

(3) Any other writing used to identify the individual as refusing to make an anatomical gift. During a terminal illness or injury, the refusal may be an oral statement or other form of communication.

(j) In the absence of contrary indications by the donor, an anatomical gift of a part is neither a refusal to give other parts nor a limitation on an anatomical gift under section 327-3 or on a removal or release of other parts under section 327-4.

(k) In the absence of contrary indications by the donor, a revocation or amendment of an anatomical gift is not a refusal to make an anatomical gift, the donor shall make the refusal pursuant to subsection (i).

§327-3 Making, revoking, and objecting to anatomical gifts, by others.

(a) Any member of the following classes of persons, in the order of priority listed, may make an anatomical gift of all or a part of the decedent's body for an authorized purpose, unless the decedent, at the time of death, has made an unrevoked refusal to make that anatomical gift:

(1) The spouse of the decedent;

(2) An adult son or daughter of the decedent;

(3) Either parent of the decedent;

(4) An adult brother or sister of the decedent;

(5) A grandparent of the decedent; and

(6) A guardian of the person of the decedent at the time of death.

(b) An anatomical gift may not be made by a person listed in subsection (a) if:

(1) A person in a prior class is available at the time of death to make an anatomical gift;

(2) The person proposing to make an anatomical gift knows of a refusal or contrary indications by the decedent; or

(3) The person proposing to make an anatomical gift knows of an objection to making an anatomical gift by a member of the person's class or a prior class.

(c) An anatomical gift by a person authorized under subsection (a) shall be made by:

(1) A document of gift signed by the person; or

(2) The person's telegraphic, recorded telephonic, or other recorded message, or other form of communication from the person that is contemporaneously reduced to writing and signed by the recipient.

(d) An anatomical gift by a person authorized under subsection (a) may be revoked by any member of the same or a prior class if, before procedures have begun for the removal of a part from the body of the decedent, the physician, surgeon, technician, or enucleator removing the part knows of the revocation.

(e) A failure to make an anatomical gift under subsection (a) is not an objection to the making of an anatomical gift.

§327-4 Authorization by medical examiner, coroner, coroner's physician, or director of health.

(a) A medical examiner, coroner, or coroner's physician, as applicable, may release and permit the removal of a part from a body within that official's custody, for transplantation or therapy, if:

(1) The official has received a request for the part from a hospital, physician, surgeon, or procurement organization;

(2) The hospital, physician, surgeon, or procurement organization certifies that the entity or person making the request has made a reasonable effort, taking into account the useful life of the part, to locate and examine the decedent's medical records and inform persons listed in section 327-3 of their option to make, or object to making, an anatomical gift;

(3) The official does not know of a refusal or contrary indication by the decedent or objection by a person having priority to act as listed in section 327-3;

(4) The removal will be by a physician, surgeon, or technician; but in the case of eyes, by one of them or by an enucleator;

(5) The removal will not interfere with any autopsy or investigation;

(6) The removal will be in accordance with accepted medical standards; and

(7) Cosmetic restoration will be done, if appropriate.

(b) If the body is not within the jurisdiction of a medical examiner, coroner, or corner's physician, the director of health may release and permit the removal of any part from the body in the director's jurisdiction for transplantation or therapy if the requirements of subsection (a) are met.

(c) An official releasing and permitting the removal of a part shall maintain a permanent record of the name of the decedent, the person making the request, the date and purpose of the request, the part requested, and the person to whom it was released.

§327-5 Routine inquiry and required request; search and notification.

(a) On or before admission to a hospital, or as soon as possible thereafter, a person designated by the hospital shall ask each patient who is at least eighteen years of age: "Are you an organ or tissue donor?" If the answer is affirmative the person shall request a copy of the document of gift. The person designated shall make available basic information regarding the option to make or refuse to make an anatomical gift. The answer to the question, an available copy of any document of gift or refusal, if any, to make an anatomical gift, and any other relevant information, shall be placed in the patient's medical record.

(b) If, at or near the time of death of a patient, there is no medical record that the patient has made or refused to make an anatomical gift, the hospital administrator or a representative designated by the administrator shall discuss the option to make or refuse to make an anatomical gift and request the making of an anatomical gift pursuant to section 327-3. The request shall be made with reasonable discretion and sensitivity to the circumstances of the family. A request is not required if the gift is not suitable, based upon accepted medical standards, for a purpose specified in section 327-6. An entry shall be made in the medical record of the patient, stating the name and affiliation of the individual making the request, and of the name, response, and relationship to the patient of the person to whom the request was made. The director of health may adopt rules to implement this subsection.

(c) The following persons shall, at the person's discretion and if time and resources permit, and if doing so would be inoffensive to anyone in the vicinity of the body, make a reasonable search of the person and the person's immediate personal effects for a document of gift or other information identifying the bearer as a donor or as an individual who has refused to make an anatomical gift:

(1) A law enforcement officer, firefighter, paramedic, or other emergency rescuer attending an individual who the searcher believes to be dead or near death; and

(2) A hospital, upon the admission of an individual at or near the time of death, if there is not immediately available any other source of that information.

(d) If a document of gift or evidence of refusal to make an anatomical gift is located by the search required by subsection (c)(1), and the individual or body to whom it relates is taken to a hospital, the hospital shall be notified of the contents and the document or other evidence shall be sent to the hospital.

(e) If, at or near the time of death of a patient, a hospital knows that an anatomical gift has been made pursuant to section 327-3 or a release and removal of a part has been permitted pursuant to section 327-4, or that a patient or an individual identified as in transit to the hospital is a donor, the hospital shall notify the donee if one is named and known to the hospital; if not, it shall notify an appropriate procurement organization. The hospital shall cooperate in the implementation of the anatomical gift or release and removal of a part.

(f) A person who fails to discharge the duties imposed by this section is not subject to criminal or civil liability but is subject to appropriate administrative sanctions.

§327-6 Persons who may become donees; purposes for which anatomical gifts may be made.

(a) The following persons may become donees of anatomical gifts for the purposes stated:

(1) A hospital, physician, surgeon, or procurement organization, for transplantation, therapy, medical or dental education, research, or advancement of medical or dental science;

(2) An accredited medical or dental school, college, or university for education, research, advancement of medical or dental science; or

(3) A designated individual for transplantation or therapy needed by that individual.

(b) An anatomical gift may be made to a designated donee or without designating a donee. If a donee is not designated or if the donee is not available or rejects the anatomical gift, the anatomical gift may be accepted by any hospital.

(c) If the donee knows of the decedent's refusal or contrary indications to make an anatomical gift or that an anatomical gift by a member of a class having priority to act is opposed by a member of the same class or a prior class under section 327-3, the donee may not accept the anatomical gift.

§327-7 Delivery of document of gift.

(a) Delivery of a document of gift during the donor's lifetime is not required for the validity of an anatomical gift.

(b) If an anatomical gift is made to a designated donee, the document of gift, or a copy, may be delivered to the donee to expedite the appropriate procedures after death. The document of gift, or a copy, may be deposited in any hospital, procurement organization, or registry office that accepts it for safekeeping or for facilitation of procedures after death. On request of an interested person, upon or after the donor's death, the person in possession shall allow the interested person to examine or copy the document of gift.

§327-8 Rights and duties at death.

(a) Rights of a donee created by an anatomical gift are superior to rights of others except with respect to autopsies under section 327-11. A donee may accept or reject an anatomical gift. If a donee accepts an anatomical gift of an entire body, the donee, subject to the terms of the gift, may allow embalming and use of the body in funeral services. If the gift is of a part of a body, the donee, upon the death of the donor and before embalming, shall cause the part to be removed without unnecessary mutilation. After removal of the part, custody of the remainder of the body vests in the person under obligation to dispose of the body.

(b) The time of death shall be determined by the physician or surgeon who attends the donor at death or, if none, the physician or surgeon who certifies the physician or surgeon who determines the time of death may participate in the procedures for removing or transplanting a part unless the document of gift designates a particular physician or surgeon pursuant to section 327-2.

(c) If there has been an anatomical gift, a technician may remove any donated parts and an enucleator may remove any donated eyes or parts of eyes, after determination of death by a physician or surgeon.

§327-9 Coordination of procurement and use.

Each hospital in this State, after consultation with other hospitals and procurement organizations, shall establish agreements or affiliations for coordination of procurement and use of human bodies and parts.

§327-10 Sale or purchase of parts prohibited.

(a) An anatomical gift authorizes any reasonable examination necessary to assure medical acceptability of the gift for the purposes intended.

(b) The provisions of this chapter are subject to the laws of this State governing autopsies.

(c) A hospital, physician, surgeon, medical examiner, the director of health, an enucleator, a technician, or other person, who acts in accordance with this chapter or with the applicable anatomical gift law of another state or attempts in good faith to do so shall not be liable for that act in a civil action or criminal proceeding.

(d) An individual who makes an anatomical gift pursuant to section 327-2 or 327-3 and the individual's estate shall not be liable for any injury or damage that may result from the making or the use of the anatomical gift.

§327-11 Examination, autopsy, liability.

(a) An anatomical gift authorizes any reasonable examination necessary to assure medical acceptability of the gift for the purposes intended.

(b) The provisions of this chapter are subject to the laws of this State governing autopsies.

(c) A hospital, physician, surgeon, medical examiner, the director of health, an enucleator, a technician, or other person, who acts in accordance with this chapter or with the applicable anatomical gift law of another state or attempts in good faith to do so shall not be liable for that act in a civil action or criminal proceeding.

(d) An individual who makes an anatomical gift pursuant to section 327-2 or 327-3 and the individual's estate shall not be liable for any injury or damage that may result from the making or the use of the anatomical gift.

§327-12 Transitional provisions.

This chapter shall apply to a document of gift, revocation, or refusal to make an anatomical gift signed by the donor or a person authorized to make or object to making an anatomical gift before, on, or after June 13, 1988.

§327-13 Uniformity of application and construction.

This chapter shall be applied and construed to effectuate its general purpose to make uniform the law with respect to the subject of this chapter among states enacting it.

§327-14. Short title.

This part may be cited as the "Uniform Anatomical Gift Act".

IDAHO

UNIFORM ANATOMICAL GIFT ACT

39-3401. Definitions.

(1) "Anatomical gift" means a donation of all or part of a human body to take effect upon or after death.

(2) "Decedent" means a deceased individual and includes a stillborn infant or fetus.

(3) "Document of gift" means a card, a statement attached to or imprinted on a motor vehicle operator's or chauffeur's license, a will, or other writing used to make an anatomical gift.

(4) "Donor" means an individual who make [makes] an anatomical gift of all or part of the individual's body.

(5) "Enucleation" means removing or processing eyes or parts of eyes.

(6) "Enucleator" means an individual who has completed a course in eye enucleation and has a certificate of competence from an agency or organization designated by the Idaho board of medicine for the purpose of providing such training.

(7) "Hospital" means a facility licensed, accredited, or approved as a hospital under the law of any state or a facility operated as a hospital by the United States government, a state, or a subdivision of a state.

(8) "Part" means an organ, tissue, eye, bone, artery, blood, fluid, or other portion of a human body.

(9) "Person" means an individual, corporation, business trust, estate, trust, partnership, joint venture, association, government, governmental subdivision or agency, or any other legal or commercial entity.

(10) "Physician" or "surgeon" means an individual licensed or otherwise authorized to practice medicine and surgery or osteopathy and surgery under the laws of any state.

(11) "Procurement organization" means a person licensed, accredited, or approved under the laws of any state for procurement, distribution, or storage of human bodies or parts.

(12) "State" means a state, territory, or possession of the United States, the District of Columbia, or the Commonwealth of Puerto Rico.

(13) "Technician" means an individual who is certified by the Idaho board of medicine to remove or process a part.

39-3401A. Duties of state department of health and welfare. [Repealed]

39-3402. Duties of state department of health and welfare.

In addition to any other duties and responsibilities, the director of the department of health and welfare shall register facilities for the storage of human bodies or human body parts which are intended for transplantation into another human. The director shall not maintain on such registry any facility which does not certify that the body part or parts to be supplied for transplantation come from a person who has been tested for acquired immunodeficiency syndrome (AIDS), AIDS related complexes (ARC), or other manifestations of human immunodeficiency virus (HIV) infection, and that the test is negative for the presence of HIV antibodies or antigens.

39-3403. Making, amending, revoking, and refusing to make anatomical gifts by individual.

(1) An individual who is at least eighteen (18) years of age may (i) make an anatomical gift for any of the purposes stated in section 39-3407 (1), Idaho Code, (ii) limit an anatomical gift to one (1) or more of those purposes, or (iii) refuse to make an anatomical gift.

(2) An anatomical gift may be made only by a document of gift signed by the donor. If the donor cannot sign, the document of gift must be signed by another individual and by two (2) witnesses, all of whom have signed at the direction and in the presence of the donor and of each other, and state that it has been so signed.

(3) If a document of gift is attached to or imprinted on a donor's motor vehicle operator's or chauffeur's license, the document of gift must comply with subsection (2) of this section. Revocation, suspension, expiration, or cancellation of the license does not invalidate the anatomical gift.

(4) A document of gift may designate a particular physician or surgeon to carry out the appropriate prodcedures [procedures]. In the absence of a designation or if the designee is not available, the donee or other person authorized to accept the anatomical gift may employ or authorize any physician, surgeon, technician, or enucleator to carry out the appropriate procedures.

(5) An anatomical gift by will takes effect upon death of the testator, whether or not the will is probated. If, after death, the will is declared invalid for testamentary purposes, the validity of the anatomical gift is unaffected.

(6) A donor may amend or revoke an anatomical gift, not made by will, only by:

(a) A signed statement;

(b) An oral statement made in the presence of two (2) individuals;

(c) Any form of communication during a terminal illness or injury addressed to a physician or surgeon; or

(d) The delivery of a signed statement to a specified donee to whom a document of gift had been delivered.

(7) The donor of an anatomical gift made by will may amend or revoke the gift in the manner provided for amendment or revocation of wills, or as provided in subsection (6).

(8) An anatomical gift that is not revoked by the donor before death is irrevocable and does not require the consent or concurrence of any person after the donor's death.

(9) An individual may refuse to make an anatomical gift of the individual's body or part by (i) a writing signed in the same manner as a document of gift, (ii) a statement attached to or imprinted on a donor's motor vehicle operator's or chauffeur's license, or (iii) any other writing used to identify the individual as refusing to make an anatomical gift. During a terminal illness or injury, the refusal may be an oral statement or other form of communication.

(10) In the absence of contrary indications by the donor, an anatomical gift or a part is neither a refusal to give other parts nor a limitation on an anatomical gift under section 39-3404, Idaho Code, or on a removal or release of other parts under section 39-3405, Idaho Code.

(11) In the absence of contrary indications by the donor, a revocation or amendment of an anatomical gift is not refusal to make another anatomical gift. If the donor intends a revocation to be refusal to make an anatomical gift, the donor shall make the refusal pursuant to subsection (9).

39-3404. Making, revoking, and objecting to anatomical gifts, by others.

(1) Any member of the following classes of persons, in the order of priority listed, may make an anatomical gift of all or a part of the decedent's body for an authorized purpose, unless the decedent, at the time of death, has made an unrevoked refusal to make that anatomical gift:

(a) The holder of an unrevoked durable power of attorney for health care:

(b) The spouse of the decedent;

(c) An adult son or daughter of the decedent;

(d) Either parent of the decedent;

(e) An adult brother or sister of the decedent;

(f) A grandparent of the decedent; and

(g) A guardian of the person of the decedent at the time of death.

(2) An anatomical gift may not be made by a person listed in subsection (1), of this section if:

(a) A person in a prior class is available at the time of death to make an anatomical gift;

(b) The person proposing to make an anatomical gift knows of a refusal or contrary indications by the decedent; or

(c) The person proposing to make an anatomical gift knows of an objection to making an anatomical gift by a member of the person's class or a prior class.

(3) An anatomical gift by person authorized under subsection (1) of this section, must be made by (i) a document of gift signed by the person or (ii) the person's telegraphic, recorded telephonic, or other recorded message, or other form of communication from the person that is contemporaneously reduced to writing and signed by the recipient.

(4) An anatomical gift by a person authorized under subsection (1) of this section, may be revoked by any member of the same or a prior class if, before procedures have begun for the removal of a part from the body of the decedent, the physician, surgeon, technician, or enucleator removing the part knows of the revocation.

(5) A failure to make an anatomical gift under subsection (1) of this section, is not an objection to the making of an anatomical gift.

39-3405. Authorization by coroner or local public health official.

(1) The coroner may release and permit the removal of a part from a body within that official's custody, for transplantation or therapy if:

(a) The official has received a request for the part from a hospital, physician, surgeon, or procurement organization;

(b) The official has made a reasonable effort, taking into account the useful life of the part, to locate and examine the decedent's medical records and inform persons listed in section 39-3404(1), Idaho Code, of their option to make, or object to making, an anatomical gift;

(c) The official does not know of a refusal or contrary indication by the decedent or objection by a person having priority to act as listed in section 39-3404(1), Idaho Code;

(d) The removal will be by a physician, surgeon, or technician; but in the case of eyes by one of them or by an enucleator;

(e) The removal will not interfere with any autopsy or investigation;

(f) The removal will be in accordance with accepted medical standards; and

(g) Cosmetic restoration will be done, if appropriate.

(2) If the body is not within the custody of the coroner, the local public health officer may release and permit the removal of any part from a body in the local public health officer's custody for transplantation or therapy of the requirements of subsection (1) of this section are met.

(3) An official releasing and permitting the removal of a part shall maintain a permanent record of the name of the decedent, the person making the request, the date and purpose of the request, the part requested, and the person to whom it was released.

39-3406. Routine inquiry and required request—Search and notification.

(1) If, at or near the time of death of a patient, there is no medical record that the patient has made or refused to make an anatomical

gift, the hospital administrator or a representative designated by the administrator shall discuss the option to make or refuse to make an anatomical gift and request the making of an anatomical gift pursuant to section 39-3401(1), Idaho Code. The request must be made with reasonable discretion and sensitivity to the circumstances of the family. A request is not required if the gift is not suitable, based upon accepted medical standards, for a purpose specified in section 39-3407, Idaho Code. An entry must be made in the medical record of the patient, stating the name and affiliation of the individual making the request, and of the name, response, and relationship to the patient of the person to whom the request was made. The director of the department of health and welfare shall adopt regulations to implement this subsection.

(2) The following persons shall make a reasonable search for a document of gift or other information identifying the bearer as a donor or as an individual who has refused to make an anatomical gift:

(a) A law enforcement officer, fireman, paramedic, or other source of that information.

(3) If a document of gift or evidence of refusal to make an anatomical gift is located by the search required by paragraph (3)(a) of this subsection, and the individual or body to whom it relates is taken to a hospital, the hospital must be notified of the contents and the document or other evidence must be sent to the hospital.

(4) If, at or near the time of death of a patient, a hospital knows that an anatomical gift has been made pursuant to section 39-3404(1), Idaho code, or a release and removal of a part has been permitted pursuant to section 39-3405, Idaho Code, or that a patient or an individual identified as in transit to the hospital is a donor, the hospital shall notify the donee if one is named and known to the hospital; if not, it shall notify an appropriate procurement organization. The hospital shall cooperate in the implementation of the anatomical gift or release and removal of a part.

(5) A person who fails to discharge the duties imposed by this section is not subject to criminal or civil liability but is subject to appropriate administrative sanctions.

39-3407. Persons who may become donees—Purposes for which anatomical gifts may be made.

(1) The following persons may become donees of anatomical gifts for the purposes stated, provided that parts for transplantation shall not be transplanted or transfused under any conditions unless accompanied by a medical certificate which states that the part comes from a person who has been tested for HIV antibodies or antigens, and that the test is negative for the presence of HIV antibodies or antigens:

(a) A hospital, physician, surgeon, or procurement organization, for transplantation, therapy, medical or dental education, research, or advancement of medical or dental science;

(b) An accredited medical or dental school, college, or university for education, research, advancement of medical or dental science; or

(c) A designated individual for transplantation or therapy needed by that individual.

(2) An anatomical gift may be made to a designated donee or without designating a donee. If a donee is not designated or if the donee is not available or rejects the anatomical gift, the anatomical gift may be accepted by any hospital.

(3) If the donee knows of the decedent's refusal or contrary indications to make an anatomical gift or that an anatomical gift by a member of a class having priority to act is opposed by a member of the same class or a prior class under section 39-3401(1), Idaho code, the donee may not accept the anatomical gift.

39-3408. Delivery of document of gift.

(1) Delivery of a document of gift during the donor's lifetime is not required for the validity of an anatomical gift.

(2) If an anatomical gift is made to a designated donee, the document of gift, or a copy, may be delivered to the donee to expedite the appropriate procedures after death. The document of gift, or a copy, may be deposited in any hospital, procurement organization, or registry office that accepts it for safekeeping or for facilitation of procedures after death. On request of an interested person, upon or after the donor's death, the person in possession shall allow the interested person to examine or copy the document of gift.

39-3409. Rights and duties at death.

(1) Rights of a donee created by an anatomical gift are superior to rights of others except with respect to autopsies under section 39-3412(1), Idaho Code. Subject to the certification requirements of section 39-2307, Idaho Code, a donee may accept or reject an anatomical gift. If a donee accepts an anatomical gift of an entire body, the donee, subject to the terms of the gift, may allow embalming and use of the body in funeral services. If the gift is of a part of a body, the donee, upon the death of the donor and before embalming, shall cause the part to be removed without unnecessary mutilation. After removal of the part, custody of the remainder of the body vests in the person under obligation to dispose of the body.

(2) The time of death must be determined by a physician or surgeon who attends the donor at death or, if none, the physician or surgeon who certifies the death. Neither the physician or surgeon who determines the time of death may participate in the procedures for removing or transplanting a part unless the document of gift designates a particular physician or surgeon pursuant to section 39-3403(4), Idaho Code.

(3) If there has been an anatomical gift, a technician may remove any donated parts and an enucleator may remove any donated eyes or parts of eyes, after determination of death by a physician or surgeon.

39-3410. Coordination of procurement and use.

Each hospital in this state, after consultation with other hospitals and procurement organizations, shall establish agreements or affiliations for coordination of procurement and use of human bodies and parts.

39-3411. Sale or purchase of parts prohibited.

(1) A person may not knowingly, for valuable consideration purchase or sell a part for transplantation or therapy, if removal of the part is intended to occur after the death of the decedent.

(2) Valuable consideration does not include reasonable payment for the removal, processing, disposal, preservation, quality control, storage, transportation, or implantation of a part.

(3) A person who violates this section is guilty of a felony and upon conviction is subject to a fine not exceeding fifty thousand dollars ($50,000) or imprisonment not exceeding five (5) years, or both.

39-3412. Examination—Autopsy—Liability.

(1) An anatomical gift authorizes any reasonable examination necessary to assure medical acceptability of the gift for the purposes intended.

(2) The provisions of this chapter are subject to the laws of this state governing autopsies.

(3) A hospital, physician, surgeon, coroner, local public health officer, enucleator, technician, or other person, who acts in accordance with this chapter or with the applicable anatomical gift law of another state or a foreign country or attempts in good faith to do so is not liable for that act in a civil action or criminal proceeding.

(4) An individual who makes an anatomical gift pursuant to section 39-3403 or 39-3404, Idaho Code, and the individual's estate are not liable for any injury or damage that may result from the making or the use of the anatomical gift.

39-3413. Forms for anatomical gift.

(1) A form substantially as follows is sufficient to comply with the provisions of this chapter for the making of an anatomical gift by a living donor, refusal to make such a gift, and the form which may be attached to a driver's license:

ANATOMICAL GIFT BY A LIVING DONOR

Pursuant to the Anatomical Gift Act, upon my death, I hereby give (check boxes applicable):

1. [ ] Any needed organs, tissues, or parts;
2. [ ] The following organs, tissues, or parts only_____;
3. [ ] For the following purposes only

_____.

(transplant-therapy-research-education)

_____   _____

Date of Birth   Signature of Donor

_____   _____

Date Signed   Address of Donor

Pursuant to the Anatomical Gift Act, I hereby refuse to make any anatomical gift.

_____   _____

Date of Birth   Signature of Declarant

_____   _____

Date of Signing   Address of Declarant

_____

Print or Type Name of Donor

Pursuant to the Anatomical Gift Act, upon my death, I hereby give (check boxes applicable):

1. [ ] Any needed organs, tissues, or parts;
2. [ ] The following organs, tissues, or parts only_____;
3. [ ] For the following purposes only

_____;

(transplant-therapy-research-education)

Refusal:

4. [ ] I refuse to make any anatomical gift.

_____

Signature

(2) A form substantially as follows is sufficient to comply with the provisions of this chapter for the making of an anatomical gift by next of kin or other authorized person:

ANATOMICAL GIFT BY NEXT OF KIN
OR GUARDIAN OF THE PERSON

Pursuant to the Uniform Anatomical Gift Act, I hereby make this anatomical gift from the body of
_____who died on _____at _____in_____.
Name of Decedent   Date   Place   City/State

The marks in the appropriate squares and the words filled into the blanks below indicate my relationship to the decedent and my wishes respecting the gift.
I survive the decedent as [ ] spouse; [ ] adult son or daughter; [ ] adult brother or sister; [ ] grandparents [ ] guardian of the person.
I hereby give (check boxes applicable):
1. {] Any needed organs, tissues, or parts;
2. [ ] The following organs, tissues, or parts only _____;
3. [ ] For the following purposes only
_____.

_____   _____
Date   Signature of Survivor
                                   _____
                                   Address of Survivor

39-3414. Transitional provisions.
This chapter applies to a document of gift, revocation, or refusal to make an anatomical gift signed by the donor or a person authorized to make or object to making an anatomical gift before, on, or after the effective date of this chapter.

39-3415. Uniformity of application and construction.
This chapter shall be applied and construed to effectuate its general purpose to make uniform the law with respect to the subject of this chapter among states enacting it.

39-3416. Severability.
If any provision of this chapter or its application thereof to any person or circumstance is held invalid, the invalidity does not affect other provisions or applications of this chapter which can be given effect without the invalid provision or application, and to this end the provisions of this chapter are severable.

39-3417. Short title.
This chapter may be cited as the "Uniform Anatomical Gift Act of 1989".

ILLINOIS

UNIFORM ANATOMICAL GIFT ACT

§301. Short Title
This Act may be cited as the Uniform Anatomical Gift Act.

§302. Definitions
(a) "Bank or storage facility" means a facility licensed, accredited or approved under the laws of any state for storage of human bodies or parts thereof.

(b) "Death" means for the purposes of the Act, the irreversible cessation of total brain function, according to usual and customary standards of medical practice.

(c) "Decedent" means a deceased individual and includes a stillborn infant or fetus.

(d) "Donor" means an individual who makes a gift of all or parts of his body.

(e) "Hospital" means a hospital licensed, accredited or approved under the laws of any state; and includes a hospital operated by the United States government, a state, or a subdivision thereof, although not required to be licensed under state laws.

(f) "Part" means organs, tissues, eyes, bones, arteries, blood, other fluids and any other portions of a human body.

(g) "Person" means an individual, corporation, government or governmental subdivision or agency, business trust, estate, trust, partnership or association or any other legal entity.

(h) "Physician" or "surgeon" means a physician or surgeon licensed or authorized to practice medicine in all of its branches under the laws of any state.

(i) "State" includes any state, district, commonwealth, territory, insular possession, and any other area subject to the legislative authority of the United States of America.

(j) "Technician" means an individual trained and certified to remove tissue, by a recognized medical training institution in the State of Illinois.

§303. Persons who may execute an anatomical gift
§3. Persons who may execute an anatomical gift.

(a) Any individual of sound mind who has attained the age of 18 may give all or any part of his or her body for any purpose specified in Section 4. Such a gift may be executed in any of the ways set out in Section 5, and shall take effect upon the individual's death without the need to obtain the consent of any survivor.

(b) If no gift has been executed under subsection (a), any of the following persons, in the order of priority stated in items (1) through (6) below, when persons in prior classes are not available and in the absence of (i) actual notice of contrary intentions by the decedent and (ii) actual notice of opposition by any member within the same priority class, may give all or any part of the decedent's body after or immediately before death for any purpose specified in Section 4:

(1) the decedent's spouse,

(2) the decedent's adult sons or daughters,

(3) either of the decedent's parents,

(4) any of the decedent's adult brothers or sisters,

(5) the guardian of the decedent at the time of his or her death,

(6) any person authorized or under obligation to dispose of the body.

If the donee has actual notice of opposition to the gift by the decedent or any person in the highest priority class in which an available person can be found, then no gift of all or any part of the decedent's body shall be accepted.

(c) For the purposes of this Act, a person will not be considered "available" for the giving of consent or refusal if:

(1) the existence of the person is unknown to the donee and is not readily ascertainable through the examination of the decedent's hospital records and the questioning of any persons who are available for giving consent;

(2) the donee has unsuccessfully attempted to contact the person by telephone or in any other reasonable manner;

(3) the person is unable or unwilling to respond in a manner which indicates the person's refusal or consent.

(d) A gift of all or part of a body authorizes any examination necessary to assure medical acceptability of the gift for the purposes intended.

(e) The rights of the donee created by the gift are paramount to the rights of others except as provided by Section 8 (d).

(f) If no gift has been executed under this Section, then no part of the decedent's body may be used for any purpose specified in Section 4 of this Act, except in accordance with the Organ Donation Request Act or the Corneal Transplant Act.

§304. Persons who may become donees; purposes for which anatomical gifts may be made
The following persons may become donees of gifts of bodies or parts thereof for the purposes stated:

(1) any hospital, surgeon, or physician, for medical or dental education, research, advancement of medical or dental science, therapy, or transplantation; or

(2) any accredited medical, chiropractic, mortuary or dental school, college or university for education, research, advancement of medical or dental science, or therapy; or

(3) any bank or storage facility, for medical or dental education, research, advancement of medical or dental science, therapy, or transplantation; or

(4) any specified individual for therapy or transplantation needed by him, or for any other purpose.

§305. Manner of executing anatomical gifts
§5. Manner of Executing Anatomical Gifts.

(a) A gift of all or part of the body under Section 3 (a) may be made by will. The gift becomes effective upon the death of the testator without waiting for probate. If the will is not probated, or if it is declared invalid for testamentary purposes, the gift, to the extent that it has been acted upon in good faith, is nevertheless valid and effective.

(b) A gift of all or part of the body under Section 3 (a) may also be made by a written, signed document other than a will. The gift becomes effective upon the death of the donor. The document, which may be a card or a valid driver's license designed to be carried on the person, must be signed by the donor in the presence of 2 witnesses who must sign the document in his presence and who thereby certify that he was of sound mind and memory and free from any undue influence and knows the objects of his bounty and affection. Such a gift may also be made by properly executing the form provided by the Secretary of State on the reverse side of the donor's driver's license pursuant to subsection (b) of Section 6-110 of The Illinois Vehicle Code. Delivery of the document of gift during the donor's lifetime is not necessary to make the gift valid.

(c) The gift may be made to a specified donee or without specifying a donee. If the latter, the gift may be accepted by the attending physician as donee upon or following death. If the gift is made to a specified donee who is not available at the time and place of death, the attending physician upon or following death, in the absence of any expressed indication that the donor desired otherwise, may accept the gift as donee. The physician who becomes a donee under this subsection shall not participate either physically or financially in the procedures for removing or transplanting a part.

(d) Notwithstanding Section 8 (b), the donor may designate in his will, card, or other document of gift the surgeon or physician to carry out the appropriate procedures. In the absence of a designation or if the designee is not available, the donee or other person authorized to accept the gift may employ or authorize any surgeon or physician for the purpose.

(e) Any gift by a person designated in Section 3 (b) shall be made by a document signed by him or made by his telegraphic, recorded telephonic, or other recorded message.

§306. Delivery of document of gift

If the gift is made by the donor to a specified donee, the will, card, or other document, or an executed copy thereof, may be delivered to the donee to expedite the appropriate procedures immediately after death. Delivery is not necessary to the validity of the gift. The will, card, or other document, or an executed copy thereof, may be deposited in any hospital, bank or storage facility, or registry office that accepts it for safekeeping or for facilitation of procedures after death. On request of any interested party upon or after the donor's death, the person in possession shall produce the document for examination.

§307. Amendment or revocation of the gift

(a) If the will, card, or other document or executed copy thereof, has been delivered to a specified donee, the donor may amend or revoke the gift by:

(1) the execution and delivery to the donee of a signed statement witnessed and certified as provided in Section 5(b)

(2) a signed card or document found on his person, or in his effects, executed at a date subsequent to the date the original gift was made and witnessed and certified as provided in Section 5 (b)

(b) Any document of gift which has not been delivered to the donee may be revoked by the donor in the manner set out in subsection (a).

(c) Any gift made by a will may also be amended or revoked in the manner provided for amendment or revocation of wills or as provided in subsection (a).

§308. Rights and duties at death
§8. Rights and Duties at Death.

(a) The donee may accept or reject the gift. If the donee accepts a gift of the entire body, he may, subject to the terms of the gift, authorize embalming and the use of the body in funeral services, unless a person named in subsection (b) of Section 3 has requested, prior to the final disposition by the donee, that the remains of said body be returned to his or her custody for the purpose of final disposition. Such request shall be honored by the donee if the terms of the gift are silent on how final disposition is to take place. If the gift is of a part of the body, the donee or technician designated by him upon the death of the donor and prior to embalming, shall cause the part to be removed without unnecessary mutilation and without undue delay in the release of the body for the purposes of final disposition. After removal of the part, custody of the remainder of the body vests in the surviving spouse, next-of-kin, or other persons under obligation to dispose of the body, in the order or priority listed in subsection (b) of Section 3 of this Act.

(b) The time of death shall be determined by a physician who attends the donor at his death, or, if none, the physician who certifies the death. The physician shall not participate in the procedures for removing or transplanting a part.

(c) A person who acts in good faith in accord with the terms of this Act and the AIDS Confidentiality Act, or the anatomical gift laws of another state or a foreign country, is not liable for damages in any civil action or subject to prosecution in any criminal proceeding for his act. Any person that participates in good faith and transplantation of any part of a decedent's body pursuant to an anatomical gift made by an individual as authorized by subsection (b) of Section 3 of this Act shall have immunity from liability, civil, criminal, or otherwise, that might result by reason of such actions. For the purpose of any proceedings, civil or criminal, the validity of an anatomical gift executed pursuant to Section 5 of this Act shall be presumed and the good faith of any person participating in the removal or transplantation of any part of a decedent's body pursuant to an anatomical gift made by the decedent or by another individual authorized by the Act shall be presumed.

(d) This Act is subject to the provisions of "An Act to revise the law in relation to coroners", approved February 6, 1874, as now or hereafter amended, to the laws of this State prescribing powers and duties with respect to autopsies, and to the statutes, rules, and regulations of this State with respect to the transportation and disposition of deceased human bodies.

(e) If the donee is provided information, or determines through independent examination, that there is evidence that the gift was exposed to the human immunodeficiency virus (HIV) or any other identified causative agent of acquired immunodeficiency syndrome (AIDS), the donee may reject the gift and shall treat the information and examination results as a confidential medical record; the donee may disclose only the results confirming HIV exposure, and only to the physician of the deceased donor. The donor's physician shall determine whether the person who executed the gift should be notified of the confirmed positive test result.

§308.1. Payment for gift
§8.1. Payment for gift.

(a) Except as provided in subsection (b), any person who knowingly pays or offers to pay any financial consideration to a donor or to any of the persons listed in subsection (b) of Section 3 for making or consenting to an anatomical gift shall be guilty of a Class A misdemeanor for the first conviction and a Class 4 felony for subsequent convictions.

(b) This Section does not prohibit reimbursement for reasonable costs associated with the removal, storage or transportation of a human body or part thereof pursuant to an anatomical gift executed pursuant to this Act.

§309. Uniformity of interpretation
This Act shall be so construed as to effectuate its general purpose to make uniform the law of those states which enact it.

§310. Repeal
Section 42a of the "Probate Act" approved July 24, 1939, as amended, is repealed.

§311. Time of taking effect
This Act shall take effect October 1, 1969.

INDIANA

UNIFORM ANATOMICAL GIFT ACT

29-2-16-1. Definitions.

Except where the context clearly indicates a different meaning, the terms used in this chapter shall be construed as follows:

(a) "Bank or storage facility" means a facility licensed, accredited or approved under the laws of any state for storage of human bodies or parts thereof.

(b) "Decedent" means a deceased individual and includes a stillborn infant or fetus.

(c) "Donor" means an individual who makes a gift of all or part of his body.

(d) "Hospital" means a hospital licensed, accredited or approved under the laws of any state: includes a hospital operated by the United States government, a state or a subdivision thereof, although not required to be licensed under state laws.

(e) "Part" means organs, tissues, eyes, bones, arteries, blood, other fluids and any other portions of a human body.

(f) "Person" means an individual, corporation, government or governmental subdivision or agency, business trust, estate, trust, partnership or association, or any other legal entity.

(g) "Physician" or "surgeon" means a physician or surgeon licensed or authorized to practice under the laws of any state.

(h) "State" includes any state, district, commonwealth, territory, insular possession and any other area subject to the legislative authority of the United States of America.

29-2-16-2. Persons who may give all or parts of a body—Exceptions.

(a) Any individual of sound mind and eighteen [18] years of age or more may give all or any part of his body for any purpose specified in section 3 [IC 29-2-16-3] of this chapter, the gift to take effect upon death.

(b) Any of the following persons, in order of priority stated when persons in prior classes are not available at the time of death, and in the absence of actual notice of contrary indications by the decedent or actual notice of opposition by a member of the same or a prior class, may give all or any part of the decedent's body for any purpose specified in section 3 of this chapter:

(1) The spouse;

(2) A son or daughter, at least eighteen [18] years of age;

(3) Either parent;

(4) A brother or sister, at least eighteen [18] years of age;

(5) A guardian of the person of the decedent at the time of his death;

(6) Any other person authorized or under obligation to dispose of the body.

(c) If the donee has actual notice of contrary indications by the decedent or that a gift by a member of a class of [is] opposed by a member of the same or a prior class, the donee shall not accept the gift. The persons authorized by subsection (b) of this section may make the gift after or immediately before death.

(d) A gift of all or part of a body authorizes any examination necessary to assure medical acceptability of the gift for the purposes intended.

(e) The rights of the donee created by the gift are paramount to the rights of others except as provided by section 7 (d) [IC 29-2-16-7(d)] of this chapter.

29-2-16-3. Persons who may become donees.

The following persons may become donees of gifts of bodies or parts thereof for the purposes stated:

(1) Any hospital, surgeon or physician for medical or dental education, research, advancement of medical or dental science, therapy or transplantation, or

(2) Any accredited medical or dental school, college or university for education, research, advancement of medical or dental science, or therapy, or

(3) Any bank or storage facility, for medical or dental education, research, advancement of medical or dental science, therapy, or transplantation, or

(4) Any specified individual for therapy or transplantation needed by him.

29-2-16-4. Method of making gifts.

(a) A gift of the body under section 2(a) [IC 29-2-16-2(a)] of this chapter may be made by will. The gift becomes effective upon the death of the testator without waiting for probate. If the will is not probated, or if it is declared invalid for testamentary purposes, the gift, to the extent that it has been acted upon in good faith, is nevertheless valid and effective.

(b) A gift of all or part of the body under section 2(a) of this chapter may also be made by document other than a will. The gift becomes effective upon the death of the donor. The document, which may be a card designed to be carried on the person, must be signed by the donor in the presence of two (2) witnesses who must sign the document in his presence. If the donor cannot sign, the document may be signed for him:

(1) At his discretion and in his presence; and

(2) In the presence of two (2) witnesses who must sign the document in his presence.

Delivery of the document of gift during the donor's lifetime is not necessary to make the gift valid.

(c) The gift may be made to a specified donee or without specifying a donee. If the latter, the gift may be accepted by the attending physician as donee upon or following death. If the gift is made to a specified donee who is not available at the time and place of death, the attending physician upon or following death, in the absence of any expressed indication that the donor desired otherwise, may accept the gift as donee. The gift of an eye or part of an eye made without specifying a donee, or made to a donee who is not available at the time and place of death and without an expression of a contrary desire, may be accepted by the attending physician as donee on behalf of an eye bank in Indiana. The physician who becomes a donee under this subsection shall not participate in the procedures for removing or transplanting a part.

(d) Notwithstanding section 7(b) [IC 29-2-16-7(b)] of this chapter, the donor may designate in his will, card, or other document of gift the surgeon or physician to carry out the appropriate procedures. In the absence of a designation or if the designee is not available, the donee or other person authorized to accept the gift may employ or authorize any surgeon or physician for the purpose. With respect to a gift of an eye or part of an eye, the eye or part may be removed for the gift, after proper certification of death by a physician and compliance with the intent of the gift as determined by reference to this chapter, by:

(1) A surgeon or physician;

(2) An embalmer or a funeral director who, before September 1, 1983, completed a course in eye enucleation and was certified as competent to enucleate eyes by an accredited school of medicine; or

(3) A person who is registered with the state board of health as an eye enucleator.

(e) An applicant for registration as an eye enucleator must submit evidence that he has successfully completed a training program in the enucleation of eyes approved by the state board of health. To be approved, a training program must:

(1) Be taught by one (1) or more surgeons or physicians;

(2) Include instruction and practice in anatomy and physiology of the eye, the maintenance of a sterile field during the removal of an eye, and the use of appropriate instruments and sterile procedures for removing the eye or part of the eye; and

(3) Comply with rules adopted by the state board of health under IC 4-22-2.

(f) The state board of health may revoke a person's registration as an eye enucleator upon a showing of good cause for revocation.

(g) A person who, in good faith reliance upon a will, card, or other document of gift, and without actual notice of the amendment, revocation, or invalidity of the will, card, or document:

(1) Takes possession of a decedent's body, or performs, or causes to be performed surgical operations upon a decedent's body; or

(2) Removes or causes to be removed organs, tissues, or other parts from a decedent's body;

is not liable in damages in any civil action brought against him for that act.

(h) Any gift by a person designated in section 2(b) of this chapter shall be made by a document signed by him or made by his telegraphic, recorded telephonic, or other recorded message.

29-2-16-5. Delivery of will, card or document.

If the gift is made by the donor to a specified donee, the will, card or other document, or an executed copy thereof, may be delivered to the donee to expedite the appropriate procedures immediately after death. Delivery is not necessary to the validity of the gift. The will, card or other document, or an executed copy thereof, may be deposited in any hospital, bank or storage facility or registry office that accepts it for safekeeping or for facilitation of procedures after death. On request of any interested party upon or after the donor's death, the person in possession shall produce the document for examination.

29-2-16-6. Amendment or revocation of gift by donor.

(a) If the will, card or other document or executed copy thereof, has been delivered to a specified donee, the donor may amend or revoke the gift by:

(1) The execution and delivery to the donee of a signed statement, or

(2) An oral statement made in the presence of two [2] persons and communicated to the donee, or

(3) a statement during a terminal illness or injury addressed to an attending physician and communicated to the donee, or

(4) A signed card or document found on his person or in his effects.

(b) Any document of gift which has not been delivered to the donee may be revoked by the donor in the manner set out in subsection (a), or by destruction, cancellation or mutilation of the document and all executed copies thereof.

(c) Any gift made by a will may also be amended or revoked in the manner provided for amendment or revocation of wills, or as provided in subsection (a).

29-2-16-7. Acceptance or rejection of gift by donee.

(a) The donee may accept or reject the gift. If the donee accepts a gift of the entire body, he may, subject to the terms of the gift, authorize embalming and the use of the body in funeral services. If the gift is of a part of the body, the donee, upon the death of the donor and prior to embalming, shall cause the part to be removed without unnecessary mutilation. After removal of the part, custody of the remainder of the body vests in the surviving spouse, next of kin, or other persons under obligation to dispose of the body.

(b) The time of death shall be determined by a physician who tends the donor at his death, or, if none, the physician who certified the death. The physician shall not participate in the procedures for removing or transplanting a part.

(c) A person who acts in good faith in accord with the terms of this chapter or with the anatomical gift laws of another state (or a foreign country) is not liable for damages in any civil action or subject to prosecution in any criminal proceeding for his act.

(d) The provisions of this chapter are subject to the laws of this state prescribing powers and duties with respect to autopsies.

29-2-16-8. Construction. —

This chapter shall be so construed as to effectuate its general purpose to make uniform the law of those states which enact it.

29-2-16-9. Short title. —

This chapter shall be cited as the "Uniform Anatomical Gift Act."

29-2-16-10. Hospital administrator to inform representative of decedent of procedures—Surrender of driver's license upon which gift made.

(a) As used in this section:

"Administrator" means a hospital administrator or a hospital administrator's designee.

"Gift" means a gift of all or any part of the human body made under this chapter.

"Representative" means a person who is:

(1) Authorized under section 2(b) [IC 29-2-16-2(b)] of this chapter to make a gift on behalf of a decedent; and

(2) Available at the time of the decedent's death when members of a prior class under section 2(b) of this chapter are unavailable.

(b) The administrator shall inform the representative of the procedures available under this chapter for making a gift whenever:

(1) An individual dies in a hospital;

(2) The hospital has not been notified that a gift has been authorized under section 2 [IC 29-2-16-2] of this chapter; and

(3) A physician determines that the individual's body may be suitable of yielding a gift.

(c) If:

(1) An individual makes an anatomical gift on the individual driver's license under IC 9-1-4-32.5; and

(2) The individual dies;

the person in possession of the individual driver's license shall immediately produce the driver's license for examination upon request, as provided in section 5 [IC 29-2-16-5] of this chapter.

(d) A gift made in response to information provided under this section must be documented as described under section 4(h) [IC 29-2-16-4(h)] of this chapter.

(e) When a representative is informed under this section about the procedures available for making a gift, the fact that the representative was so informed must be noted in the decedent's medical record.

IOWA

UNIFORM ANATOMICAL GIFT LAW

§ 142A.1. Definitions.

1. "Bank or storage facility" means a facility licensed, accredited, or approved under the laws of any state for storage of human bodies or parts thereof.

2. "Decedent" means a deceased individual and includes a stillborn infant or fetus.

3. "Donor" means an individual who makes a gift of all or part of his body.

4. "Hospital" means a hospital licensed under the laws of this state, or licensed, accredited, or approved under the laws of any other state and includes a hospital operated by the United States government, a state, or a subdivision thereof, although not required to be licensed under state laws.

5. "Part" includes organs, tissues, eyes, bones, arteries, blood, other fluids and other portions of a human body, and "part" includes "parts".

6. "Person" means an individual, corporation, government or governmental subdivision or agency, business trust, partnership, association, or any other legal entity.

7. "Physician" or "surgeon" means a physician, surgeon, or osteopathic physician and surgeon, licensed or authorized to practice under the laws of any state.

8. "State" includes any state, district, commonwealth, territory, insular possession, and any other area subject to the legislative authority of the United States of America.

§ 142A.2. Persons who may execute an anatomical gift.

1. Any individual of sound mind and eighteen years of age or more may give all or any part of the individual's body for any purposes specified in section 142A.3, the gift to take effect upon death.

2. Any of the following persons, in order of priority stated, when persons in prior classes are not available at the time of death, and in the absence of actual notice of contrary indications by the decedent, or actual notice of opposition by a member of the same or a prior class, may give all or any part of the decedent's body for any purposes specified in section 142A.3:

   a. The spouse.

   b. An adult son or daughter.

   c. Either parent.

   d. An adult brother or sister.

   e. A guardian of the person of the decedent at the time of the decedent's death.

   f. Any other person authorized or under obligation to dispose of the body. The persons authorized by this subsection may make the gift after death or immediately before death.

3. If the donee has actual notice of contrary indications by the decedent, or that a gift by a member of a class is opposed by a member of the same or a prior class, the donee shall not accept the gift.

4. A gift of all or part of a body authorizes any examination necessary to assure medical acceptability of the gift for the purposes intended.

5. The rights of the donee created by the gift are paramount to the rights of others except as provided by section 142A.7, subsection 4.

§ 142A.3. Persons who may become donees, and purposes for which anatomical gifts may be made.

The following persons may become donees of gifts of bodies or parts thereof for the purposes stated:

1. Any hospital, surgeon, or physician, for medical or dental education, research, advancement of medical or dental science, therapy, or transplantation.

2. Any accredited medical or dental school, college, or university, for education, research, advancement of medical or dental science, or therapy.

3. Any bank or storage facility, for medical or dental education, research, advancement of medical or dental science, therapy, or transplantation.

4. Any specified individual for therapy or transplantation needed by the individual.

§ 142A.4. Manner of executing anatomical gifts.

1. A gift of all or part of the body under section 142A.2, subsection 1, may be made by will. The gift becomes effective upon the death of the testator without waiting for probate. If the will is not probated, or if it is declared invalid for testamentary purposes, the gift, to the extent that it has been acted upon in good faith, is nevertheless valid and effective.

2. A gift of all or part of the body under section 142A.2, subsection 1, may also be made by a document other than a will. The gift becomes effective upon the death of the donor. The document, which may be a card designed to be carried on the person, must

be signed by the donor, in the presence of two witnesses who must sign the document in the donor's presence. If the donor cannot sign, the document may be signed for the donor at the donor's direction and in the donor's presence, and in the presence of two witnesses who must sign the document in the donor's presence. Delivery of the document of gift during the donor's lifetime is not necessary to make the gift valid.

3. The gift may be made to a specified donee or without specifying a donee. If the latter, the gift may be accepted by the attending physician as donee upon or following death. If the gift is made to a specified donee who is not available at the time and place of death, the attending physician upon or following death, in the absence of any expressed indication that the donor desired otherwise, may accept the gift as donee. The physician who becomes a donee under this subsection shall not participate in the procedures for removing or transplanting a part, except as provided in section 142A.7, subsection 2.

4. Notwithstanding section 142A.7, subsection 2, the donor may designate in the donor's will, card or other document of gift the surgeon or physician to carry out the appropriate procedures. In the absence of a designation, or if the designee is not available, the donee or other person authorized to accept the gift may employ or authorize any surgeon or physician for the purpose.

5. Any gift by a person designated in section 142A.2, subsection 2, shall be made by a document signed by the person, or made by the person's telegraphic, recorded telephonic or other recorded message.

§ 142A.5. Delivery of document of gift.

If the gift is made by the donor to a specified donee, the will, card, or other document, or an executed copy thereof, may be delivered to the donee to expedite the appropriate procedures immediately after death, but delivery is not necessary to the validity of the gift. The will, card, or other document, or an executed copy thereof, may be deposited in any hospital, bank, or storage facility, or registry office that accepts documents for safekeeping or for facilitation of procedures after death. On request of any interested party upon or after the donor's death, the person in possession shall produce the document for examination.

§ 142A.6. Amendment or revocation of the gift.

1. If the will, card, or other document, or executed copy thereof, has been delivered to a specified donee, the donor may amend or revoke the gift by:

   a. The execution and delivery to the donee of a signed statement.

   b. An oral statement made in the presence of two persons and communicated to the donee.

   c. A statement during a terminal illness or injury addressed to an attending physician and communicated to the donee.

   d. A signed card or document found on the donor's person or in the donor's effects.

2. Any document of gift which has not been delivered to the donee may be revoked by the donor in the manner set out in subsection 1, or by destruction, cancellation, or mutilation of the document and all executed copies thereof.

3. Any gift made by a will may also be amended or revoked in the manner provided for amendment or revocation of wills, or as provided in subsection 1.

4. An anatomical gift is not amendable or revocable by a person other than the donor.

§ 142A.7. Rights and duties at death.

1. The donee may accept or reject the gift. If the donee accepts a gift of the entire body, the donee may, subject to the terms of the gift, authorize embalming and the use of the body in funeral services. If the gift is of a part of the body, the donee, upon the death of the donor and prior to embalming, shall cause the part to be removed without unnecessary mutilation. After removal of the part, custody of the remainder of the body vests in the surviving spouse, next of kin, or other persons under obligation to dispose of the body.

2. The time of death shall be determined by a physician who attends the donor at the donor's death, or, if none, the physician who certifies the death. This physician shall not participate in the procedures for removing or transplanting a part, the enucleation of eyes being the exception. A licensed funeral director, as defined in chapter 156, upon successfully completing a course in eye enucleation and receiving a certificate of competence from the department of ophthalmology, college of medicine, of the University of Iowa, may enucleate the eyes of a donor.

3. A person who acts in good faith in accordance with the terms of this chapter, or under the anatomical gift laws of another state, is not liable for damages in any civil action or subject to prosecution in any criminal proceeding for the person's act.

4. The provisions of this chapter are subject to the laws of this state prescribing powers and duties with respect to autopsies.

§ 142A.8. Service but not a sale.

The procurement, processing, distribution or use of whole blood, plasma, blood products, blood derivatives and other human tissues such as corneas, bones or organs for the purpose of injecting, transfusing or transplanting any of them into the human body is declared to be, for all purposes, the rendition of a service by every person participating therein and, whether or not any remuneration is paid therefor, is declared not to be a sale of such whole blood, plasma, blood products, blood derivatives or other tissues, for any purpose, subsequent to July 1, 1969. However, any person or entity that renders such service warrants only under this section that due care has been exercised and that acceptable professional standards of care in providing such service according to the current state of the medical arts have been followed. Strict liability, in tort, shall not be applicable to the rendition of such service.

§ 142A.9. Uniformity of interpretation.
This chapter shall be so construed as to effectuate its general purpose to make uniform the law of those states which enact it.

§ 142A.10. Short title.
This chapter may be cited as the "Uniform Anatomical Gift Act".

KANSAS

UNIFORM ANATOMICAL GIFT ACT

§ 65-3201 to 65-3208.

History: L. 1968, ch. 63, §§ 1 to 8; Repealed, L. 1969, ch. 301, § 10; July 1.

§ 65-3209. Definitions.

(a) "Bank or storage facility" means a facility licensed, accredited, or approved under the laws of any state for storage of human bodies or parts thereof.

(b) "Decedent" means a deceased individual and includes a stillborn infant or fetus.

(c) "Donor" means an individual who makes a gift of all or part of his body.

(d) "Hospital" means a hospital licensed, accredited, or approved under the laws of any state; includes a hospital operated by the United States government, a state, or a subdivision thereof, although not required to be licensed under state laws.

(e) "Part" means organs, tissues, eyes, bones, arteries, blood, other fluids and any other portions of a human body.

(f) "Person" means an individual, corporation, government or governmental subdivision or agency, business trust, estate, trust, partnership or association, or any other legal entity.

(g) "Physician" or "surgeon" means a physician or surgeon licensed or authorized to practice under the laws of any state.

(h) "State" includes any state, district, commonwealth, territory, insular possession, and any other area subject to the legislative authority of the United States of America.

§ 65-3210. Persons who may execute an anatomical gift.

(a) Any individual of sound mind and eighteen (18) years of age or more may give all or any part of his body for any purpose specified in K.S.A. 65-3211, the gift to take effect upon death.

(b) Any of the following persons, in order of priority stated, when persons in prior classes are not available at the time of death, and in the absence of actual notice of contrary indications by the decedent or actual notice of opposition by a member of the same or a prior class, may give all or any part of the decedent's body for any purpose specified in K.S.A. 65-3211:

(1) the spouse,

(2) an adult son or daughter,

(3) either parent,

(4) an adult brother or sister,

(5) a guardian of the person of the decedent at the time of his death,

(6) any other person authorized or under obligation to dispose of the body.

(c) If the donee has actual notice of contrary indications by the decedent or that a gift by a member of a class is opposed by a member of the same or a prior class, the donee shall not accept the gift. The persons authorized by subsection (b) may make the gift after or immediately before death.

(d) A gift of all or part of a body authorizes any examination necessary to assure medical acceptability of the gift for the purposes intended.

(e) The rights of the donee created by the gift are paramount to the rights of others except as provided by K.S.A. 65-3215(d).

§ 65-3211. Persons who may become donees; purpose for which anatomical gifts may be made.

The following persons may become donees of gifts of bodies or parts thereof for the purposes stated:

(1) any hospital, surgeon, or physician, for medical or dental education, research, advancement of medical or dental science, therapy, or transplantation; or

(2) any accredited medical or dental school, college or university for education, research, advancement of medical or dental science, or therapy; or

(3) any bank or storage facility, for medical or dental education, research, advancement of medical or dental science, therapy, or transplantation; or

(4) any specified individual for therapy or transplantation needed by him.

§ 65-3212. Manner of executing anatomical gifts.

(a) A gift of all or part of the body under K.S.A. 65-3201(a) may be made by will. The gift becomes effective upon the death of the testator without waiting for probate. If the will is not probated, or if it is declared invalid for testamentary purposes, the gift, to the extent that it has been acted upon in good faith, is nevertheless valid and effective.

(b) A gift of all or part of the body under K.S.A. 65-3210(a) may also be made by document other than a will. The gift becomes effective upon the death of the donor. The document, which may be a card designed to be carried on the person, must be signed by the donor in the presence of two (2) witnesses who must sign the document in his presence. If the donor cannot sign, the document may be signed for him at his direction and in his presence in the presence of two (2) witnesses who must sign the document in his presence. Delivery of the document of gift during the donor's lifetime is not necessary to make the gift valid.

(c) The gift may be made to a specified donee or without specifying a donee. If the latter, the gift may be accepted by the attending physician as donee upon or following death. If the gift is made to a specified donee who is not available at the time and place of death, the attending physician upon or following death, in the absence of any expressed indication that the donor desired otherwise, may accept the gift as donee. The physician who becomes a donee under this subsection shall not participate in the procedures for removing or transplanting a part.

(d) Notwithstanding K.S.A. 65-3215(b), the donor may designate in his will, card, or other document of gift the surgeon or physician to carry out the appropriate procedures. In the absence of a designation or if the designee is not available, the donee or other person authorized to accept the gift may employ or authorize any surgeon or physician for the purpose.

(e) Any gift by a person designated in K.S.A. 65-3210(b) shall be made by a document signed by him or made by his telegraphic, recorded telephonic, or other recorded message.

§ 65-3213. Delivery of document of gift.

If the gift is made by the donor to a specified donee, the will, card, or other document, or an executed copy thereof, may be delivered to the donee to expedite the appropriate procedures immediately after death. Delivery is not necessary to the validity of the gift. The will, card, or other document, or an executed copy thereof, may be deposited in any hospital, bank or storage facility, or registry office that accepts it for safekeeping or for facilitation of procedures after death. On request of any interested party upon or after the donor's death, the person in possession shall produce the document for examination.

§ 65-3214. Amendment or revocation of the gift.

(a) If the will, card, or other document or executed copy thereof, has been delivered to a specified donee, the donor may amend or revoke the gift by:

(1) the execution and delivery to the donee of a signed statement, or

(2) an oral statement made in the presence of two (2) persons and communicated to the donee, or

(3) a statement during a terminal illness or injury addressed to an attending physician and communicated to the donee, or

(4) a signed card or document found on his person or in his effects.

(b) Any document of gift which has not been delivered to the donee may be revoked by the donor in the manner set out in subsection (a) or by destruction, cancellation, or mutilation of the document and all executed copies thereof.

(c) Any gift made by a will may also be amended or revoked in the manner provided for amendment or revocation of wills or as provided in subsection (a).

§ 65-3215. Rights and duties at death.

(a) The donee may accept or reject the gift. If the donee accepts a gift of the entire body, he may, subject to the terms of the gift, authorize embalming and the use of the body in funeral services. If the gift is of a part of the body, the donee, upon the death of the donor and prior to embalming, shall cause the part to be removed without unnecessary mutilation. After removal of the part, custody of the remainder of the body vests in the surviving spouse, next of kin, or other persons under obligation to dispose of the body.

(b) The time of death shall be determined by a physician who attends the donor at his death, or, if none, the physician who certifies the death. The physician shall not participate in the procedures for removing or transplanting a part.

(c) A person who acts in good faith in accord with the terms of this act or the anatomical gift laws of another state or a foreign country is not liable for damages in any civil action or subject to prosecution in any criminal proceeding for his act.

(d) The provisions of this act are subject to the laws of this state prescribing powers and duties with respect to autopsies.

§ 65-3216. Uniformity of interpretation.

This act shall be so construed as to effectuate its general purpose to make uniform the law of those states which enact it.

§ 65-3217. Short title.

This act may be cited as the uniform anatomical gift act.

§ 65-3218. Hospitals to develop protocols for identifying potential donors of body parts; family of potential donor to be informed of option to donate parts of deceased's body; factors protocols may consider.

(a) Each hospital in this state shall develop a protocol for identifying potential donors of body parts. The protocol shall require that any potential donor's next of kin or other individual who may execute an anatomical gift pursuant to K.S.A. 65-3210 and amendments thereto, at or near the time of notification of death, be asked whether the potential donor had authorized the donation of any body parts. If not, the family shall be informed of the option to donate parts of the deceased's body pursuant to the uniform anatomical gift act. With the approval of the designated next of kin or other individual who may execute an anatomical gift pursuant to K.S.A. 65-3210 and amendments thereto, the hospital shall then notify an organ and tissue procurement organization and cooperate in the procurement of the anatomical gift or gifts. The protocol shall encourage reasonable discretion and sensitivity to the family circumstances in all discussion regarding donations of body parts. The protocol may take into account the deceased individual's religious beliefs or obvious nonsuitability for donation of body parts. The protocol may take into account the hospital's ability to maintain a potential donor in a condition which would allow for retrieval of body parts. If an organ and tissue procurement organization does not exist in the region, the hospital shall contact an organ or a tissue procurement organization, as appropriate. Laws pertaining to notification of the coroner shall be complied with in all cases of reportable deaths.

(b) This section shall be part of and supplemental to the uniform anatomical gift act.

KENTUCKY

ANATOMICAL GIFT

311.165. Definitions for KRS 311.165 to 311.235.

(1) "Bank or storage facility" means a facility licensed, accredited or approved under the laws of any state for storage of human bodies or parts thereof;

(2) "Decedent" means a deceased individual and includes a stillborn infant or fetus;

(3) "Donor" means an individual who makes a gift of all or part of his body;

(4) "Hospital" means a hospital licensed, accredited, or approved under the laws of any state; includes a hospital operated by the United States government, a state, or a subdivision thereof, although not required to be licensed under state laws:

(5) "Part" means organs, tissues, eyes, bones, arteries, blood, other fluids and any other portions of a human body;

(6) "Person" means an individual, corporation, government or governmental subdivision or agency, business trust, estate, trust, partnership or association, or any other legal entity;

(7) "Physician" or "Surgeon" means a physician or surgeon licensed or authorized to practice under the laws of any state;

(8) "State" includes any state, district, commonwealth, territory, insular possession, and any other area subject to the legislative authority of the United States of America.

311.175. Persons who may execute an anatomical gift.

(1) Any individual of sound mind and eighteen (18) years of age or more may give all or any part of his body for any purpose specified in KRS 311.185, the gift to take effect upon death.

(2) Any of the following persons, in order of priority stated, when persons in prior classes are not available at the time of death, and in the absence of actual notice of contrary indications by the decedent or actual notice of opposition by a member of the same or a prior class, may give all or any part of the decedent's body for any purpose specified in KRS 311.185;

    (a) The spouse,

    (b) An adult son or daughter,

    (c) Either parent,

    (d) An adult brother or sister,

    (e) A guardian of the persons of the decedent at the time of his death,

    (f) Any other person authorized or under obligation to dispose of the body.

(3) If the donee has actual notice of contrary indications by the decedent or that gift by a member of a class is opposed by a member of the same or a prior class, the donee shall not accept the gift. The persons authorized by subsection (2) of this section may make the gift after or immediately before death.

(4) A gift of all or part of a body authorizes any examination necessary to assure medical acceptability of the gift for the purposes intended.

(5) The rights of the donee created by the gift are paramount to the rights of others except as provided by subsection (4) of KRS 311.225.

311.185. Persons who may become donees—Purposes for which anatomical gifts may be made.

The following persons may become donees of gifts of bodies or parts thereof for the purposes stated:

(1) Any hospital, surgeon, or physician, for medical or dental education, research, advancement of medical or dental science, therapy, or transplantation; or

(2) Any accredited medical or dental school, college or university for education, research, advancement of medical or dental science, or therapy; or

(3) Any bank or storage facility, for medical or dental education, research, advancement of medical or dental science, therapy, or transplantation; or

(4) Any specified individual for therapy or transplantation needed by him.

311.187. Removal of cornea or corneal tissue from decedent whose death defined as a coroner's case—Conditions—Who may remove.

(1) In any case in which a patient is in need of a cornea or corneal tissue for a transplant, the coroner, medical examiner, or his appropriately qualified designee with training in ophthalmologic techniques may, upon the request of any person authorized under KRS 311.185, provide or authorize the removal of the cornea or corneal tissue by a qualified physician under the following conditions:

    (a) The decedent has been defined as a "coroner's case" as set forth by KRS 72.405(2), an autopsy has been ordered pursuant to KRS 72.410, and the cornea or corneal tissue are suitable for transplant;

    (b) No objection by the next of kin is known by the coroner or medical examiner; and

    (c) The removal of the cornea or corneal tissue will not interfere with the subsequent course of an investigation or autopsy or alter the post mortem facial appearance.

(2) The medical examiner, coroner, or his appropriately qualified designee or any persons authorized under KRS 311.185 shall not be held liable in any civil or criminal action for failure to obtain consent of the next of kin.

(3) An individual certified by a department of ophthalmology in an accredited school of medicine as having received competent training, may remove corneas for gift after proper certification of death by a physician and in compliance with the provisions of KRS 311.175.

311.195. Manner of executing anatomical gifts.

(1) A gift of all or part of the body under subsection (1) of KRS 311.175 may be made by will. The gift becomes effective upon the death of the testator without waiting for probate. If the will is not probated, or if it is declared invalid for testamentary purposes, the gift, to the extent that it has been acted upon in good faith, is nevertheless valid and effective.

(2) A gift of all or part of the body under subsection (1) of KRS 311.175 may also be made by document other than a will. The gift becomes effective upon the death of the donor. The document, which may be a card designed to be carried on the person, must be signed by the donor in the presence of two (2) witnesses who must sign the document in his presence. If the donor cannot sign, the document may be signed for him at his direction and in his presence in the presence of two (2) witnesses who must sign the document in his presence. Delivery of the document of gift during the donor's lifetime is not necessary to make the gift valid.

(3) A gift of all or part of the body under KRS 186.412 may also be made by a statement provided for on all Kentucky operators' licenses. The gift becomes effective upon the death of the owner. The statement must be signed by the owner of the motor vehicle or motorcycle license in the presence of two (2) witnesses, who must sign the statement in the presence of the donor. Delivery of the license during the donor's lifetime is not necessary to make the gift valid. The gift shall become invalidated upon expiration, cancellation, revocation, or suspension of the license, and the gift must be renewed upon renewal of each license.

(4) The gift may be made to a specified donee or without specifying a donee. If the latter, the gift may be accepted by the attending physician as donee upon or following death. If the gift is made to a specified donee who is not available at the time and place of death, the attending physician upon or following death, in the absence of any expressed indication that the donor desired otherwise, may accept the gift as donee. The physician who becomes a donee under this subsection shall not participate in the procedures for removing or transplanting a part.

(5) Notwithstanding subsection (2) of KRS 311.225, the donor may designate in his will, card, or other document of gift the surgeon or physician to carry out the appropriate procedures. In the absence of a designation or if the designee is not available, the donee or other person authorized to accept the designee is not available, the donee or other person authorized to accept the gift may employ or authorize any surgeon or physician for the purpose.

(6) Any gift by a person designated in subsection (2) of KRS 311.175 shall be made by a document signed by him or made by his telegraphic, recorded telephonic or other recorded message.

311.205. Delivery of document of gift.

If the gift is made by the donor to a specified donee, the will, card, or other document, or an executed copy thereof, may be delivered to the donee to expedite the appropriate procedures immediately after death. Delivery is not necessary to the validity of the gift. The will, card, or other document, or an executed copy thereof, may be deposited in any hospital, bank or storage facility or registry office that accepts it for safekeeping or for facilitation of procedures after death. On request of any interested party upon or after the donor's death, the person in possession shall produce the document for examination.

311.215. Amendment or revocation of the gift.

(1) If the will, card, or other document or executed copy thereof, has been delivered to a specified donee, the donor may amend or revoke the gift by:
   (a) The execution and delivery to the donee of a signed statement, or
   (b) An oral statement made in the presence of two (2) persons and communicated to the donee, or
   (c) A statement during a terminal illness or injury addressed to an attending physician and communicated to the donee, or
   (d) A signed card or document found on his person or in his effects.

(2) Any document of gift which has not been delivered to the donee may be revoked by the donor in the manner set out in subsection (1) of this section, or by destruction, cancellation, or mutilation of the document and all executed copies thereof.

(3) Any gift made by a will may also be amended or revoked in the manner provided for amendment or revocation of wills, or as provided in subsection (1) of this section.

311.225. Rights and duties at death.

(1) The donee may accept or reject the gift. If the donee accepts a gift of the entire body, he may, subject to the terms of the gift, authorize embalming and the use of the body in funeral services. If the gift is of a part of the body, the donee, upon the death of the donor and prior to embalming, shall cause the part to be removed without unnecessary mutilation, After removal of the part, custody of the remainder of the body vests in the surviving spouse, next of kin, or other persons under obligation to dispose of the body.

(2) The time of death shall be determined by a physician who tends the donor at his death, or, if none, the physician who certifies

the death. The physician shall not participate in the procedures for removing or transplanting a part.

(3) A person who acts in good faith in accord with the terms of KRS 311.165 to 311.235 or with the anatomical gift laws of another state is not liable for damages in any civil action or subject to prosecution in any criminal proceeding for his act.

(4) The provisions of KRS 311.165 to 311.235 are subject to the laws of this state prescribing powers and duties with respect to autopsies.

311.235. Uniformity of interpretation.

(1) KRS 311.165 to 311.235 shall be so construed as to effectuate its general purpose to make uniform the law of those states which enact it.

(2) KRS 311.165 to 311.235 may be cited as the Uniform Anatomical Gift Act.

311.241. Hospitals to establish organ procurement protocol—Notification to federally certified organ procurement organization of potential availability of organ and identity of potential donor.

(1) Each hospital licensed under the provisions of KRS Chapter 216B shall, as a condition of licensure, establish an organ procurement for transplant protocol, in consultation with a federally certified organ procurement organization, which encourages organ donation and identifies potential organ donors.

(2) When an individual has died or has been identified by a medical hospital staff member as having a terminal condition and is further identified as a potential organ donor and meets the criteria set forth in the hospital's organ procurement for transplant protocol, the hospital administrator or his official designee shall then notify the federally certified organ procurement organization of the potential availability of the organ. The notification of the federally certified organ procurement organization as to the identity of a potential organ donor shall be documented in such patient's medical record. Any identified contraindication to organ donation shall be documented in the patient's medical record.

311.243. Family of donor not financially liable for cost of evaluation of donor suitability or retrieval of organ.

The family of any individual whose organ is donated for transplantation shall not be financially liable for any cost related to the evaluation of donor organ suitability and any cost of retrieval of the organ.

311.245. Duty of hospital and allied health personnel to make known patient's intent to donate organ.

All hospital physicians, nurses, and other allied health personnel shall make every reasonable effort to convey to the appropriate hospital unit the intent of any hospitalized patient to make a donation of all or any part of his body, as provided in KRS 311.175, in order that necessary documents may be executed under the provisions of this chapter.

311.247. Duty of law enforcement and medical personnel in accident and coroners' cases.

Law enforcement and medical personnel involved with the investigation of accidents and coroners' cases shall make a reasonable effort to ascertain if the victim has elected to give all or any part of his body as provided in KRS 311.175 and shall make a reasonable effort to send that information on to the coroner, medical examiner, or hospital personnel.

LOUISIANA

ANATOMICAL GIFT ACT

§ 2351. Definitions.

(1) "Bank or storage facility" means a facility licensed or approved under the laws of any state for storage of human bodies or parts thereof, for use in medical education, research, therapy, or transplantation to individuals.

(2) "Decedent" means an individual of any age and includes a stillborn infant.

(3) "Hospital" means a hospital licensed, accredited, or approved under the laws of any state and includes a hospital operated by the United States government, a state, or a subdivision thereof, although not required to be licensed under state laws.

(4) "Part" of a body includes organs, tissues, eyes, bones, arteries, blood, other fluids and other portions of bodies, and "part" includes "parts."

(5) "Person" means individual, corporation, government or governmental subdivision or agency, business trust, estate, trust, partnership or association, or any other legal entity.

(6) "Physician" or "surgeon" means a physician or surgeon licensed to practice under the laws of any state.

(7) "State" includes any state, district, commonwealth, territory, insular possession, and any other area subject to the legislative authority of the United States of America.

(8) "Technician" means any individual who has successfully completed a course in eye enucleation for ophthalmic medical assistants approved by the American Association of Ophthalmology and possesses documentary proof of qualifications.

§ 2352. Persons who may execute an anatomical gift.

A. Any individual who is competent to execute a will may give all or any part of his body for any of the purposes specified in R.S. 17:2353, the gift to take effect after death. The rights of the donee are superior to the rights of the surviving spouse and next of kin.

B. Unless he has knowledge that contrary directions have been given by the decedent, any of the following persons, in the order of priority stated, may give all or any part of a decedent's body for any of the purposes specified in R.S. 17:2353:

(1) The spouse if one survives; if not,

(2) An adult son or daughter,

(3) Either parent,

(4) An adult brother or sister,

(5) The guardian of the person of the decedent at the time of his death,

(6) Any other person authorized or under obligation to dispose of the body.

If there is no surviving spouse, and an adult son or daughter is not immediately available at the time of death, the gift may be made by either parent; if neither an adult son or daughter nor a parent is immediately available, it may be made by any adult brother or sister; but the donee shall not accept the gift if he or his agent has received notice that there is controversy within the class of relatives enabled under the above priorities to make the gift. The persons authorized by this subsection to make the gift may execute the document of gift either after death or immediately before death during a terminal illness or injury.

C. Any gift of all or part of a body is deemed to authorize such examination as may be necessary to assure medical acceptability of gift for the purposes intended.

D. No person shall disclose, disseminate or make public the fact of the making or acceptance of a gift authorized under the provisions of this Part without the prior specific consent of the donor, or if he is unable, that of the person authorized to make gifts under the provisions of Subsection (B) hereof in the order therein prescribed, unless otherwise required by law. Any person who makes any such disclosure as contemplated herein in violation of the provisions of this subsection shall be subject to absolute liability for damages in an amount of not less than five thousand dollars nor more than ten thousand dollars in a civil action instituted pursuant hereto by the person whose authorization therefor had not been obtained.

§ 2353. Persons who may become donees; purposes for which anatomical gifts may be made.

The following persons may become donees of gifts of bodies or parts thereof for the purposes stated:

(1) Any hospital, surgeon, or physician, for medical or dental education, research, advancement of medical or dental science, therapy, or transplantation to individuals;

(2) Any accredited medical or dental school, college, or university engaged in medical or dental education or research for educational, research, or medical or dental science purposes;

(3) Any person operating a bank or storage facility;

(4) Any specific donee, for therapy or transplantation needed by him.

§ 2354. Manner of executing anatomical gifts.

A. A gift of all or part of the body under this Part may be made by will, in which case the gift becomes effective at the death of the testator without waiting for probate. If the will is not probated, or if it is declared invalid for testamentary purposes, the gift, to the extent that it has been acted upon in good faith, is nevertheless valid and effective.

B. A gift of all or part of the body under this Part may also be made by a document other than a will. The document must be signed by the donor, in the presence of two witnesses who in turn shall sign the document in his presence. If the donor cannot sign in person, the document may be signed for him at his direction and in his presence, and in the presence of two witnesses who shall sign the document in his presence. Delivery of the document of gift during the donor's lifetime is not necessary to make the gift valid. The gift becomes effective at the death of the donor.

C. The document of gift may consist of a properly executed card carried on the donor's person or in his effects. The document of gift also may be printed on the reverse side of an operator's or chauffeur's license as provided by R.S. 32:410.

D. The gift may be made either to a named donee or without the naming of a donee. If the latter, the gift may be accepted by and utilized under the direction of the attending physician at or following death. If the gift is made to a named donee who is not reasonably available at the time and place of death, and the gift is evidenced by a properly executed card or other writing carried on the donor's person or in his effects, the attending physician at or following death, in reliance upon the card or writing, and in the absence of any expressed indication that the donor desired otherwise, may accept and utilize the gift as the agent of the donee for any purpose authorized in R.S. 17:2353. The agent possesses and may exercise all of the rights and is entitled to all of the immunities of the donee under this Part.

E. Except as provided in R.S. 17:2357(B), the donor may designate in his will or other document of gift the surgeon, physician or technician to implement the appropriate procedures. In the absence of such designation, or if the designee is not reasonably available, the donee or other person authorized to accept the gift may employ or authorize any licensed surgeon, physician or technician to implement the appropriate procedures herein authorized.

F. Any gift by a person designated in Subsection (B) of R.S. 17:2352, shall be by a document signed by the person authorized by that section in the presence of two witnesses who shall sign the document in his presence.

G. Except as provided in R.S. 17:2357(b), in the situation relative to a gift of one's eye or eyes, the donor may designate in his will or other document of gift the surgeon, physician or technician to implement the enucleation of his eye or eyes. In the absence of such designation by the donor or if such designee is unavailable, the donee or other person authorized to accept the gift may employ or authorize any surgeon, physician, any state licensed funeral director, embalmer, technician, or trained medical school student; provided that the funeral director, embalmer, or trained medical school student has successfully completed an eye enucleation course in any accredited medical school in the United States.

§ 2354.1. Coroner's consent for eye enucleation.

A. A physician, technician, or other authorized person trained in eye enucleation may remove the eyes of a decedent immediately following certification of death provided:

(1) There is written authorization by a person empowered to execute an anatomical gift as provided in R.S. 17:2352(B); or

(2) There is authorization by the parish coroner; and

(3) The eyes will be donated to an authorized donee of gifts of bodies or parts thereof as defined in R.S. 17:2353 for the purposes of advancing medical science or for the replacement or rehabilitation of eyes in living persons.

B. Neither the coroner, physician, surgeon, technician, hospital, bank or storage facility, nor the donee, who acts in good faith to comply with this Section shall be liable in any civil action to a claimant who alleges that his authorization for use of the eyes was required.

The provisions of this Subsection shall not be construed as limiting or restricting the liability of a coroner, physician, surgeon, technician, hospital, bank, storage facility or the donee as provided by R.S. 17:2357(C).

§ 2354.2. Coroner's consent for kidney removal.

A. A physician or surgeon may remove the kidneys of a decedent immediately following certification of death provided:

(1) There is written authorization by a person empowered to execute an anatomical gift as provided in R.S. 17:2352(B); or

(2) There is authorization by the parish coroner; and

(3) The kidneys will be or are intended to be donated to an authorized donee of gifts of bodies or parts thereof as defined in R.S. 17:2353 for the purpose of advancing medical science or for the replacement of kidneys in living persons.

B. Neither the coroner, physician, surgeon, technician, hospital, bank or storage facility, nor the donee, who acts in good faith to comply with this Section, shall be liable in any civil action to a claimant who alleges that his authorization for use of the kidneys was required.

The provisions of this Subsection shall not be construed as limiting or restricting the liability of a coroner, physician, surgeon, technician, hospital, bank, storage facility or the donee as provided in R.S. 17:2357(C).

§ 2354.3. Coroner's consent for heart, lungs, liver, soft tissue, or bone removal.

A. A physician or surgeon may remove the heart, lungs, liver, soft tissue, or bone of a decedent immediately following certification of death provided:

(1) There is written authorization by a person empowered to execute an anatomical gift as provided in R.S. 17:2352(B); or

(2) There is authorization by the parish coroner; and

(3) The heart, lungs, liver, soft tissue, or bone will be donated to an authorized donee of gifts of bodies or parts thereof as defined in R.S. 17:2353 for the purpose of advancing medical science or for the replacement of the heart, lungs, liver, soft tissue, or bone in living persons.

B. (1) Neither the coroner, physician, surgeon, technician, hospital, bank or storage facility, nor the donee, who acts in good faith to comply with this Section shall be liable in any civil action to a claimant who alleges that his authorization for use of the heart, lungs, liver, soft tissue, or bone was required.

(2) The provisions of this Subsection shall not be construed as limiting or restricting the liability of a coroner, physician, surgeon, technician, hospital, bank or other storage facility, or the donee as provided by R.S. 17:2357(C).

§ 2354.4. Duties of hospital administrator; training; coordination.

A. As used in this Section:

(1) "Administrator" means the chief operating officer of a hospital.

(2) "Death" shall have the meaning provided in R.S. 9:111.

(3) "Hospital" means any institution, place, building, or agency, public or private, whether for profit or not, devoted primarily to the maintenance and operation of facilities for ten or more individuals for the diagnosis, treatment, or care of persons admitted for overnight stay or longer who are suffering from illness, injury, infirmity, or deformity or other physical condition for which obstetrical, medical, or surgical services would be available and appropriate. The term "hospital" does not include the following:

(a) Physicians' offices or clinics where patients are not regularly kept as bed patients for twenty-four hours or more;

(b) Nursing homes as defined by and regulated under the provisions of R.S. 40:2009.1 through R.S. 40:2009.12;

(c) Persons, schools, institutions, or organizations engaged in the care and treatment of mentally retarded children and which are required to be licensed by the provisions of R.S. 28:421 through R.S. 28:427; or

(4) "Suitable candidate" means a patient who is certified by the attending physician, at or immediately before the time of death, to be a suitable donor for any organ or tissue donation based on accepted medical standards, and who has been released by the coroner in those instances required by law.

B. When death occurs in a hospital, to a person determined to be a suitable candidate for organ or tissue donation based on accepted medical standards, the hospital administrator or designated representative shall request the appropriate person described in Subsection H of this Section to consent to the gift of any part of the decedent's body as an anatomical gift.

C. No request shall be required, pursuant to this Section, when the requesting person has actual notice of contrary intention by the decedent or those persons described in Subsection H of this Section according to the priority stated therein, or reason to believe that an anatomical gift is contrary to the decedent's religious beliefs.

D. (1) A nonprofit organ or tissue bank or retrieval organization shall notify said hospital administrator in writing that any donation can be properly obtained and fully utilized in a manner consistent with accepted medical standards. Such notice shall provide that the nonprofit organ or tissue bank or retrieval organization will be responsible for all costs and charges of the hospital relating to obtaining the donated organ or tissue. The time within which the notice is to be effective shall be specified.

(2) Requests under this Section shall be limited to nonprofit organ or tissue banks or retrieval organizations.

E. Upon approval of the proper individual specified in Subsection H of this Section, the hospital administrator or designated representative shall notify an appropriate organ or tissue bank, or retrieval organization and cooperate in the procurement of the anatomical gift.

F. When a request is made, pursuant to Subsection B of this Section, the person making the request shall complete a certificate of request for an anatomical gift, on a form to be supplied by the secretary of the Department of Health and Human Resources. The certificate shall include the following:

(1) A statement indicating that a request for an anatomical gift was made.

(2) The name and affiliation of the person making the request.

(3) An indication of whether consent was granted and, if so, what organs and tissues were donated.

(4) The name of the person granting or refusing the request, and his relationship to the decedent.

G. A copy of the certificate described in Subsection F of this Section shall be included in the decedent's medical records.

H. The following persons shall be requested to consent to a gift, in the order of priority stated:

(1) The spouse if one survives; if not,

(2) An adult son or daughter,

(3) Either parent,

(4) An adult brother or sister,

(5) The curator or tutor of the person of the decedent at the time of his death,

(6) Any other person authorized or under obligation to dispose of his body.

I. When a donation is requested, consent or refusal need only be obtained from the person in the highest priority class available after best efforts have been exercised to contact those persons in a higher priority class. If there is more than one person within an above named class, then the consent to the donation shall be made by all members of that class reasonably available for consultation.

J. The secretary of the Department of Health and Human Resources shall:

(1) Establish rules concerning the procedures to be employed in making the request.

(2) Compile and disseminate a list of those nonprofit organ or tissue banks or retrieval organizations authorized to receive donations under this Section.

(3) Establish rules to implement appropriate procedures to facilitate proper coordination among hospitals, organ and tissue banks, and retrieval organizations.

K. (1) Neither the physician, administrator, surgeon, technician, hospital, organ and tissue bank, retrieval organization, nor the donee, who acts in good faith to comply with this Section shall be liable in any civil action to a claimant who alleges that his consent for the donation was required.

(2) The provisions of R.S. 17:2354(B), R.S. 17:2354.2(B), R.S. 17:2354.3(B)(1) and (2) and R.S. 9:2797 are applicable to this Section.

§ 2355. Delivery of document of gift.

If the gift is made by the donor to a named donee, the will or other document, or a copy thereof, may be delivered to him to expedite the appropriate procedures immediately after death, but such delivery is not necessary to validity of the gift. The document may also be deposited in any hospital or registry office that accepts such documents for safekeeping or for facilitation of procedures after death. Upon request of any interested party at or after the donor's death, the person in possession must produce the document for examination.

§ 2356. Revocation of the gift.

A. If the document of gift has been delivered to a named donee, it may be revoked by either:

(1) The execution and delivery to the donee or his agent of a revocation in writing signed by the donor, or

(2) An oral statement of revocation made in the presence of two persons, communicated to the donee or his agent, or

(3) A statement during a terminal illness addressed to the attending physician and communicated to the donee, or

(4) A card or writing, signed by the donor and carried on his person or in his effects, revoking the gift.

B. Any document of gift which has not been delivered to the donee may be revoked in the manner set out in Subsection (A) of this section or by destruction, cancellation, or mutilation of the document.

C. Any gift made by a will may be revoked or amended in the manner provided for revocation or amendment of wills.

D. An anatomical gift may not be amended or revoked by any person other than the donor, except that when the gift is of the entire body, the body shall be returned after removal of all the useable organs to the surviving spouse or the next of kin upon the request of either.

§ 2357. Rights and duties at death.

A. The donee may accept or reject the gift. If the donee accepts, and if the gift is of the entire body, the donee or his agent, if he deems it desirable, may authorize embalming and funeral services. If the gift is of a part of the body, the donee or his agent, immediately after the death of the donor and prior to embalming, may cause the part included in the gift to be removed without unnecessary mutilation. After removal of the part, custody of the remainder of the body shall be transferred promptly to the surviving spouse or next of kin or other persons under obligation to dispose of the body.

B. The time of death shall be determined by the physician who attends the donor at his death, or, if none, the physician who certifies the death. The physician shall not be a participant in the procedures for removing the part or transplanting it.

C. The donee, agent of a donee, other person authorized to accept and utilize the gift, or any person authorized by the donor or donee to perform the surgical operation to remove parts covered by the gift is not liable for damages in any civil action or subject to prosecution in any criminal proceeding for his act if he acts in good faith and without actual knowledge of revocation of the gift and in accord with the terms of a gift under this Part, in accord with a document carried by the donor as provided in this Part, or in accord with the laws of the state in which the document of gift was executed.

D. The provisions of this Part are subject to the laws of this state prescribing powers and duties with respect to autopsies.

§ 2358. Uniformity of interpretation.

This Part shall be so construed as to effectuate its general purpose to make uniform the law of those states which enact it.

§ 2359. Short title.

This Part may be cited as the Anatomical Gift Act.

MAINE

CHAPTER 710
UNIFORM ANATOMICAL GIFT ACT

§ 2901. Definitions

1. Bank or storage facility. "Bank or storage facility" means a facility licensed, accredited or approved under the laws of any state for storage of human bodies or parts thereof.

2. Decedent. "Decedent" means a deceased individual and includes a stillborn infant or fetus.

3. Donor. "Donor" means an individual who makes a gift of all or part of his body.

4. Hospital. "Hospital" means a hospital licensed, accredited or approved under the laws of any state and includes a hospital operated by the United States Government, a state or a subdivision thereof, although not required to be licensed under state laws.

5. Part. "Part" includes organs, tissues, eyes, bones, arteries, blood, other fluids and other portions of a human body, and "part" includes "parts".

6. Person. "Person" means an individual, corporation, government or governmental subdivision or agency, business trust, estate, trust, partnership or association or any other legal entity.

7. Physician or surgeon. "Physician" or "surgeon" means a physician or surgeon licensed or authorized to practice under the laws of any state.

8. State. "State" includes any state, district, commonwealth, territory, insular possession, and any other area subject to the legislative authority of the United States of America.

§ 2902. Persons who may execute an anatomical gift

1. Individuals. Any individual of sound mind and of legal age may give all or any part of his body for any purposes specified in section 2903, the gift to take effect upon death.

2. Others. Any of the following persons, in order of priority stated, when persons in prior classes are not available at the time of death, and in the absence of actual notice of contrary indications by the decedent, or actual notice of opposition by a member of the same or a prior class, may give all or any part of the decedent's body for any purposes specified in section 2903:

    A. The spouse;

    B. An adult son or daughter;

    C. Either parent;

    D. An adult brother or sister;

    E. A guardian of the person of the decedent at the time of his death;

    F. Any other person authorized or under obligation to dispose of the body.

3. Notice to donee. If the donee has actual notice of contrary indications by the decedent, or that a gift by a member of a class is opposed by a member of the same or a prior class, the donee shall not accept the gift. The persons authorized by subsection 2 may make the gift after death or immediately before death.

4. Examination. A gift of all or part of a body authorizes any examination necessary to assure medical acceptability of the gift for the purposes intended.

5. Rights. The rights of the donee created by the gift are paramount to the rights of others, except as provided by section 2907, subsection 4.

§ 2903. Persons who may become donees, and purposes for which anatomical gifts may be made

The following persons may become donees of gifts of bodies or parts thereof for the purposes stated:

1. Medical. Any hospital, surgeon or physician, for medical or dental education, research, advancement of medical or dental science, therapy or transplantation; or

2. School. Any accredited medical or dental school, college or university for education, research, advancement of medical or dental science or therapy; or

3. Storage facility. Any bank or storage facility, for medical or dental education, research, advancement of medical or dental science, therapy or transplantation; or

4. Specified individuals. Any specified individual for therapy or transplantation needed by him.

§ 2904. Manner of executing anatomical gifts

1. Will. A gift of all or part of the body under section 2902, subsection 1 may be made by will. The gift becomes effective upon the death of the testator without waiting for probate. If the will is not probated, or if it is declared invalid for testamentary purposes, the gift, to the extent that it has been acted upon in good faith, is nevertheless valid and effective.

2. Other documents. A gift of any part of the body under section 2902, subsection 1, may be made by document other than a will. The gift becomes effective upon the death of the donor and upon acceptance by the donee. The document, which may be a card designed to be carried on the person, must be signed by the donor, in the presence of 2 witnesses who must sign the document in his presence. If the donor cannot sign, the document may be signed for him at his direction and in his presence, and in the

presence of 2 witnesses who must sign the document in his presence. Delivery of the document of gift during the donor's lifetime is not necessary to make the gift valid.

3. Donee. The gift may be made to a specified donee or without specifying a donee. If the latter, the gift may be accepted by the attending physician as donee upon or following death. If the gift is made to a specified donee who is not available at the time and place of death, the attending physician, upon or following death in the absence of any expressed indication that the donor desired otherwise, may accept the gift as donee. The physician who becomes a donee under this subsection shall not participate in the procedures for removing or transplanting a part.

4. Designee. Notwithstanding section 2907, subsection 2, the donor may designate in his will, card or other document of gift the surgeon or physician to carry out the appropriate procedures; provided that eye enucleations may also be performed by a person who has successfully completed a course of training either taught by an ophthalmologist, or given by the New England Eye Bank, and that the person is then examined and certified as qualified to perform eye enucleations by an ophthalmologist licensed to practice in Maine. The course shall include instruction and practice in anatomy and physiology of the eye, maintaining a sterile field during the procedure, use of the appropriate instruments and sterile procedures for removing the corneal button and preserving it in a preservation fluid. In the absence of a designation, or if the designee is not available, the donee or other person authorized to accept the gift may employ or authorize any surgeon or physician for the purpose.

5. How made. Any gift by a person designated in section 2902, subsection 2 shall be made by a document signed by him, or made by his telegraphic, recorded telephonic or other recorded message.

This subsection includes, but is not limited to, gifts made pursuant to section 2910. Any gift pursuant to section 2910, by a person designated in section 2902, subsection 2, shall be made by a document signed by him, by a telegraphic, recorded telephonic or other recorded message, or by a telephonic message witnessed by at least 2 people in which case the witnesses shall document the telephonic message in writing.

§ 2905. Delivery of document of gift

If the gift is made by the donor to a specified donee, the will, card or other document, or an executed copy thereof, may be delivered to the donee to expedite the appropriate procedures immediately after death, but delivery is not necessary to the validity of the gift. The will, card or other document, or an executed copy thereof, may be deposited in any hospital, bank or storage facility or registry office that accepts them for safekeeping or for facilitation of procedures after death. On request of any interested party upon or after the donor's death, the person in possession shall produce the document for examination.

§ 2906. Amendment or revocation of the gift

1. Amendment. If the will, card or other document or executed copy thereof has been delivered to a specified donee, the donor may amend or revoke the gift by:

A. The execution and delivery to the donee of a signed statement; or

B. An oral statement made in the presence of 2 persons and communicated to the donee; or

C. A statement during a terminal illness or injury addressed to an attending physician and communicated to the donee; or

D. A signed card or document found on his person or in his effects.

2. Revocation. Any document of gift which has not been delivered to the donee may be revoked by the donor in the manner set out in subsection 1 or by destruction, cancellation or mutilation of the document and all executed copies thereof.

3. Other methods. Any gift made by a will may also be amended or revoked in the manner provided for amendment or revocation of wills, or as provided in subsection 1.

§ 2907. Rights and duties at death

1. Accepted or rejected. The donee may accept or reject the gift. If the donee accepts a gift of the entire body, he may, subject to the terms of the gift, authorize embalming and the use of the body in funeral services. If the gift is of a part of the body, the donee, upon the death of the donor and prior to embalming, shall cause the part to be removed without unnecessary mutilation. After removal of the part, custody of the remainder of the body vests in the surviving spouse, next of kin or other persons under obligation to dispose of the body.

2. Time of death. The time of death shall be determined by a physician who attends the donor at his death, or, if none, the physician who certifies the death. This physician shall not participate in the procedures for removing or transplanting a part.

3. Good faith. A person who acts in good faith in accord with the terms of this chapter, or under the anatomical gift laws of another state or a foreign country, is not liable for damages in any civil action or subject to prosecution in any criminal proceeding for his act.

4. Applicability of other laws. This chapter is subject to the laws of this State prescribing powers and duties with respect to autopsies and to the provisions of chapter 711, the Medical Examiner Act.

§ 2908. Uniformity of interpretation

This chapter shall be so construed as to effectuate its general purpose to make uniform the law of those states which enact it.

§ 2909. Short title

This chapter may be cited as the Uniform Anatomical Gift Act.

MARYLAND

ANATOMICAL GIFT ACT

§4-501. Definitions.

(a) In this subtitle the following words have the meanings indicated.

(b) Body or part of body.— "Body" or "part of body" includes organs, tissues, bones, blood, and other body fluids.

(c) Licensed hospital. — "Licensed hospital" includes any hospital licensed by the State Department of Health and Mental Hygiene under the laws of the State, and any hospital operated by the United States government, although not required to be licensed under the laws of the State.

(d) Next of kin. — "Next of kin" includes spouse.

(e) Person. — "Person" means any individual, corporation, government or governmental agency or subdivision, estate, trust, partnership or association, or any other legal entity.

(f) Physician or surgeon. —"Physician" or "surgeon" means any physician or surgeon licensed to practice under the laws of the state.

§4.502. Legislative policy; purpose of subtitle.

(a) Legislative policy. —Because of the rapid medical progress in the field of tissue and organ preservation, the transplantation of tissue, and tissue culture, and because it is in the public interest to aid the development of this field of medicine, it is the policy and purpose of the General Assembly of Maryland in enacting this subtitle to encourage and aid the development of reconstructive medicine and surgery and the development of medical research by facilitating authorizations for premortem and postmortem donations of tissue and organs.

(b) Purpose of subtitle. —It is the purpose of this subtitle to regulate only the gift of a body or parts of a body to be made after the death of a donor.

§4.503. Execution of documents of anatomical gift.

(a) Competence of donor. —Any individual who is 18 years of age or over and who is competent to execute a will may give all or any part of his body for any one or more of the purposes specified in this subtitle. The gift takes effect after death of the donor.

(b) Persons who may make gift. —Unless he has knowledge that contrary directions have been given by the decedent, the following persons, in the order of priority stated, may give all or any part of a body of a decedent for any one or more of the purposes specified in this subtitle:

(1) The spouse, if one survives;

(2) An adult son or daughter;

(3) Either parent;

(4) An adult brother or sister;

(5) The guardian of the person of the decedent at the time of his death;

(6) Any other person or agency authorized or under obligation to dispose of the body.

If there is no surviving spouse and an adult son or daughter is not immediately available at the time of death of a decedent, the gift may be made by either parent. If a parent of decedent is not immediately available, the gift may be made by any adult brother or sister of decedent. If there is known to be a controversy within the class of persons first entitled to make the gift, the gift may not be accepted. The persons authorized by this subsection to make the gift may execute the document of gift either after death or during a terminal illness.

(c) Method of making gift. —If the gift is made by a person designated in §4.503 (b) of this section, it shall be by a document signed by him or by his telegraphic, recorded telephonic, or other recorded message.

(d) Examination for medical acceptance. —A gift of all or part of a body authorizes any examination of the body, or any other procedure, necessary to assure medical acceptability of the gift for the purposes intended.

(e) Rights of donee. —Except as provided in § 4-507 of this subtitle, the rights of the donee created by the gift are paramount to the rights of others.

§4-504. Persons eligible to become donees of anatomical gifts.

(a) General. —The persons listed in this section are eligible to receive gifts of human bodies or parts of them for the purposes stated.

(b) Hospital, surgeon, or physician. —Any licensed hospital, surgeon, or physician may receive a gift for medical education, research, advancement of medical science, therapy, or transplantation to individuals.

(c) Medical school. —An accredited medical school, college, or university engaged in medical education or research may receive a gift for therapy, educational research, or medical science purposes.

(d) Storage of blood or human organs. —Any licensed person operating a bank or storage facility for blood, arteries, eyes, pituitaries, or other human parts may receive a gift for use in medical education, research, therapy, or transplantation needed by him.

§4-505. Methods of making anatomical gifts.

(a) Gift by will. —A gift of all or part of the body for purposes of this subtitle may be made by will, in which case the gift becomes effective immediately upon death of the testator without waiting for probate. If the will is not probated, or if it is declared invalid for testamentary purposes, the gift, to the extent that it has been acted upon in good faith, is nevertheless valid and effective.

(b) Gift of document. —A gift of all or part of the body for purposes of this subtitle also may be made by document other than a will. The document must be signed by the donor in the presence of two witnesses, who, in turn, shall sign the document in the presence of the donor. If the donor cannot sign in person, the document may be signed for him, at his direction and in his presence, and in the presence of two witnesses, who, in turn, shall sign the document in the presence of the donor. Delivery of the document or gift during the lifetime of the donor is not necessary to make the gift valid. The document may consist of a properly executed card carried on the person of the donor or in his effects. The document and card may conform substantially to the following form:

ANATOMICAL GIFT BY A LIVING DONOR

I am at least 18 years of age and make this anatomical gift to take effect upon my death. The marks in the appropriate squares and words filled into the blanks below indicate my desires.

1. I give:__my body;__any needed organs or parts;__the following organs or parts_____
2. To the following person, agency, or institution:__any person, tissue bank, or institution authorized by law;
__ the Anatomy Board of Maryland;
__ the following named physician, hospital, tissue bank or other medical institution_____
3. For the following purposes:__any purposes authorized by law;__transplantation;__therapy;__medical research and education.

Dated_____City and State_____Signed by the Donor in the presence of the following who sign as witnesses:

_____   _____
Witness   Signature of Donor

_____   _____
Witness   Address of Donor

(c) Designation of donee; acceptance of gift by attending physician. —The gift may be made either to a named donee, or without the naming of a donee. If the latter, the gift may be accepted by and utilized at the discretion of the attending physician at or following death. If the gift is made to a named donee who is not readily available at the time and place of death, and if the gift is evidenced by a properly executed card or other document carried on the person of the donor, or in his effects, the attending physician at or following death, in reliance upon the card or other document, may accept and utilize the gift in his discretion, as the agent of the donee. The agent possesses and may exercise all rights and is entitled to all immunities of the donee under this subtitle.

(d) Designation of surgeon to carry out procedures. —The donor may designate in his will or other document of gift the surgeon, physician, or technician to carry out the appropriate procedures. In the event the designee is not available, or in the absence of a designation, the donee or other person authorized to accept the gift may employ or authorize any licensed surgeon, licensed physician, or technician for the purpose.

(e) Validity of document of gift executed in another state. —A document of gift executed in another state and in accord with the laws of that state or executed in a territory or possession of the United States under the control and dominion of the federal government exclusively, and in accord with a federal law is valid as a document of gift within the state, even if the document does not substantially conform to the requirements of §4-505 (b) of this subtitle.

§4-506. Delivery of will or document of gift to donee.

(a) Delivery to expedite procedure. —Immediately after death if the gift is made to a named donee, the will or other document or an attested true copy of it may be delivered to him to expedite the appropriate procedure, but delivery is not necessary to validate the gift.

(b) Production of will. —Upon request of the named donee or his agent after the death of the donor, the person in possession shall produce the will or other document of gift for examination.

§4-507. Revocation of gift.

(a) Revocation of delivered document. —Any document of gift which has been delivered to the donee may be revoked by
    (1) The execution and delivery to the donee or his agent of a revocation in writing, signed by the donor,
    (2) An oral statement of revocation witnessed by two persons, and communicated to the donee or his agent,

(3) A statement during a terminal illness addressed to the attending physician and communicated to the donee, or his agent, or

(4) A card or other writing signed by the donor and carried on his person or his effects, revoking the gift.

(b) Revocation of undelivered document. —Any document of gift which has not been delivered to the donee may be revoked in the manner set out in subsection (a) of this section, or by destruction, cancellation, or mutilation of the document.

(c) Revocation of will. —Any gift made by a will may be revoked in the manner set out in subsection (a) of this section, or in the manner provided for revocation or amendment of wills.

§4-508. Rights of next of kin and donee; time of death; civil or criminal liability; autopsies.

(a) Acceptance or rejection of gift; custody of body of decedent; determining time of death. —The donee may accept or reject the gift. If the gift is only a part of the body, promptly following the removal of the part named, custody of the remaining parts of the body shall be transferred to the next of kin or other person or agency authorized or under obligation to dispose of the body. The time of death shall be determined by the physician in attendance upon the terminal illness of the donor or certifying his death, and the physician may not be a member of the team of physicians which transplants the part to another individual.

(b) No civil or criminal liability for unknowingly violating subtitle. —A person who, in good faith and acting in reliance upon an authorization made under the provisions of this subtitle or under the anatomical gift laws of another state or foreign country and without notice of revocation, takes possession of, performs surgical operations upon, or removes tissue, substances, or parts from the human body or refuses the gift, or a person who unknowingly fails to carry out the wishes of the donor according to the provisions of this subtitle or under the anatomical gift laws of another state or foreign country, is not subject to prosecution in any criminal proceedings or liable for damages in a civil action brought against him for the act or failure to act.

(c) Effect of laws concerning autopsies. —The provisions of this subtitle are subject to the laws prescribing powers and duties with respect to autopsies and are not in contravention of them.

§4-509. When Chief Medical Examiner or his deputy or assistant may provide organ for transplant.

(a) Requirements. —In any case where a patient is in immediate need for an internal organ as a transplant, the Chief Medical Examiner, the deputy chief medical examiner, or an assistant medical examiner may provide the organ upon the request of the transplanting surgeon under the following conditions:

(1) The medical examiner has charge of a decedent who may provide a suitable organ for the transplant;

(2) A reasonable, unsuccessful search has been made by the treating physician and the hospital where the patient is located to contact the next of kin;

(3) No known objection by the next of kin is foreseen by the medical examiner; and

(4) The organ for transplant will not interfere with the subsequent course of an investigation or autopsy.

(b) Liability of medical examiner. —The Chief Medical Examiner, the deputy chief medical examiner, and an assistant chief medical examiner are not liable for civil action if the next of kin is located subsequently and contends that authorization of that kin was required, if the Chief Medical Examiner has obtained a written statement from the treating physician or the hospital where the patient was located that a reasonable unsuccessful search was conducted for the next of kin prior to the removal of the tissue for transplantation.

§4-509.01. When Chief Medical Examiner or his deputy or assistant may provide cornea for transplant.

(a) Requirements. —In any case where there is a need for corneal tissue for a transplant or research, the Chief Medical Examiner, the deputy chief medical examiner, or an assistant medical examiner shall provide the cornea upon the request of the Medical Eye Bank of Maryland, Incorporated, or the Lions of District 22-C Eye Bank and Research Foundation, Incorporated, subject to the provisions of subsection (b) of this section, and under the following conditions:

(1) The medical examiner has charge of a decedent who may provide a suitable cornea for the transplant or research;

(2) An autopsy will be required;

(3) No objection by the next of kin is known by the medical examiner;

(4) No religious objection made by the decedent before death is known by the medical examiner; and

(5) Removal of the cornea for transplant will not interfere with the subsequent course of an investigation or autopsy or alter the postmortem facial appearance.

(b) Distribution of corneal tissue. Corneal tissue provided under subsection (a) of this section shall be distributed as follows:

(1) If the decedent died in Prince George's County, Montgomery county, Charles County, Calvert County, or St. Mary's County, the corneal tissue shall be distributed to the Lions of District 22-C Eye Bank and Research Foundation, Incorporated; or

(2) If the decedent died in any other county or in Baltimore City, the corneal tissue shall be distributed to the Medical Eye Bank of Maryland, Incorporated.

(c) Liability of medical examiner, Medical Eye Bank of Maryland, etc.—The Chief Medical Examiner, the deputy chief medical examiner, an assistant medical examiner, the Medical Eye Bank of Maryland, Incorporated, or the Lions of District 22-C Eye Bank and Research Foundation, Incorporated, are not liable for civil action if the next of kin subsequently contends that authorization of that kin was required.

§4-510. Gifts completed during lifetime of donor.

The provisions of this subtitle do not apply to gifts of parts of the body if the gifts are made during the lifetime of the donor with the intention that the part of the body is delivered to the donee during the lifetime of the donor.

§4-511. Validity of authority or instrument executed prior to July 1, 1968.

Nothing in this subtitle invalidates any authority or instrument executed prior to July 1, 1968.

§4-512. Short title.

This subtitle may be cited as the Maryland Anatomical Gift Act.

MASSACHUSETTS

PROMOTION OF ANATOMICAL SCIENCE

§7. Definitions.

In sections eight to fourteen, inclusive, unless the context otherwise requires, the following words shall have the following meanings:

"Acute hospital", any hospital licensed under section fifty-one of chapter one hundred and eleven, and the teaching hospital of the University of Massachusetts medical school, which contain a majority of medical-surgical, pediatric, obstetric, and maternity beds as defined by the department of public health.

"Bank or storage facility", a facility licensed, accredited or approved by the department of public health.

"Commissioner", the commissioner of the department of public health.

"Decedent", a deceased individual and includes a stillborn infant or fetus.

"Department", the department of public health.

"Donor", an individual who makes a gift of all or part of his body.

"Hospital", a hospital licensed, accredited or approved under the laws of any state and includes a hospital operated by the United States government, a state or a subdivision thereof, although not required to be licensed under state laws.

"Part", includes organs, tissues, skin, eyes, bones, arteries, blood, other fluids and other portions of a human body and "part" includes "parts".

"Person", an individual, corporation, government or governmental subdivision or agency, business trust, estate, trust, partnership or association or any other legal entity.

"Physician" or "surgeon", a physician or surgeon licensed or authorized to practice under the laws of any state.

"State", includes any state, district, commonwealth, territory, insular possession, and any other area subject to the legislative authority of the United States of America.

§8. Gifts of Human Bodies, Organs, and Tissues, Who May Make; Rights Created.

(a) A person of sound mind and who is eighteen years of age or older may make a gift of all or any part of his body for any purposes specified in section nine, said gift to take effect upon his death, or in the case of a living donor at such time prior to his death as he may specify in accordance with the requirements of subsection (b) of section ten, so long as such donation does not jeopardize in any way the life and health of the donor.

(b) On or before the occurrence of death in an acute hospital, the director or other person in charge of such hospital, or his designated representative, including, but not limited to, the physician responsible for the care of the patient, shall inform any of the persons listed below in the order of priority stated, when persons in prior classes are not available, of the opportunity of authorizing a gift of all or part of the decedent's body for the purposes of organ and tissue transplantation as specified in section nine; provided, however, that (1) no actual notice of contrary intentions by such persons has been received, (2) such information shall not cause undue emotional stress to the next of kin and (3) consent to such transplantation would yield an organ or tissue donation suitable for use in accordance with medical criteria as defined by physicians engaged in clinical transplantation therapy and as established by rules and regulations promulgated by the department which shall contain standards consistent with the standards set forth in the Manual of the New England Organ Bank. The order of priority of such persons shall be:

(1) the spouse,

(2) an adult son or daughter,

(3) either parent,

(4) an adult brother or sister,

(5) a guardian of the person of the decedent at the time of his death,

(6) any other person authorized or under obligation to dispose of the body.

(c) The director or person in charge of such hospital or his designated representative shall record in a book kept for such purpose (1) the names of those patients for whom consent to an anatomical gift had been granted, (2) the organs or tissues donated, (3) the name of the person granting consent, and (4) the relationship of such person to the decedent.

(d) If the donee has actual notice of contrary indications by the decedent, or that a gift authorized by a member of a class is opposed by a member of the same or a prior class, the donee shall not accept the gift. The persons authorized by subsection (b) may make the gift after death or immediately before death.

(e) A gift of all or part of a body authorizes premortem tests, and any other examination necessary to assure medical acceptability of the gift for the purposes intended by the donor.

(f) The rights of the donee created by the gift are paramount to the rights of others except as provided by subsection (d) of section thirteen.

(g) The commissioner shall issue an annual report summarizing and evaluating the data collected pursuant to subsection (c).

§9. Who May Become Donees of Anatomical Gifts.

The following persons may become donees of gifts of bodies or parts thereof for the purposes stated:

(1) any hospital, surgeon, or physician, for medical or dental education, research, advancement of medical or dental science, therapy or transplantation; or

(2) any accredited medical or dental school, college, or university for education, research, advancement of medical or dental science or therapy; or

(3) any bank or storage facility for medical or dental education, research, advancement of medical or dental science, therapy or transplantation; or

(4) any specified individual for therapy or transplantation needed by him.

§10. Gift May Be Made by Will or Other Instrument; When Effective; Execution; Donee When None Specified.

(a) A gift of all or part of the body under subsection (a) of section eight may be made by will. Such gift shall become effective upon the death of the testator. If the will is not probated, or if it is declared invalid for testamentary purposes, such gift, to the extent that it has been acted upon in good faith, shall be nevertheless valid and effective.

(b) A gift of all or part of the body under subsection (a) of section eight may also be made by a document other than a will. Such gift shall become effective upon the death of the donor.

In the case of a gift of a living donor intended for transplantation, the donor shall authorize such gift in a document signed by the donor and also by at least two of the physicians who are to participate in the transplantation operation and who shall have previously examined the donor in connection with his gift. In all cases other than those involving the gift of a living donor, the document may be a card designed to be carried on the person which shall be signed by the donor in the presence of two competent witnesses who shall attest to and subscribe the document in said donor's presence. If the donor, cannot sign, the document may be signed for him at his direction and in his presence, and in the presence of two witnesses who must sign the document in his presence. Delivery of such document during the donor's lifetime is not necessary to make the gift valid.

(c) The gift may be made to a specified donee or without specifying a donee. If no donee is specified, the gift may be accepted by the attending physician as donee upon the death of the donor. If the gift is made to a specified donee who is not available at the time and place of death, the attending physician upon the death of the donor, in the absence of any expressed indication that the donor desired otherwise, may accept the gift as donee. The physician who becomes a donee under this subsection shall not participate in the procedures for removing or transplanting a part.

(d) Notwithstanding subsection (b) of section thirteen, the donor may designate in his will, card or other document of gift the surgeon or physician to carry out the appropriate procedures; provided, however, that eye enucleations may be performed also by a technician who has successfully completed a course of training acceptable to the Eye Bank of the Massachusetts Eye and Ear Infirmary. In the absence of a designation, or if the designee is not available, the donee or other person authorized to accept the gift may employ or authorize any surgeon or physician for said purpose.

(e) Any gift by a person designated in subsection (b) of section eight shall be made by a document signed by him, or made by his telegraphic, recorded telephonic or other recorded message.

§11. Gift Instrument May Be Delivered to Donee or Deposited for Safekeeping; Production on or after Donor's Death.

If the gift is made by the donor to a specified donee, the will, card, or other document, or an executed copy thereof, may be delivered to the donee to expedite the appropriate procedures immediately after death, but delivery is not necessary to the validity of the gift. The will, card or other document, or an executed copy thereof, may be deposited in any hospital, bank or storage facility or registry office that accepts them for safekeeping or for facilitation of procedures after death. On request of any interested party upon or after the donor's death, the person in possession shall produce the document for examination.

§12. Amendment or Revocation of Gift.

(a) If the will, card or other document or executed copy thereof has been delivered to a specified donee, the donor may amend or revoke the gift by:

(1) the execution and delivery to the donee of a signed statement, or

(2) an oral statement made in the presence of two persons and communicated to the donee, or

(3) a statement during a terminal illness or injury addressed to an attending physician and communicated to the donee, or

(4) a signed card or document found on his person or in his effects.

(b) Any document of gift which has not been delivered to the donee may be revoked by the donor in the manner set out in subsection (a) or by destruction, cancellation, or mutilation of the document and all executed copies thereof.

(c) Any gift made by a will may also be amended or revoked in the manner provided for amendment or revocation of wills, or as provided in subsection (a).

§13. Donee May Accept or Reject Gift; Procedure upon Acceptance; Who Shall Determine Time of Death; Persons Acting in Good Faith Shall Not Be Liable, etc.

(a) The donee may accept or reject the gift. If the donee accepts a gift of the entire body, he may, subject to the terms of the gift, authorize embalming and the use of the body in funeral services. If the gift is of a part of the body, the donee, upon the death of the donor and prior to embalming, shall cause the part to be removed without unnecessary mutilation. After removal of the part, custody of the remainder of the body vests in the surviving spouse, next of kin or other persons under obligation to dispose of the body. If the donee is responsible for the disposition of the body, he shall dispose of it in accordance with the terms specified by the donor, or if no such terms are specified, he shall have said body decently buried or cremated.

(b) The time of death shall be determined by a physician who attends the donor at his death, or, if none, the physician who certified the death. This physician shall not participate in the procedures for removing or transplanting a part.

(c) A person who acts in good faith in accordance with the terms of sections seven to thirteen, inclusive, or under the anatomical gift laws of another state or a foreign country shall not be liable for damages in any civil action or be subject to prosecution in any criminal proceeding for his act.

(d) The provisions of sections seven to thirteen, inclusive, shall be subject to the laws of the commonwealth relative to autopsies.

§14. Cornea, Removal for Transplant Purposes; Procedure; Penalty for Violation.

Upon request of the New England Eye Bank, an unincorporated nonprofit association registered with the attorney general, located at the Massachusetts Eye and Ear Infirmary, a medical examiner or a physician acting under his direction may provide the cornea of a decedent to said New England Eye Bank under the following conditions: (a) the body of the decedent is under the jurisdiction of the medical examiner authorizing the removal of the cornea and an autopsy is required in accordance with the provisions of chapter thirty-eight; (b) a period of one hour has elapsed after the medical examiner or physician acting under his direction has notified said eye bank and said eye bank has received such notification that the cornea of the decedent is available for transplant, and during such period said eye bank has made a good faith effort to notify decedent's spouse or next of kin that such transplant is proposed; (c) no objections to the donation have been made known by the decedent prior to his death or by the decedent's spouse or next of kin to said medical examiner or physician; (d) the removal of the cornea for transplant will not interfere with a subsequent investigation or autopsy; and (e) the removal of the cornea will not alter the decedent's facial appearance. The time of such notification by said medical examiner or physician acting under his direction to said eye bank, shall be entered into a log kept specifically for such purpose and such log shall be available for inspection upon request during regular business hours, by a spouse or next of kin of a decedent whose cornea has been removed.

No medical examiner, physician or said eye bank, acting under the provisions of this section, shall be liable in any criminal or civil action brought as a result of a removal of a decedent's cornea if such good faith effort to notify decedent's spouse or next of kin of such transplant has been made.

MICHIGAN

ANATOMICAL GIFTS

333.10101. Definitions.

Sec. 10101. As used in this part:

(a) "Bank or storage facility" means a facility licensed, accredited, or approved under the laws of any state for storage of human bodies or physical parts thereof.

(b) "Decedent" means a deceased individual and includes a stillborn infant or fetus.

(c) "Donor" means an individual who makes a gift of all or a physical part of his or her body.

(d) "Hospital" means a hospital licensed, accredited, or approved under the laws of any state. It includes a hospital operated by the United States government, a state or a subdivision thereof, although not required to be licensed under state laws.

(e) "Person" means an individual, corporation, government or governmental subdivision or agency, business trust, estate, trust, partnership or association, or any other legal entity.

(f) "Physical part" means organs, tissues, eyes, bones, arteries, blood, other fluids, and any other portions of a human body.

(g) "Physician" or "surgeon" means a physician or surgeon licensed or authorized to practice under the laws of any state.

(h) "State medical school" means the university of Michigan school of medicine, the Michigan state university college of human medicine, the Michigan state university college of osteopathic medicine, or the Wayne state university school of medicine.

333.10102. Persons who may donate body or any physical part thereof; objections; examinations; rights of donee.

Sec. 10102. (1) An individual of sound mind and 18 years of age or more may give all or any physical part of the individual's body for any purpose specified in section 10103, the gift to take effect upon death.

(2) Any of the following persons, in order of priority stated, when persons in prior classes are not available at the time of death, and in the absence of actual notice of contrary indications by the decedent or actual notice of opposition by a member of the same or a prior class, may give all or any physical part of the decedent's body for any purpose specified in section 10103:

(a) The spouse.

(b) An adult son or daughter.

(c) Either parent.

(d) An adult brother or sister.

(e) A guardian of the person of the decedent at the time of the death.

(f) Any other person authorized or under obligation to dispose of the body.

(3) If the donee has actual notice of contrary indications by the decedent or that a gift by a member of a class is opposed by a member of the same or a prior class, the donee shall not accept the gift. The persons authorized by subsection (2) may make the gift after or immediately before death.

(4) A gift of all or a physical part of a body authorizes any examination necessary to assure medical acceptability of the gift for the purposes intended.

(5) The rights of the donee created by the gift are paramount to the rights of others except as provided by section 10108 (4).

333.10102a. Anatomical gifts; requests; hospital organ donation log sheet; summary; request policy; rules; withholding or medical care.

Sec. 10102a. (1) Subject to section 10102(3) and subsections (2) to (7), the person designated pursuant to subsection (7) shall, at or near the death of a patient whose body, according to accepted medical standards, is suitable for donation or for the donation of physical parts, request 1 of the persons listed in section 10102(2), in the order of priority stated, to consent to the gift of all or any physical part of the decedents; body.

(2) The person designated pursuant to subsection (7) shall not make a request for consent pursuant to subsection (1) if 1 or more of the following conditions exist:

(a) The person designated pursuant to subsection (7) has actual notice of contrary indications by the patient or decedent.

(b) The person designated pursuant to subsection (7) has actual notice of opposition by a person listed in section 10102(2) unless a person in a prior class under that section is available for a request to be made.

(c) The person designated pursuant to subsection (7) has knowledge that the gift of all or a physical part of a body is contrary to the religious beliefs of the decedent.

(3) Each hospital shall maintain a hospital organ donation log sheet on a form provided by the department. The organ donation log sheet shall include all of the following information:

(a) The name and age of the patient or decedent for whom a request is made pursuant to this section.

(b) A list of patients or decedents for whom a request was not made pursuant to this section and the reason for not making the request, as set forth in subsection (2).

(c) An indication that a request for consent to a gift of all or a physical part of a body has been made.

(d) An indication of whether or not consent was granted.

(e) If consent was granted, an indication of which physical parts of the body were donated, or whether the entire body was donated.

(f) The name and signature of the person making the request.

(4) After making a request for a gift pursuant to subsection (1), the person designated pursuant to subsection (7) shall complete the hospital's organ donation log sheet.

(5) A summary of the information contained in the organ donation log sheets annually shall be transmitted by each hospital to the department. The summary shall include all of the following:

(a) The number of deaths.

(b) The number of requests made.

(c) The number of consents granted.

(d) The number of bodies or physical parts donated in each category as specified on the organ donation log sheet.

(6) A gift made pursuant to a request required by this section shall be executed pursuant to this part.

(7) The chief executive officer of each hospital shall develop and implement a policy regarding requests made pursuant to this section. The policy shall provide, at a minimum, for all of the following:

(a) The designation of persons who shall make requests under this section.

(b) That if a patient's religious preference is known, a clergy of that denomination shall, if possible, be made available upon request to the person to whom a request under this section is made.

(c) The development of a support system which facilitates the making of requests under this section.

(d) The maintenance of the organ donation log sheet required by subsection (3).

(8) The director may promulgate rules to establish minimum training standards for persons required to make requests pursuant to this section and to revise the organ donation log sheet required by subsection (3).

(9) This section shall not be construed to authorize the withdrawal or withholding of medical care for a patient who is a possible donor and who is near death.

333.10103. Persons who may become donees of gift of bodies or physical parts thereof.

Sec. 10103. The following persons may become donees of gifts of bodies or physical parts thereof for the purposes stated:

(a) Any hospital, surgeon, or physician for medical or dental education, research, advancement of medical or dental science, therapy, or transplantation.

(b) Any accredited medical or dental school, college, or university for education, research, advancement of medical or dental science, or therapy.

(c) Any bank or storage facility for medical or dental education, research, advancement of medical or dental science, therapy, or transplantation.

(d) Any specified individual for therapy or transplantation needed by that individual.

(e) Any approved or accredited school of optometry, nursing, or veterinary medicine.

333.10104. Gift by will or document other than will; specified and non-specified donees; foreign documents.

Sec. 10104. (1) A gift of all or a physical part of the body under section 10102(1) may be made by will. The gift becomes effective upon the death of the testator without waiting for probate. If the will is not probated, or if it is declared invalid for testamentary purposes, the gift, to the extent that it has been acted upon in good faith, is nevertheless valid and effective.

(2) A gift of all or a physical part of the body under section 10102(1) may also be made by document other than a will. The gift becomes effective upon the death of the donor. The document, which may be a card designed to be carried on the person, shall be signed by the donor in the presence of 2 witnesses who shall sign the document in the donor's presence. If the donor cannot sign, the document may be signed for the donor at his or her direction and in his or her presence in the presence of 2 witnesses who shall sign the document in the donor's presence. Delivery of the document of gift during the donor's lifetime is not necessary to make the gift valid. A document which conforms substantially to the following form is sufficient for the purposes of this subsection:

Uniform Donor Card

Of_____

    Print or type name of donor

In the hope that I may help others, I hereby make this anatomical gift if medically acceptable, to take effect upon my death. The words and marks below indicate my desires.

I give: (a)_____any needed organs or physical parts

      (b)_____ only the following organs or physical parts

_____

Specify the organ(s) or physical part(s)

For the purposes of transplantation, therapy, medical research or education;

(c)_____my body for anatomical study if needed. Limitations or special wishes, if any:_____
Signed by the donor and the following 2 witnesses in the presence of each other:

_____   _____
Signature of donor   Date of birth of donor

_____   _____
Date signed   City and state

_____   _____
Witness   Witness

(3) The gift may be made to a specified donee or without specifying a donee. If the latter, the gift may be accepted by the attending physician as donee upon or following death. If the gift is made to a specified donee who is not available at the time and place of death, the attending physician upon or following death, in the absence of any expressed indication that the donor desired otherwise, may accept the gift as donee. The physician who becomes a donee under this subsection shall not participate in the procedures for removing or transplanting a physical part.

(4) Notwithstanding section 10108(4), the donor may designate in his or her will, card, or other document of gift the surgeon or physician to carry out the appropriate procedures. In the absence of a designation or if the designee is not available, the donee or other person authorized to accept the gift may employ or authorize any surgeon or physician for the purpose.

(5) Any gift by a person designated in section 10102(2) shall be made by a document signed by the person or made by the person's telegraphic, recorded telephonic, or other recorded message.

(6) A document of gift executed in another state or foreign country and in accord with the laws of that state or country is valid as a document of gift in this state, although the document does not conform substantially to the form set forth in subsection (2).

333.10105. Eye enucleation.

Sec. 10105. In the absence of designation of a physician or surgeon by either the donor or the donee of an eye or a physical part thereof of a decedent, or because the physician or surgeon is not readily available to excise the eye or physical part thereof as specified in a donor card or will, a licensed physician or a person who is certified by a state medical school may perform the operation and arrange for placement of the gift in the nearest eye bank. A state medical school may certify a person as qualified to perform the operation required for the removal of an eye or a physical part thereof only after successfully completing a comprehensive course in eye enucleation organized and conducted by the state medical school or who has successfully completed a similar course offered by a nationally accredited medical school located outside this state.

333.10106. Delivery of will, card or other document; safekeeping; examination.

Sec. 10106. If the gift is made by the donor to a specified donee, the will, card, or other document, or an executed copy thereof, may be delivered to the donee to expedite the appropriate procedures immediately after death. Delivery is not necessary to the validity of the gift. The will, card, or other document, or an executed copy thereof, may be deposited in any hospital, bank or storage facility, or registry office that accepts it for safekeeping or for facilitation of procedures after death. On request of any interested party upon or after the donor's death, the person in possession shall produce the document for examination.

333.10107. Amendment or revocation of gift.

Sec. 10107. (1) If the will, card, or other document or executed copy thereof, has been delivered to a specified donee, the donor may amend or revoke the gift by any of the following methods:

(a) The execution and delivery to the donee of a signed statement.

(b) An oral statement made in the presence of 2 persons and communicated to the donee.

(c) A statement during a terminal illness or injury addressed to an attending physician and communicated to the donee.

(d) A signed card or document found on the donor's person or in the donor's effects.

(2) Any document of gift which has not been delivered to the donee may be revoked by the donor in the manner set out in subsection (1), or by destruction, cancellation, or mutilation of the document and all executed copies thereof.

(3) Any gift made by a will may also be amended or revoked in the manner provided for amendment or revocation of wills, or as provided in subsection (1).

333.10108. Acceptance or rejection of gift; removal of physical part and custody of remainder; liability; autopsy laws.

Sec. 10108. (1) The donee may accept or reject the gift. If the donee accepts a gift of the entire body, the surviving spouse, next of kin, or other persons having authority to direct and arrange for the funeral and burial or other disposition of the body, subject to the terms of the gift, may authorize embalming and the use of the body in funeral services. If the gift is a physical part of the body, the donee, upon the death of the donor and prior to embalming, shall cause the physical part to be removed without unnecessary mutilation. After removal of the physical part, custody of the remainder of the body vests in the surviving spouse, next of kin, or such other persons having authority to direct and arrange for the funeral and burial or other disposition of the remainder of the body. The holder of a license for the practice of mortuary science under article 18 of the occupational code, Act.

No. 299 of the Public Acts of 1980, being sections 339.1801 to 339.1812 of the Michigan Compiled Laws, who acts pursuant to the directions of persons alleging to have authority to direct and arrange for the funeral and burial or other disposition of the remainder of the body, is relieved of any liability for the funeral and for the burial or other disposition of the remainder of the body. A holder of a license for the practice of mortuary science under that act may rely on the instructions and directions of any person alleging to be either a donee or a person authorized under this part to donate a body or any physical part thereof. A holder of a license for the practice of mortuary science under that act is not liable for removal of any physical part of a body donated under this part.

(2) The time of death shall be determined by a physician who attends the donor at the death, or, if none, the physician who certifies the death. The attending or certifying physician shall not participate in the procedures for removing or transplanting a physical part.

(3) A person, including a hospital, who acts in good faith in accord with the terms of this part or with the anatomical gift laws of another state or a foreign country is not liable for damages in any civil action or subject to prosecution in any criminal proceeding for the act.

(4) This part is subject to the laws of this state prescribing powers and duties with respect to autopsies.

333.10109. Construction of part.

Sec. 10109. This part shall be construed to effectuate its general purpose to make uniform the law of those states which enact it.

MINNESOTA

UNIFORM ANATOMICAL GIFT ACT

§ 525.921. Definitions.

Subdivision 1. For the purposes of sections 525.921 to 525.93 the terms defined in this section have the meanings given them.

Subd. 2. "Bank or storage facility" means a facility licensed, accredited, or approved under the laws of any state for storage of human bodies or parts thereof.

Subd. 3. "Decedent" means a deceased individual and includes a stillborn infant or fetus.

Subd. 4. "Donor" means an individual who makes a gift of all or part of the individual's body.

Subd. 5. "Hospital" means a hospital licensed, accredited, or approved under the laws of any state; includes a hospital operated by the United States government, a state, or a subdivision thereof, although not required to be licensed under state laws.

Subd. 6. "Part" means organs, tissues, eyes, bones, arteries, blood, other fluids and any other portions of a human body.

Subd. 7. "Person" means an individual, corporation, government or governmental subdivision or agency, business trust, estate, trust, partnership or association, or any other legal entity.

Subd. 8. "Physician" or "surgeon" means a physician or surgeon licensed or authorized to practice medicine under the laws of any state.

Subd. 9. "State" includes any state, district, commonwealth, territory, insular possession, and any other area subject to the legislative authority of the United States of America.

§ 525.922. Persons who may execute an anatomical gift.

Subdivision 1. Any individual of sound mind and 18 years of age or more, or any minor, with written consent of both parents, a legal guardian, or the parent or parents with legal custody may give all or any part of the individual's body for any purpose specified in section 525.923, the gift to take effect upon death.

Subd. 2. Any of the following persons, in order of priority stated, when persons in prior classes are not available at the time of death, and in the absence of actual notice of contrary indications by the decedent or actual notice of opposition by a member of the same or a prior class, may give all or any part of the decedent's body for any purpose specified in section 525.923:

(a) the spouse,

(b) an adult son or daughter,

(c) either parent,

(d) an adult brother or sister,

(e) a guardian of the person of the decedent at the time of death,

(f) any other person authorized or under obligation to dispose of the body.

Subd. 3. If the donee has actual notice of contrary indications by the decedent or that a gift by a member of a class is opposed by a member of the same or a prior class, the donee shall not accept the gift. The persons authorized by subdivision 2 may make the gift after or immediately before death.

Subd. 4. A gift of all or part of a body authorizes any examination necessary to assure medical acceptability of the gift for the purposes intended.

Subd. 5. The rights of the donee created by the gift are paramount to the rights of others except as provided by Minnesota Statutes 1967, section 390.11.

§ 525.923. Persons who may become donees; purposes for which anatomical gifts may be made.

The following persons may become donees of gifts of bodies or parts thereof for the purposes stated:

(1) any hospital, surgeon, or physician, for medical or dental education, research, advancement of medical or dental science, therapy, or transplantation; or

(2) any accredited medical or dental school, college or university for education, research, advancement of medical or dental science, therapy, or transplantation; or

(3) any bank or storage facility, for medical or dental education, research, advancement of medical or dental science, therapy, or transplantation; or

(4) any specified individual for therapy or transplantation needed by the individual; or

(5) any approved chiropractic college for education, research or advancement of chiropractic science.

§ 525.924. Manner of executing anatomical gifts.

Subdivision 1. A gift of all or part of the body under section 525.922, subdivision 1, may be made by will. The gift becomes effective upon the death of the testator without waiting for probate. If the will is not probated, or if it is declared invalid for testamentary purposes, the gift, to the extent that it has been acted upon in good faith, is nevertheless valid and effective.

Subd. 2. A gift of all or part of the body under section 525.922, subdivision 1, may also be made by document other than a will. The gift becomes effective upon the death of the donor. The document, which may be a card designed to be carried on the person, must be signed by the donor in the presence of two witnesses who must sign the document in the donor's presence. If the donor cannot sign, the document may be signed for the donor at the donor's direction and in the donor's presence in the presence of two witnesses who must sign the document in the donor's presence. Delivery of the document of gift during the donor's lifetime is not necessary to make the gift valid.

Subd. 2a. A gift of all or part of the body under section 525.922, subdivision 1, may be made by a minor, in a document other than a will. The gift becomes effective upon the death of the donor. The document, which may be a card designed to be carried on the person, must: (1) be signed by the minor donor and both of the minor donor's parents, a legal guardian, or the parent or parents with legal custody; (2) give the minor donor's date of birth; (3) give the address of the minor donor; and (4) contain the following words: "In hope that I may help others to live, I hereby make this anatomical gift, if medically acceptable, to take effect upon my death. I give (organ name) for the purpose of transplantation." If the minor cannot sign, the card may not be signed for the minor. Delivery of the gift document during the minor donor's lifetime is not necessary to make the gift valid.

Subd. 3. The gift may be made to a specified donee or without specifying a donee. If the latter, the gift may be accepted by the attending physician as donee upon or following death. If the gift is made to a specified donee who is not available at the time and place of death, the attending physician upon or following death, in the absence of any expressed indication that the donor desired otherwise, may accept the gift as donee. The physician who becomes a donee under this subdivision shall not participate in the procedures for removing or transplanting a part.

Subd. 4. Notwithstanding section 525.927, subdivision 2, the donor may designate in a will, card, or other document of gift the surgeon or physician to carry out the appropriate procedures. In the absence of a designation or if the designee is not available, the donee or other person authorized to accept the gift may employ or authorize any surgeon or physician for the purpose.

Subd. 5. Any gift by a person designated in section 525.922, subdivision 2, shall be made by a document signed by the person or made by telegraphic, recorded telephonic, or other recorded message.

Subd. 6. In respect to a gift of an eye, a person licensed to practice mortuary science under chapter 149, or any other person who has completed a course in eye enucleation conducted and certified by the department of ophthalmology of any accredited college of medicine, and holds a valid certificate of competence for completing the course, may enucleate eyes for a gift after pronouncement of death by a physician. A written release authorizing the enucleation must be obtained prior to the performance of the procedure. The release shall be obtained from a relative or other person in the order of priority stated in section 525.922, subdivision 2. A mortician or other person acting in accordance with the provisions of this subdivision shall not have any liability, civil or criminal, for the eye enucleation.

Subd. 7. The designation "donor" on the front side of a donor's driver's license or nonqualification certificate, pursuant to the provisions of section 171.07, subdivision 5, shall constitute sufficient legal authority for the removal of all body organs or parts, upon the death of the donor for the purpose of transplantation.

§ 525.925. Delivery of document of gift.

Subdivision 1. If the gift is made by the donor to a specified donee, the will, card, or other document, or an executed copy thereof, may be delivered to the donee to expedite the appropriate procedures immediately after death. Delivery is not necessary to the validity of the gift. The will, card, or other document, or an executed copy thereof, may be deposited in any hospital, bank or storage facility, or registry office that accepts it for safekeeping or for facilitation of procedures after death. On request of any interested party upon or after the donor's death, the person in possession shall produce the document for examination.

Subd. 2. A card, or other document, or an executed copy thereof, may be filed with the local registrar of vital statistics in the city or county of the donor's residence. The local registrar upon filing or recording the same shall transmit to the state registrar of vital statistics on or before the tenth of each month a copy thereof. The applicable provisions of the uniform vital statistics act shall apply to the filing and recording of the instrument referred to in this subdivision.

§ 525.926. Amendment or revocation of the gift.

Subdivision 1. If the will, card, or other document or executed copy thereof, has been delivered to a specified donee, the donor may amend or revoke the gift by:

    (a) the execution and delivery to the donee of a signed statement, or

    (b) an oral statement made in the presence of two persons and communicated to the donee, or

    (c) a statement during a terminal illness or injury addressed to an attending physician and communicated to the donee, or

    (d) a signed card or document found on the donor's person or in the donor's effects.

Subd. 2. Any document of gift which has not been delivered to the donee may be revoked by the donor in the manner set out in subdivision 1 or by destruction, cancellation, or mutilation of the document and all executed copies thereof.

Subd. 3. Any gift made by a will may also be amended or revoked in the manner provided for amendment or revocation of wills or as provided in subdivision 1. If an amendment or revocation of the gift is made in conformity with subdivision 1, such amendment or revocation shall not affect any other part of the will.

§ 525.927. Rights and duties at death.

Subdivision 1. The donee may accept or reject the gift. The donee, on accepting a gift of the entire body, may, subject to the terms of the gift, authorize embalming and the use of the body in funeral services. If the gift is of a part of the body, the donee, upon the death of the donor and prior to embalming, shall cause the part to be removed without unnecessary mutilation. After removal of the part, custody of the remainder of the body vests in the surviving spouse, next of kin, or other persons under obligation to dispose of the body.

Subd. 2. The time of death shall be determined by a physician who attends the donor at death, or, if none, the physician who certifies the death. The physician shall not participate in the procedures for removing or transplanting a part.

Subd. 3. A person who acts in good faith in accord with the terms of sections 171.07, subdivisions 5; 171.12, subdivision 5; and 525.921 to 525.93, or the anatomical gift laws of another state or a foreign country is not liable for damages in any civil action or subject to prosecution in any criminal proceeding for the act.

§ 525.928. Parts for transplantation.

The use of any part of a body for the purpose of transplantation in the human body shall be construed, for all purposes whatsoever, as a rendition of a service by each and every person participating therein and shall not be construed as a sale of such part for any purpose whatsoever.

§ 525.929. Uniformity of interpretation.

Sections 525.921 to 525.93 shall be so construed as to effectuate it general purpose to make uniform the law of those states which enact it.

§ 525.93. Short title.

Sections 525.921 to 525.93 may be cited as the uniform anatomical gift act.

§ 525.94. Establishment of protocol to obtain organs for transplantation.

Subdivision 1. Requirement to establish organ procurement protocol. A hospital licensed under sections 144.50 to 144.58 must establish written protocols for the identification of potential organ donors for transplantation to:

(1) assure that families of potential organ donors are made aware of the option of organ and tissue donation and their option to decline;

(2) require that an organ procurement agency be notified of potential organ donors; and

(3) establish medical criteria and practical considerations concerning the suitability and feasibility of organ donation for transplantations.

For purposes of this subdivision, the term "organ" or "tissue" includes but is not limited to a human kidney, liver, heart, lung, pancreas, skin, bone, ligament, tendon, eye, and cornea.

Subd. 2. Notification requirement. If an individual dies in a hospital or is identified by an appropriate hospital staff member as having a terminal condition and is further identified as a suitable candidate for organ or tissue donation based on medical criteria established in the written protocol, in accordance with the hospital's protocol, the hospital administrator or the administrator's designated representative shall notify any of the following persons listed below in order of priority, of the option of organ or tissue donation and their option to decline:

(1) the spouse;

(2) an adult child;

(3) either parent;

(4) an adult brother or sister; or

(5) a guardian of the decedent's person at the time of death.

The hospital administrator or the designated representative shall attempt to locate the person's driver's license, organ donation card, or other documentation of the person's desire to be an organ donor. If documentation of the person's desire to be a donor is located, it constitutes consent if there is no objection from the relative or guardian in clauses (1) to (5) or if no relative or guardian can be located.

If a person listed in clauses (1) to (5) wishes to consent to the gift of all or part of the decedent's body for transplantation, consent may be obtained by either the hospital administrator's representative or the organ procurement agency's representative. Consent or refusal must be obtained only from the available person highest on the list in clauses (1) to (5).

Subd. 3. Documentation. Notification under subdivision 2, as well as any identified contradiction to organ donation, must be documented in the patient's medical record, which must include the name of the person notified and the person's relationship to the decedent.

Subd. 4. Financial liability. The family of an individual whose organ is donated for transplantation is not financially liable for costs related to the evaluation of donor organ suitability or retrieval of the organ.

Subd. 5. Compliance with uniform anatomical gift act. A gift made pursuant to the request required under this section must be executed according to the uniform anatomical gift act.

Subd. 6. Training. The commissioner of health shall work with hospital representatives and other interested persons to develop guidelines for training hospital employees who may notify persons of the option to make an anatomical gift and the procedure to be used in executing the gift and for ensuring that each tissue or organ is tested for possible disease before being made available for transplantation.

MISSISSIPPI

THE ANATOMICAL GIFT LAW

§ 41-39-31. Title.
Sections 41-39-31 to 41-39-51 may be cited as "the Anatomical Gift Law."

§ 41-39-33. Definitions.
As used in sections 41-39-31 to 41-39-51, the following terms shall have the meaning indicated:

(a) "Person" means individual, corporation, government or governmental agency or subdivision, estate, trust, partnership or association, or any other legal entity.

(b) "Body or part of body" includes organs, tissues, bones, blood and other body fluids, and "part" includes "parts."

(c) "Licensed hospital" includes any hospital licensed by the state board of health under the laws of this state and any hospital operated by the United States Government although not required to be licensed under the laws of the state of Mississippi.

(d) "Licensed physician or surgeon" means any physician or surgeon who is certified by the state board of health as being qualified to remove and preserve parts of a body pursuant to this chapter.

(e) "Technician" means an individual other than a physician or surgeon who is certified by the state board of health as being qualified to remove and preserve parts of a body pursuant to this chapter.

(f) "Accredited school of mortuary science" means a mortuary science program in a state junior college approved by the state junior college commission and the vocational technical division of the Mississippi Department of Education.

§ 41-39-35. Persons authorized to make donations.
(a) Any individual who is eighteen (18) years of age or over and who is competent to execute a will may give all or any part of his body for any one or more of the purposes specified in sections 41-39-31 to 41-39-51, the gift to take effect after death.

(b) Unless he has knowledge that contrary directions have been given by the decedent, the following persons, in the order of priority stated, may give all or any part of a decedent's body for any one or more of the purposes specified in sections 41-39-31 to 41-39-51:

(1) The spouse, if one survives.

(2) An adult son or daughter.

(3) Either parent.

(4) An adult brother or sister.

(5) The guardian of the person of the decedent at the time of his death.

(6) Any other person or agency authorized or under obligation to dispose of the body.

If there is no surviving spouse and an adult son or daughter is not immediately available at the time of death of a decedent, the gift may be made by either parent.

If a parent of decedent is not immediately available, the gift may be made by an adult brother or sister of decedent. If there is known to be a controversy within the class of persons first entitled to make the gift, the gift will not be accepted. The persons authorized herein to make the gift may execute the document of gift either after death or during a terminal illness. The decedent may be a minor or a stillborn infant.

If the gift is made by a person designated above, it shall be by written or telegraphic consent.

§ 41-39-37. Persons eligible to receive donations.
The following persons are eligible to receive gifts of human bodies or parts thereof for the purposes stated:

(1) Any licensed hospital, surgeon or physician, for medical education, research, advancement of medical science, therapy or transplantation to individuals.

(2) Any accredited medical school, college or university engaged in medical education or research, for therapy, educational research or medical science purposes.

(3) Any person operating a bank or storage facility for blood, arteries, eyes, pituitaries, or other human parts, for use in medical education, research, therapy or transplantation to individuals.

(4) Any specified donee, for therapy or transplantation needed by him.

(5) Any accredited school of mortuary science.

§ 41-39-39. Manner of effecting donation.
(1) A gift of all or part of the body for purposes of sections 41-39-39 to 41-39-51 may be made by will, in which case the gift becomes effective immediately upon death of the testator without waiting for probate. If the will is not probated, or if it is declared invalid for testamentary purposes, the gift, to the extent that it has been acted upon in good faith, is nevertheless valid and effective.

(2) A gift of all or part of the body for purposes of sections 41-39-31 to 41-39-51 may also be made by document other than a will. The document must be signed by the donor in the presence of two (2) witnesses who, in turn, shall sign the document in

the donor's presence. If the donor cannot sign in person, the document may be signed for him, at his direction and in his presence, and in the presence of two (2) witnesses who, in turn, shall sign the document in the donor's presence. The gift becomes effective immediately upon death of donor.

Delivery of the document of gift during the donor's lifetime is not necessary to make the gift valid. The document may consist of a properly executed card carried on the donor's person or in his effects. The document and/or card shall conform substantially to the following form:

"CERTIFICATE OF AUTHORIZATION FOR POST-MORTEM STUDY AND EXAMINATION OR REMOVAL OF TISSUES OR ORGANS

I, the undersigned, this _____ day of _____, 19____, desiring that my _____ be made available after my demise for:

(1) Any licensed hospital, surgeon or physician, for medical education, research, advancement of medical science, therapy or transplantation to individuals;

(2) Any accredited medical school, college or university engaged in medical education or research, for therapy, educational research or medical science purposes or any accredited school of mortuary science;

(3) Any person operating a bank or storage facility for blood, arteries, eyes, pituitaries, or other human parts, for use in medical education, research, therapy or transplantation to individuals;

(4) The donee specified below, for therapy or transplantation needed by him or her, do hereby donate my _____ for said purpose to _____ (Name) at _____ (Address).

I hereby authorize a licensed physician, surgeon or certified technician or the state anatomy board to remove and preserve for use my _____ for said purpose.

Witnessed this _____ day of _____, 19___.

_____
(Donor)

_____
(Name and Address)

_____
(Address)

_____
(Name and Address)

_____
(Telephone)

(3) The gift may be made either to a named donee or without the naming of a donee. If the latter, the gift may be accepted by and utilized at the discretion of the attending physician at or following death.

If the gift is made to a named donee who is not readily available at the time and place of death, and if the gift is evidenced by a properly executed card or other document carried on the donor's person or in his effects, the attending physician at or following death may, in reliance upon the card or other document, accept and utilize the gift in his discretion as the agent of the donee. The agency possesses and may exercise all of the rights and is entitled to all of the immunities of the donee under sections 41-39-31 to 41-39-51.

If the gift is made to a named donee, the will or other document or an attested true copy thereof may be delivered to him to expedite the appropriate procedure immediately after death, but such delivery is not necessary to validity of the gift. Upon request of the named donee or his agent on or after the donor's death, the person in possession shall produce for examination the will or other document of gift.

(4) The donor may designate in his will or other document of gift the surgeon, physician or technician to carry out the appropriate procedures. In the event of the nonavailability of such designee, or in the absence of a designation, the donee or other person authorized to accept the gift may employ or authorize any licensed physician, licensed surgeon or technician for the purpose.

(5) A document of gift executed in another state and in accord with the laws of that state thereunto pertaining, or executed in a territory or possession of the United States under the control and dominion of the federal government exclusively and in accord with a federal law thereunto pertaining, shall be deemed valid as a document of gift within the state of Mississippi, notwithstanding that said document does not substantially conform to the requirements of this section.

§ 41-39-41. Revocation.

(a) Any document of gift which has been delivered to the donee may be revoked by either:

(1) the execution and delivery to the donee or his agent of a revocation in writing, signed by the donor, or

(2) an oral statement of revocation witnessed by two persons, and communicated to the donee or his agent, or

(3) a statement during a terminal illness addressed to the attending physician and communicated to the donee or his agent, or

(4) a card or other writing signed by the donor and carried on his person or in his effects revoking the gift.

(b) Any document of gift which has not been delivered to the donee may be revoked in the manner set out above or by destruction, cancellation or mutilation of the document.

(c) Any gift made by a will may be revoked in the manner set out in subsection (a) above or in the manner provided for revocation or amendment of wills.

§ 41-39-43. Acceptance or rejection of gift; determination of time of death.

The donee may accept or reject the gift. When the gift is only a part of the body, promptly following the removal of the part named, custody of the remaining parts of the body shall be transferred to the next of kin or other person or agency authorized or under obligation to dispose of the body. The time of death shall be determined by the physician in attendance upon the donor's terminal illness or certifying his death. Said physician shall not be a member of the team of physicians which transplants the part to another individual.

§ 41-39-45. Civil liability.

Any person who, in good faith and acting in reliance upon and authorization made under the provisions of sections 41-39-31 to 41-39-51 and without notice of revocation thereof, takes possession of, performs surgical operations upon, removes tissue, substances or parts from the human body, or refuses such a gift, and any person who unknowingly fails to carry out the wishes of the donor according to the provisions of said sections shall not be liable for damages in a civil action brought against him for such act.

§ 41-39-47. Effect of laws respecting autopsies.

The provisions of sections 41-39-31 to 41-39-51 are subject to the laws of this state prescribing powers and duties with respect to autopsies, and are not in contravention thereof.

§ 41-39-49. Application to gifts intended to be made during donor's lifetime.

The provisions of sections 41-39-31 to 41-39-51 shall not apply to gifts of parts of the body when said gifts are made during the lifetime of the donor with the intention that said part of the body be delivered to the donee during the lifetime of the donor.

§ 41-39-51. Effect on prior authority or instrument.

Nothing in sections 41-39-31 to 41-39-51 shall invalidate any authority or instrument executed prior to April 6, 1970.

§ 41-39-53. Identification of donors on driver's license; duties of public safety commissioner.

(1) The commissioner of public safety is hereby directed to adopt and implement a program whereby anatomical organ donors may be so identified by an appropriate decal, sticker or other marking to be affixed to the driver's license of such person.

(2) The commissioner shall provide space on every application for a driver's license or renewal thereof in which the applicant may indicate his desire to have such marking on his driver's license. In addition, any person whose license has not expired or who has already obtained a license may have such marking affixed by the commissioner upon request.

(3) The commissioner shall publish the existence of such program along with information regarding the procedures for having such marking affixed by the commissioner upon request.

(4) The commissioner shall notify his counterparts in each of the other states as to the existence of the program and the significance of the marking.

(5) No provision of this section shall be construed to modify or repeal any provisions of the Anatomical Gift Law, Sections 41-39-31 et seq., and the actual donation of such anatomical organ shall be in conformity with and subject to all provisions of the Anatomical Gift Law.

§ 41-39-11. Use of chemical analysis in criminal investigations.

(1) In respect to a gift of an eye as provided for in this chapter, a person licensed for the practice of funeral service under the provisions of sections 73-11-41 et seq., who has successfully completed a course in eye enucleation and has received a certificate of competence from the state board of health, may enucleate eyes for such gift after the proper certification of death by a physician and compliance with the extent of such gift as defined within sections 41-39-31 through 41-39-53. No such properly certified funeral service licensee acting in accordance with the terms of this chapter shall have any liability, civil or criminal, for such eye enucleation.

(2) The state board of health shall promulgate such rules as are necessary to provide for the proper certification of such funeral service licensees and for the implementation of this section.

MISSOURI

UNIFORM ANATOMICAL GIFT ACT

194.210. Definitions.

As used in sections 194.210 to 194.290, the following words and terms mean:

(1) "Bank or storage facility", a facility licensed, accredited, or approved under the laws of any state for storage of human bodies or parts thereof:

(2) "Decedent", a deceased individual and includes a stillborn infant or fetus;

(3) "Donor", an individual who makes a gift of all or part of his body;

(4) "Hospital", a hospital licensed, accredited, or approved under the laws of any state and includes a hospital operated by the United States government, a state, or a subdivision thereof, although not required to be licensed under state laws.

(5) "Part", organs, tissues, eyes, bones, arteries, blood, other fluids and any other portions of a human body;

(6) "Person", an individual, corporation, government or governmental subdivision or agency, business trust, estate, trust, partnership or association, or any other legal entity;

(7) "Physician" or "surgeon", a physician or surgeon licensed or authorized to practice under the laws of any state;

(8) "State" includes any state, district, commonwealth, territory, insular possession, and any other area subject to the legislative authority of the United States of America.

194.220. Persons who may execute an anatomical gift.

1. Any individual of sound mind who is at least eighteen years of age may give all or any part of his body for any purpose specified in section 194.230, the gift to take effect upon death.

2. Any of the following persons, in order of priority stated, when persons in prior classes are not available at the time of death, and in the absence of actual notice of contrary indications by the decedent or actual notice of opposition by a member of the same or a prior class, may give all or any part of the decedent's body for any purpose specified in section 194.230:

(1) The spouse,

(2) An adult son or daughter,

(3) Either parent,

(4) An adult brother or sister,

(5) A guardian of the person of the decedent at the time of his death,

(6) Any other person authorized or under obligation to dispose of the body, including an attorney in fact acting under authority of a durable power of attorney that expressly refers to making a gift of all or part of the principal's body under the Uniform Anatomical Gift Act.

3. If the donee has actual notice of contrary indications by the decedent or that a gift by a member of a class is opposed by a member of the same or a prior class, the donee shall not accept the gift. The persons authorized by subsection 2 of this section may make the gift after or immediately before death.

4. A gift of all or part of a body authorizes any examination necessary to assure medical acceptability of the gift for the purposes intended.

5. The rights of the donee created by the gift are paramount to the rights of others except as provided by subsection 4 of section 194.270.

194.230. Persons who may become donees—purposes for which anatomical gifts may be made.

The following persons may become donees of gifts of bodies or parts thereof for the purposes stated:

(1) Any hospital, surgeon, or physician, for medical or dental education, research, advancement of medical or dental science, therapy, or transplantation; or

(2) Any accredited medical or dental school, college or university or the state anatomical board for education, research, advancement of medical or dental science, or therapy; or

(3) Any bank or storage facility, for medical or dental education, research, advancement of medical or dental science, therapy or transplantation; or

(4) Any specified individual for therapy or transplantation needed by him.

194.233. Anatomical gifts—hospital to make request, to whom, when verification in patient's record—hospital not liable for cost of retrieval.

1. The chief executive officer of each hospital in this state shall designate one or more trained persons to request anatomical gifts which persons shall not be connected with determination of death. The hospital official may designate a representative of an organ or tissue procurement organization to request consent.

2. When there is a patient who is a suitable candidate for organ or tissue donation based on hospital accepted criteria the designee shall request consent to a donation from the persons authorized to give consent as specified in subdivision (1), (2), (3), or (4) of

subsection 2 of section 194.220. The request shall be made in the order of priority stated in subsection 2 of section 194.220.

3. No request shall be required if the hospital designee has actual notice of contrary indications by the decedent or by a member of a prior class specified in subsection 2 of section 194.220.

4. Consent shall be obtained by the methods specified in section 194.240.

5. Where a donation is requested, the designee shall verify such request in the patient's medical record. Such verification of request for organ donation shall include a statement to the effect that a request for consent to an anatomical gift has been made, and shall further indicate thereupon whether or not consent was granted, the name of the person granting or refusing the consent, and his or her relationship to the decedent.

6. Upon the approval of the designated next of kin or other individual, as set forth in subsection 2 of section 194.220, the hospital shall then notify an organ or tissue procurement organization and cooperate in the procurement of the anatomical gift or gifts pursuant to applicable provisions of sections 194.210 to 194.290.

7. No hospital shall have an obligation to retrieve the organ or tissue donated pursuant to this section.

194.240. Methods of executing anatomical gifts—person to carry out procedures.

1. A gift of all or part of the body under subsection 1 of section 194.220 may be made by will. The gift becomes effective upon the death of the testator without waiting for probate. If the will is not probated, or if it is declared invalid for testamentary purposes, the gift, to the extent that it has been acted upon in good faith, is nevertheless valid and effective.

2. A gift of all or part of the body under subsection 1 of section 194.220 may also be made by document other than a will. The gift becomes effective upon the death of the donor. The document, which may be a card designed to be carried on the person, must be signed by the donor in the presence of two witnesses who must sign the document in his presence or before a notary or other official authorized to administer oaths generally. If the donor cannot sign, the document may be signed for him at his direction and in his presence in the presence of two witnesses who must sign the document in his presence. Delivery of the document of gift during the donor's lifetime is not necessary to make the gift valid.

3. The gift may be made to a specified donee or without specifying a donee. If the latter, the gift may be accepted by the attending physician as donee upon or following death. If the gift is made to a specified donee who is not available at the time and place of death, the attending physician upon or following death, in the absence of any expressed indication that the donor desired otherwise, may accept the gift as donee. The physician who becomes a donee under this subsection shall not participate in the procedures for removing or transplanting a part.

4. Notwithstanding the provisions of subsection 2 of section 194.270, the donor may designate in his will, card, or other document of gift the surgeon or physician to carry out the appropriate procedures. In the absence of a designation or if the designee is not available, the donee or other person authorized to accept the gift may employ or authorize any surgeon or physician to carry out the appropriate procedures. For the purpose of removing an eye or part thereof, any medical technician employed by a hospital, physician or eye bank and acting under supervision may perform the appropriate procedures. Any medical technician authorized to perform such procedure shall successfully complete the course prescribed in section 194.295 for embalmers.

5. Any gift by a person designated in subsection 2 of section 194.220 shall be made by a document signed by him or made by his telegraphic, recorded telephonic, or other recorded message.

6. A gift of part of the body under subsection 1 of section 194.220 may also be made by a statement on a form which shall be provided on the reverse side of all Missouri motor vehicle operators' and chauffeurs' licenses. The statement to be effective shall be signed by the owner of the operator's or chauffeur's license in the presence of two witnesses, who shall sign the statement in the presence of the donor. The gift becomes effective upon the death of the donor. Delivery of the license during the donor's lifetime is not necessary to make the gift valid. The gift shall become invalidated upon expiration, cancellation, revocation, or suspension of the license, and the gift must be renewed upon renewal of each license. Pertinent medical information which may affect the quality of the gift may be included in the statement of gift.

194.250. Delivery of document of gift.

If the gift is made by the donor to a specified donee, the will, card, or other document, or an executed copy thereof, may be delivered to the donee to expedite the appropriate procedures immediately after death. Delivery is not necessary to the validity of the gift. The will, card, or other document, or an executed copy thereof, may be deposited in any hospital, bank or storage facility or registry office that accepts it for safekeeping or for facilitation of procedures after death. On request of any interested party upon or after the donor's death, the person in possession shall produce the document for examination.

194.260. Amendment or revocation of the gift.

1. If the will, card, or other document or executed copy thereof, has been delivered to a specified donee, the donor may amend or revoke the gift by:

(1) The execution and delivery to the donee of a signed statement, or

(2) An oral statement made in the presence of two persons and communicated to the donee, or

(3) A statement during a terminal illness or injury addressed to an attending physician and communicated to the donee, or

(4) A signed card or document found on his person or in his effects.

2. Any document of gift which has not been delivered to the donee may be revoked by the donor in the manner set out in subsection 1, or by destruction, cancellation, or mutilation of the document and all executed copies thereof.

3. Any gift made by a will may also be amended or revoked in the manner provided for amendment or revocation of wills, or as provided in subsection 1.

194.270. Rights and duties at death.

1. The donee may accept or reject the gift. If the donee accepts a gift of the entire body, he may, subject to the terms of the gift, authorize embalming and the use of the body in funeral services. If the gift is of a part of the body, the donee, upon the death of the donor and prior to embalming, shall cause the part to be removed without unnecessary mutilation. After removal of the part, custody of the remainder of the body vests in the surviving spouse, next of kin, or other persons under obligation to dispose of the body.

2. The time of death shall be determined by a physician who tends the donor at his death, or, if none, the physician who certifies the death. The physician shall not participate, directly or indirectly, in the procedures for removing or transplanting a part or be a relative within the fourth degree of consanguinity of any donee of a body or part thereof which is removed or transplanted.

3. A person who acts without negligence and in good faith in accord with the terms of this act or with the anatomical gift laws of another state or a foreign country is not liable for damages in any civil action or subject to prosecution in any criminal proceeding for his act.

4. The provisions of this act are subject to the laws of this state prescribing powers and duties with respect to autopsies.

194.280. Uniformity of interpretation.

Sections 194.210 to 194.290 shall be so construed as to effectuate its general purpose to make uniform the laws of those states which enact it.

194.290. Short title.

Sections 194.210 to 194.290 may be cited as the "Uniform Anatomical Gift Act".

MONTANA

ANATOMICAL GIFT ACT

Part 1 General Provisions

72-17-101. Short title.
This chapter may be cited as the "Uniform Anatomical Gift Act".

72-17-102. Definitions.
As used in this chapter the following definitions apply:
(1) "Anatomical gift" means a donation of all or part of a human body to take effect upon or after death.
(2) "Decedent" means a deceased individual and includes a stillborn infant or fetus.
(3) "Department" means the department of health and environmental sciences provided for in Title 2, chapter 15, part 21.
(4) "Document of gift" means a card, a statement attached to or imprinted on a motor vehicle operator's license, a will, or other writing used to make an anatomical gift.
(5) "Donor" means an individual who makes a gift of all or part of the individual's body.
(6) "Enucleator" means an individual who is certified pursuant to 72-17-311 to remove or process eyes or parts of eyes.
(7) "Hospital" means a facility licensed, accredited, or approved under the laws of any state or a facility operated as a hospital by the United States government, a state, or a subdivision of a state.
(8) "Ophthalmologist" means a licensed physician or surgeon who specializes in the treatment or correction of diseases of the eye.
(9) "Part" means an organ, tissue, eye, bone, artery, blood, fluid, or other portion of a human body.
(10) "Person" means an individual, corporation, government, governmental subdivision or agency, business trust, estate, trust, partnership, joint venture, association, or any other legal or commercial entity.
(11) "Physician" or "surgeon" means an individual licensed or otherwise authorized to practice medicine and surgery or osteopathy and surgery under the laws of any state.
(12) "Procurement organization" means a person licensed, accredited, or approved under the laws of any state for procurement, distribution, or storage of human bodies or parts.
(13) "State" means a state, territory, or possession of the United States, the District of Columbia, or the Commonwealth of Puerto Rico.
(14) "Technician" means an individual who is certified by the state board of medical examiners to remove or process a part.

72-17-103. Uniformity of interpretation.
This chapter shall be so construed as to effectuate its general purpose to make uniform the law of those states which enact it.

72-17-104. Repealed.

72-17-105 through 72-17-107 reserved.

72-17-108. Coordination of procurement and use.
Each hospital in this state, after consultation with other hospitals and procurement organizations, shall establish agreements or affiliations for coordination of procurement and use of human bodies and parts.

Part 2 Execution and Operation of Anatomical Gift

72-17-201. Making, amending, revoking, and refusing to make anatomical gifts by an individual.
(1) An individual who is at least 18 years of age may:
   (a) make an anatomical gift for any of the purposes stated in 72-17-202;
   (b) limit an anatomical gift to one or more of those purposes; or
   (c) refuse to make an anatomical gift.
(2) An anatomical gift may be made only by a document of gift signed by the donor. If the donor cannot sign, the document of gift must be signed by another individual and by two witnesses, all of whom have signed at the direction and in the presence of the donor and of each other, and must state that it has been so signed.
(3) If a document of gift is attached to or imprinted on a donor's motor vehicle operator's license, the document of gift must comply with subsection (2). Revocation, suspension, expiration, or cancellation of the license does not invalidate the anatomical gift.
(4) A document of gift may designate a particular physician or surgeon to carry out the appropriate procedures. In the absence of a designation or if the designee is not available, the donee or other person authorized to accept the anatomical gift may employ

or authorize any physician, surgeon, technician, or enucleator to carry out the appropriate procedures.

(5) An anatomical gift by will takes effect upon the death of the testator, whether or not the will is probated. If, after the testator's death, the will is declared invalid for testamentary purposes, the validity of the anatomical gift is unaffected.

(6) A donor may amend or revoke an anatomical gift not made by will only by:

(a) a signed statement;

(b) an oral statement made in the presence of two individuals;

(c) any form of communication during a terminal illness or injury addressed to a physician or surgeon; or

(d) the delivery of a signed statement to a specified donee to whom a document of gift had been delivered.

(7) The donor of an anatomical gift made by will may amend or revoke the gift in the manner provided for amendment or revocation of wills, or as provided in subsection (6).

(8) An anatomical gift that is not revoked by the donor before death is irrevocable and does not require the consent or concurrence of any person after the donor's death.

(9)(a) An individual may refuse to make an anatomical gift of the individual's body or part by:

(i) a writing signed in the same manner as a document of gift;

(ii) a statement attached to or imprinted on a donor's motor vehicle operator's license; or

(iii) any other writing used to identify the individual as refusing to make an anatomical gift.

(b) During a terminal illness or injury, the refusal may be an oral statement or other form of communication.

(10) In the absence of contrary indications by the donor, an anatomical gift of a part is neither a refusal to give other parts nor a limitation on an anatomical gift under 72-17-214 or on a removal or release of other parts under 72-17-215.

(11) In the absence of contrary indications by the donor, a revocation or amendment of an anatomical gift is not a refusal to make another anatomical gift. If the donor intends a revocation to be a refusal to make an anatomical gift, the donor shall make the refusal pursuant to subsection (9).

72-17-202. Persons who may become donees—purposes for which anatomical gifts may be made.

(1) The following persons may become donees of anatomical gifts for the purpose stated:

(a) a hospital, surgeon, physician, or procurement organization for medical or dental education, research, advancement of medical or dental science, therapy, or transplantation;

(b) an accredited medical or dental school, college, or university for education, research, advancement of medical or dental science; or

(c) a designated individual for therapy or transplantation needed by that individual.

(2) An anatomical gift may be made to a designated donee or without designating a donee. If a donee is not designated or if the donee is not available or rejects the anatomical gift, the anatomical gift may be accepted by a hospital.

(3) If the donee knows of the decedent's refusal or contrary indications to make an anatomical gift or that an anatomical gift by a member of a class having priority to act is opposed by a member of the same class or a prior class under 72-17-214, the donee may not accept the anatomical gift.

72-17-203 through 72-17-206. Repealed.

72-17-207. Examination—autopsy—liability.

(1) An anatomical gift authorizes any reasonable examination necessary to assure medical acceptability of the gift for the purposes intended.

(2) The provisions of this chapter are subject to the laws of this state governing autopsies.

(3) A hospital, physician, surgeon, coroner, enucleator, technician, nurse, or other person who acts in accordance with this chapter or with the applicable anatomical gift act of another state or attempts in good faith to do so is not liable for that act in a civil action or criminal proceeding.

(4) An individual who makes an anatomical gift pursuant to 72-17-201 or 72-17-214 and the individual's estate are not liable for any injury or damage that may result from the making or use of the anatomical gift.

72-17-208. Delivery of document of gift.

(1) Delivery of a document of gift during the donor's lifetime is not required for the validity of an anatomical gift.

(2) If an anatomical gift is made to a designated donee, the document of gift, or a copy, may be delivered to the donee to expedite the appropriate procedures after death. The document of gift, or a copy, may be deposited in any hospital, procurement organization, or registry office that accepts it for safekeeping or for facilitation of procedures after death. On request of an interested person, upon or after the donor's death, the person in possession shall allow the interested person to examine or copy the document of gift.

72-17-209. Repealed.

72-17-210. Renumbered 72-17-301 by Code Commissioner, 1983.

72-17-211. Repealed.

72-17-212. Repealed.

72-17-213. Routine inquiry and required request—search and notification.

(1) If, at or near the time of death of a patient, there is no medical record that the patient has made or refused to make anatomical gift, the hospital administrator or a representative designated by the administrator shall discuss the option to make or refuse to make an anatomical gift and request the making of an anatomical gift pursuant to 72-17-214(1). The request must be made with reasonable discretion and sensitivity to the circumstances of the family. A request is not required if the gift is not suitable, based upon accepted medical standards, for a purpose specified in 72-17-202 or if there are medical or emotional conditions under which the request would contribute to severe emotional distress. An entry must be made in the medical record of the patient, stating the name and affiliation of the individual making the request and the name, response, and relationship to the patient of the person to whom the request was made. The department shall adopt rules to implement this subsection.

(2) The following persons shall make a reasonable search for a document of gift or other information identifying the bearer as a donor or as an individual who has refused to make an anatomical gift:

(a) a law enforcement officer, fireman, paramedic, or other emergency rescuer finding an individual whom the searcher believes is dead or near death; and

(b) a hospital, upon the admission of an individual at or near the time of death, if there is not immediately available any other source of that information.

(3) If a document of gift or evidence of refusal to make an anatomical gift is located by the search required by subsection (3)(a) and the individual or body to whom it relates is taken to a hospital, the hospital must be notified of the contents and the document or other evidence must be sent to the hospital.

(4) If, at or near the time of death of a patient, a hospital knows that an anatomical gift has been made pursuant to 72-17-214(1) or a release and removal of a part has been permitted pursuant to 72-17-215, or that a patient or an individual identified as in transit to the hospital is a donor, the hospital shall notify the donee if one is named and known to the hospital; if not, it shall notify an appropriate procurement organization. The hospital shall cooperate in the implementation of the anatomical gift or release and removal of a part.

(5) A person who fails to discharge the duties imposed by this section is not subject to criminal or civil liability but is subject to appropriate administrative sanctions.

72-17-214. Making, revoking, and objecting to anatomical gifts by others.

(1) Any member of the following classes of persons, in the order of priority listed, may make an anatomical gift of all or a part of the decedent's body for an authorized purpose, unless the decedent, at the time of death, had made an unrevoked refusal to make that anatomical gift:

(a) the spouse of the decedent;

(b) an adult son or daughter of the decedent;

(c) either parent of the decedent;

(d) an adult brother or sister of the decedent;

(e) a grandparent of the decedent; and

(f) a guardian of the person of the decedent at the time of death.

(2) An anatomical gift may not be made by a person listed in subsection (1) if:

(a) a person in a prior class is available at the time of death to make an anatomical gift;

(b) the person proposing to make an anatomical gift knows of a refusal or contrary indications by the decedent; or

(c) the person proposing to make an anatomical gift knows of an objection to making an anatomical gift by a member of the person's class or a prior class.

(3) An anatomical gift by a person authorized under subsection (1) must be made by:

(a) a document of gift signed by the person; or

(b) the person's telegraphic, recorded telephonic, or other recorded message, or other form of communication from the person that is contemporaneously reduced to writing and signed by the recipient.

(4) An anatomical gift by a person authorized under subsection (1) my be revoked by any member of the same or a prior class if, before procedures have begun for the removal of a part from the body of the decedent, the physician, surgeon, technician, or enucleator removing the part knows of the revocation.

(5) A failure to make an anatomical gift under subsection (1) is not an objection to the making of an anatomical gift.

72-17-215. Authorization by coroner or local public health official.

(1) The coroner may release and permit the removal of a part from a body within that official's custody, for transplantation or therapy, if:

(a) the official has made a reasonable effort, taking into account the useful life of the part, to locate and examine the decedent's medical records and inform persons listed in 72-17-214(1) of their option to make, or object to making, an anatomical gift;

(c) the official does not know of a refusal or contrary indication by the decedent or objection by a person having priority to act as listed in 72-17-214(1);

    (d) the removal will be by a physician, surgeon, or technician; but in the case of eyes, by one of them or by an enucleator;

    (e) the removal will not interfere with any autopsy or investigation;

    (f) the removal will be in accordance with accepted standards; and

    (g) cosmetic restoration will be done, if appropriate.

(2) If the body is not within the custody of the coroner, the local public health officer may release and permit the removal of any part from a body in the local public health officer's custody for transplantation or therapy if the requirements of subsection (1) are met.

(3) An official releasing and permitting the removal of a part shall maintain a permanent record, of the name of the decedent, the person making the request, the date and purpose of the request, the part requested, and the person to whom it was released.

Part 3 Regulation—Qualifications

72-17.301. Rights and duties at death.

(1) Rights of a donee created by an anatomical gift are superior to rights of others under 72-17-214(1), except with respect to autopsies. A donee may accept or reject an anatomical gift. If the donee accepts an anatomical gift of the entire body, the donee, subject to the terms of the gift, may allow embalming and the use of the body in funeral services. If the gift is of a part of the body, the donee, upon the death of the donor and before embalming, shall cause the part to be removed without unnecessary mutilation. After removal of the part, custody of the remainder of the body vests in the person under obligation to dispose of the body.

(2) The time of death must be determined by a physician or surgeon who attends the donor at death or, if none, the physician or surgeon who certifies the death. Neither the physician or surgeon who attends the donor at death nor the physician or surgeon who determines the time of death may participate in the procedures for removing or transplanting a part unless the document of gift designates a particular physician or surgeon pursuant to 72-17-201(4).

(3) If there has been an anatomical gift, a technician may remove any donated parts and an enucleator may remove any donated eyes or parts of eyes after determination of death by a physician or surgeon.

72-17-302. Sale or purchase of parts prohibited.

(1) A person may not knowingly, for valuable consideration, purchase or sell a part for transplantation or therapy, if removal of the part is intended to occur after the death of the decedent.

(2) Valuable consideration does not include reasonable payment for the removal, processing, disposal, preservation, quality control, storage, transportation, or implantation of a part.

(3) A person who violates this section is guilty of a felony and upon conviction is subject to a fine not exceeding $50,000 or imprisonment not exceeding 5 years, or both.

72-17-303 through 72-17-310 reserved.

72-17-311. Eye enucleations—enucleators—qualifications.

(1) Eye enucleations for purposes of anatomical gifts may be performed:

    (a) by a licensed physician or surgeon; or

    (b) by an enucleator trained in eye enucleation.

(2) An acceptable course in eye enucleation must include the anatomy and physiology of the eye, instruction in maintaining a sterile field during the enucleation procedure, and use of appropriate instruments and sterile procedures for removal and preservation of corneal tissue.

(3) Certification of satisfactory completion of a course in eye enucleation must be provided by the ophthalmologist who teaches the course. This certification qualifies an enucleator to perform eye enucleations for a period of 3 years from the date of completion of the course.

72-17-312. Approval of eye banks.

Any bank or storage facility that furnishes to the department written evidence of its membership and certification and reports and recommendations for future compliance, granted by the eyebank association of America, is approved for receipt and storage of eye tissue for the term of such membership and certification and is eligible during such term to be a donee of eye tissue pursuant to 72-17-202.

NEBRASKA

UNIFORM ANATOMICAL GIFT ACT

§ 71-4801. Terms, defined.

As used in sections 71-4801 to 71-4812, unless the context otherwise requires:

(1) Bank or storage facility means a facility licensed, accredited or approved under the laws of any state for storage of human bodies or parts thereof;

(2) Decedent means a deceased individual and includes a stillborn infant or fetus;

(3) Donor means an individual who makes a gift of all or part of his body;

(4) Hospital means a hospital licensed, accredited or approved under the laws of any state and includes a hospital operated by the United States government, a state, or a subdivision thereof, although not required to be licensed under state laws;

(5) Part includes organs, tissues, eyes, bones, arteries, blood, other fluids and other portions of a human body, and parts includes parts;

(6) Person means an individual, corporation, government or governmental subdivision or agency, business trust, estate, trust, partnership or association or any other legal entity;

(7) Physician or surgeon means a physician or surgeon licensed or authorized to practice under the laws of any state; and

(8) State includes any state, district, commonwealth, territory, insular possession, and any other area subject to the legislative authority of the United States of America.

§ 71-4802. Persons who may execute anatomical gift; when.

(1) Any individual of sound mind and nineteen years of age or more may give all or any part of his body for any purposes specified in section 71-4803, the gift to take effect upon death.

(2) Any of the following persons, in order of priority stated, when persons in prior classes are not available at the time of death, and in the absence of actual notice of contrary indications by the decedent, or actual notice of opposition by a member of the same or a prior class, may give all or any part of the decedent's body for any purposes specified in section 71-4803:

(a) The spouse,

(b) An adult son or daughter,

(c) Either parent,

(d) An adult brother or sister;

(e) A guardian of the person of the decedent at the time of his death, and

(f) Any other person authorized or under obligation to dispose of the body.

The persons authorized by this subsection may make the gift after death or immediately before death.

(3) If the donee has actual notice of contrary indications by the decedent, or that a gift by a member of a class is opposed by a member of the same or a prior class, the donee shall not accept the gift.

(4) A gift of all or part of a body authorizes any examination necessary to assure medical acceptability of the gift for the purposes intended.

(5) The rights of the donee created by the gift are paramount to the rights of others except as provided by subdivision (4) of section 71-4807.

§ 71-4803. Persons who may become donees; purposes for which anatomical gifts may be made.

The following persons may become donees of gifts of bodies or parts thereof for the purposes stated:

(1) Any hospital, surgeon, or physician, for medical or dental education, research, advancement of medical or dental science, therapy or transplantation;

(2) Any accredited medical or dental school, college or university for education, research, advancement of medical or dental science or therapy;

(3) The State Anatomical Board, any bank or storage facility, for medical or dental education, research, advancement of medical or dental science, therapy or transplantation; or

(4) Any specified individual for therapy or transplantation needed by him.

§ 71-4804. Manner of executing anatomical gifts.

(1) A gift of all or part of the body under subsection (1) of section 71-4802 may be made by will. The gift becomes effective upon the death of the testator without waiting for probate. If the will is not probated or if it is declared invalid for testamentary purposes, the gift, to the extent that it has been acted upon in good faith, is nevertheless valid and effective.

(2) A gift of all or part of the body under subsection (1) of section 71-4802 may also be made by document other than a will. The gift becomes effective upon the death of the donor. The document, which may be a card designed to be carried on the person, must be signed by the donor, in the presence of two witnesses who must sign the document in his or her presence. If the donor cannot sign, the document may be signed for him or her at his or her direction and in his or her presence and in the presence of

two witnesses who must sign the document in his or her presence. Delivery of the document of gift during the donor's lifetime is not necessary to make the gift valid.

(3) A gift of all or part of the body under subsection (1) of section 71-4802 may also be made by an indication on a motor vehicle operator's license pursuant to sections 60-493 to 60-495. The gift shall become effective upon the death of the owner.

(4) The gift may be made to a specified donee or without specifying a donee. If the latter, the gift may be accepted by the attending physician as donee upon or following death. If the gift is made to a specified donee who is not available at the time and place of death, the attending physician upon or following death, in the absence of any expressed indication that the donor desired otherwise, may accept the gift as donee. Any physician who becomes a donee under this subsection shall not participate in the procedures for removing or transplanting any part of the body except as provided in subsection (2) of section 71-4807.

(5) Notwithstanding subsection (2) of section 71-4807, the donor may designate in his or her will, card, or other document of gift the surgeon or physician to carry out the appropriate procedures. In the absence of a designation or if the designee is not available, the donee or other person authorized to accept the gift may employ or authorize any surgeon or physician for the purpose.

(6) Any gift by a person designated in subsection (2) of section 71-4802 shall be made by a document signed by him or her or made by his or her telegraphic, recorded telephonic, or other recorded message.

§ 71-4805. Document of gift; delivery.

If the gift is made by the donor to a specified donee, the will, card or other document, or an executed copy thereof, may be delivered to the donee to expedite the appropriate procedures immediately after death, but delivery is not necessary to the validity of the gift. The will, card or other document, or an executed copy thereof, may be deposited in any hospital, medical or dental school, State Anatomical Board, bank or storage facility or registry office that accepts them for safekeeping or for facilitation of procedures after death. On request of any interested party upon or after the donor's death, the person in possession shall produce the document for examination.

§ 71-4806. Gifts; amendment; revocation.

(1) If the will, card or other document or executed copy thereof, has been delivered to a specified donee, the donor may amend or revoke the gift by:

   (a) The execution and delivery to the donee of a signed statement;
   (b) An oral statement made in the presence of two persons and communicated to the donee;
   (c) A statement during a terminal illness or injury addressed to an attending physician and communicated to the donee; or
   (d) A signed card or document found on his person or in his effects.

(2) Any document of gift which has not been delivered to the donee may be revoked by the donor in the manner set out in subsection (1) of this section or by destruction, cancellation, or mutilation of the document and all executed copies thereof.

(3) Any gift made by a will may also be amended or revoked in the manner provided for amendment or revocation of wills, or as provided in subsection (1) of this section.

§ 71-4807. Rights and duties at death.

(1) The donee may accept or reject the gift. If the donee accepts a gift of the entire body, he or she may, subject to the terms of the gift, authorize embalming and the use of the body in funeral services. If the gift is of a part of the body, the donee, upon the death of the donor and prior to embalming, shall cause the part to be removed without unnecessary mutilation. After removal of the part, custody of the remainder of the body vests in the surviving spouse, next of kin, or other persons under obligation to dispose of the body.

(2) The time of death shall be determined by a physician who attends the donor at his or her death or, if none, the physician who certifies the death. This physician shall not participate in the procedures for removing or transplanting a part, except the enucleation of eyes. An appropriately qualified designee of a physician with training in ophthalmologic techniques or a licensed funeral director or mortician, as defined in section 71-1325, upon (a) successfully completing a course in eye enucleation and (b) receiving a certificate of competence from the Department of Ophthalmology, College of Medicine of the University of Nebraska, may enucleate the eyes of the donor.

(3) A person who acts in good faith in accord with the terms of the Uniform Anatomical Gift Act or under the anatomical gift laws of another state shall not be liable for damages in any civil action or subject to prosecution in any criminal proceeding for his or her act.

(4) The Uniform Anatomical Gift Act shall be subject to the laws of this state prescribing powers and duties with respect to autopsies.

§ 71-4808. Blood and human tissues; who may consent to donate.

Any individual of sound mind and seventeen years of age or more may consent to donate whole blood and any individual of sound mind and nineteen years of age or more may consent to donate other human tissues such as corneas, bones, or organs, for the purpose of injecting, transfusing, or transplanting such blood or other human tissues in the human body. No person seventeen or eighteen years of age shall receive compensation for any donation of whole blood without parental permission or authorization.

§ 71-4809. Legal liability; policy of state.

The availability of scientific knowledge, skills and materials for the transplantation, injection, transfusion or transfer of human tissue, organs, blood and components thereof is important to the health and welfare of the people of this state. The imposition of legal liability without fault upon the persons and organizations engaged in such scientific procedures inhibits the exercise of sound medical judgment and restricts the availability of important scientific knowledge, skills and materials. It is therefore the public policy of this state to promote the health and welfare of the people by limiting the legal liability arising out of such scientific procedures to the instances of negligence or willful misconduct.

§ 71-4810. Legal liability; exemption; exceptions.

No physician, surgeon, hospital, blood bank, tissue bank, licensed funeral director or mortician, or other person or entity who donates, obtains, prepares, transplants, injects, transfuses or otherwise transfers, or who assists or participates in obtaining, preparing, transplanting, injecting, transfusing or transferring any tissue, organ, blood or component thereof from one or more human beings, living or dead, to another human being, shall be liable in damages as a result of any such activity, save and except that each such person or entity shall remain liable in damages for his or its own negligence or willful misconduct.

§ 71-4811. Act, how construed.

Sections 71-4801 to 71-4812 shall be construed as to effectuate its general purpose to make uniform the law of those states which enact it.

§ 71-4812. Act, how cited.

Sections 71-4801 to 71-4812 may be cited as the Uniform Anatomical Gift Act.

§ 71-4813. Eye tissue; pituitary gland; removal; when authorized.

When an autopsy is performed by the physician authorized by the county coroner to perform such autopsy, the physician or an appropriately qualified designee with training in ophthalmologic techniques, as provided for in subsection (2) of section 71-4807, may remove eye tissue of the decedent for the purpose of transplantation. The physician may also remove the pituitary gland for the purpose of research and treatment of hypopituitary dwarfism and of other growth disorders. Removal of the eye tissue or the pituitary gland shall only take place if the:

(1) Autopsy was authorized by the county coroner;

(2) County coroner receives permission from the person having control of the disposition of the decedent's remains pursuant to section 71-1339; and

(3) Removal of eye tissue or of the pituitary gland will not interfere with the course of any subsequent investigation or alter the decedent's post mortem facial appearance.

The removed eye tissue or pituitary gland shall be transported to the Director of Health or any desired institution or health facility as prescribed by section 71-1341.

NEVADA

ANATOMICAL GIFTS (UNIFORM ACT)

§ 451.500. Short title.
NRS 451.500 to 451.590, inclusive, may be cited as the Uniform Anatomical Gift Act.

§ 451.503. Applicability of act.
NRS 451.500 to 451.590, inclusive, apply to a document of gift, revocation or refusal to make an anatomical gift signed by the donor or a person authorized to make or object to making an anatomical gift before, on or after October 1, 1989.

§ 451.505. Uniformity of application and construction.
NRS 451.500 to 451.590, inclusive, must be applied and construed to effectuate their general purpose to make uniform the law with respect to the subject of the Uniform Anatomical Gift Act among states enacting it.

§ 451.510. Definitions.
Unless the context otherwise requires, as used in NRS 451.500 to 451.590, inclusive, the words and terms defined in NRS 451.513 to 451.553, inclusive, have the meanings ascribed to them in those sections.

§ 451.513. "Anatomical gift" defined.
"Anatomical gift" means a donation of all or part of a human body to take effect upon or after death.

§ 451.515. "Bank or storage facility" defined.
Repealed. (See chapter 200, Statutes of Nevada 1989, 431)

§ 451.520. "Decedent" defined.
"Decedent" means a deceased person and includes a stillborn infant or fetus.

§ 451.523. "Document of gift" defined.
"Document of gift" means a card, a statement attached to or imprinted on a motor vehicle operator's or chauffeur's license, a will, or other writing used to make an anatomical gift.

§ 451.525. "Donor" defined.
"Donor" means a person who makes an anatomical gift of all or part of his body.

§ 451.527. "Enucleator" defined.
"Enucleator" means a person who is authorized by NRS 451.583 to enucleate an eye of a dead person.

§ 451.530. "Hospital" defined.
"Hospital" means a facility licensed, accredited or approved as a hospital under the laws of the State of Nevada or a facility operated as a hospital by the United States Government, the state or a subdivision of the state.

§ 451.535. "Part" defined.
"Part" means an organ, tissue, eye, bone, artery, blood, fluid or other portion of a human body.

§ 451.540. "Person" defined.
"Person" includes a government, a governmental agency and a political subdivision of a government.

§ 451.545. "Physician" defined.
"Physician" means a person licensed or otherwise authorized to practice medicine and surgery or osteopathy and surgery under the laws of any state.

§ 451.547. "Procurement organization" defined.
"Procurement organization" means a person licensed, accredited or approved under the laws of the State of Nevada for procurement, distribution or storage of human bodies or parts.

§ 451.550. "State" defined.
"State" means a state, territory or possession of the United States, the District of Columbia or the Commonwealth of Puerto Rico.

§ 451.553. "Technician" defined.
"Technician" means a person who, under the supervision of a licensed physician, removes or processes a part.

§ 451.555. Making, amending, revoking and refusing to make gifts: By person.
1. Any person who is at least 18 years of age may:
    (a) Make an anatomical gift for any of the purposes stated in subsection 1 of NRS 451.560;
    (b) Limit an anatomical gift to one or more of those purposes; or
    (c) Refuse to make an anatomical gift.
2. An anatomical gift may be made only by a document of gift signed by the donor. If the donor cannot sign, the document of gift must be signed by another person and by two witnesses, all of whom have signed at the direction and in the presence of the donor and of each other and state that it has been so signed.
3. If a document of gift is attached to or imprinted on a donor's motor vehicle operator's or chauffeur's license, the document of gift must comply with subsection 2. Revocation, suspension, expiration or cancellation of the license does not invalidate the anatomical gift.
4. A document of gift may designate a particular physician to carry out the appropriate procedures. In the absence of a designation or if the designee is not available, the donee or other person authorized to accept the anatomical gift may employ or authorize any physician, technician or enucleator to carry out the appropriate procedures.
5. An anatomical gift by will takes effect upon death of the testator, whether or not the will is probated. If, after death, the will is declared invalid for testamentary purposes, the validity of the anatomical gift is unaffected.
6. A donor may amend or revoke an anatomical gift, not made by will, only by:
    (a) A signed statement;
    (b) An oral statement made in the presence of two persons;
    (c) Any form of communication during a terminal illness or injury addressed to a physician; or
    (d) The delivery of a signed statement to a specified donee to whom a document of gift had been delivered.
7. The donor of an anatomical gift made by will may amend or revoke the gift in the manner provided for amendment or revocation of wills in chapter 133 of NRS or as provided in subsection 6.
8. An anatomical gift that is not revoked by the donor before death is irrevocable and does not require the consent or concurrence of any person after the donor's death.
9. A person may refuse to make an anatomical gift of his body or part by:
    (a) A writing signed in the same manner as a document of gift;
    (b) A statement attached to or imprinted on his motor vehicle operator's or chauffeur's license; or
    (c) Any other writing used to identify him as refusing to make an anatomical gift.
During a terminal illness or injury, the refusal may be an oral statement or other form of communication.
10. In the absence of contrary indications by the donor, an anatomical gift of a part is neither a refusal to give other parts nor a limitation on an anatomical gift under NRS 451.557.
11. In the absence of contrary indications by the donor, a revocation or amendment of an anatomical gift is not a refusal to make another anatomical gift. If the donor intends a revocation to be a refusal to make an anatomical gift, he shall make the refusal pursuant to subsection 9.

§ 451.557. Making, revoking and objecting to gifts: By others.
1. Any member of the following classes of persons, in the order of the priority listed, may make an anatomical gift of all or a part of the decedent's body for an authorized purpose, unless the decedent, at the time of death, has made an unrevoked refusal to make that anatomical gift:
    (a) The spouse of the decedent;
    (b) An adult son or daughter of the decedent;
    (c) Either parent of the decedent;
    (d) An adult brother or sister of the decedent;
    (e) A grandparent of the decedent; and
    (f) A guardian of the person of the decedent at the time of death.
The legal procedure for authorization must be defined and established by the committee on anatomical dissection established by the University of Nevada System.
2. An anatomical gift may not be made by a person listed in subsection 1 if:
    (a) A person in a prior class is available at the time of death to make an anatomical gift;
    (b) The person proposing to make an anatomical gift knows of a refusal or contrary indications by the decedent; or
    (c) The person proposing to make an anatomical gift knows of an objection to making an anatomical gift by a member of the person's class or a prior class.
3. An anatomical gift by a person authorized under subsection 1 must be made by:
    (a) A document of gift signed by him; or

(b) His telegraphic, recorded telephonic or other recorded message, or other form of communication from him that is contemporaneously reduced to writing and signed by the recipient.

4. An anatomical gift by a person authorized under subsection 1 may be revoked by any member of the same or a prior class if, before procedures have begun for the removal of a part from the body of the decedent, the physician, technician or enucleator removing the part knows of the revocation.

5. A failure to make an anatomical gift under subsection 1 is not an objection to the making of an anatomical gift.

§ 451.560. Qualifications of donee; purpose for which gifts may be made.

1. The following persons may become donees of anatomical gifts for the purposes stated:

(a) A hospital, physician, dentist or procurement organization, for transplantation, therapy, medical or dental education, research or advancement of medical or dental science;

(b) An accredited medical or dental school, college or university, for education, research or advancement of medical or dental science; or

(c) A designated person, for transplantation or therapy needed by that person.

2. An anatomical gift may be made to a designated donee or without designating a donee. If a donee is not designated or if the donee is not available or rejects the anatomical gift, the anatomical gift may be accepted by any hospital or procurement organization.

3. If the donee knows of the decedent's refusal or contrary indications to make an anatomical gift or that an anatomical gift by a member of a class having priority to act is opposed by a member of the same class or a prior class under subsection 1 of NRS 451.557, the donee shall not accept the anatomical gift.

§ 451.565. Manner of making anatomical gift.

Repealed. (See chapter 200, Statutes of Nevada 1989, at page 438.)

§ 451.570. Delivery of document of gift.

1. Delivery of a document of gift during the donor's lifetime is not required for the validity of an anatomical gift.

2. If an anatomical gift is made to a designated donee, the document of gift, or a copy, may be delivered to the donee to expedite the appropriate procedures after death. The document of gift, or a copy, may be deposited in any hospital, procurement organization or registry office that accepts it for safekeeping or for facilitation of procedures after death. On request of a person listed in subsection 1 of NRS 451.557, upon or after the donor's death, the person in possession shall allow the person making the request to examine or copy the document of gift.

§ 451.573. Permission of donor may be attached to driver's license or identification card; immunity of department and representatives from damages or criminal prosecution.

1. A person who makes a gift of all or part of his body may attach written permission for a physician to carry out the appropriate procedures on a driver's license or an identification card issued by the department of motor vehicles and public safety.

2. The department and its representatives are not liable for damages in a civil action or subject to prosecution in any criminal proceeding on account of any entry on or document attached to a driver's license or an identification card issued by the department.

§ 451.575. Amendment or revocation of gift.

Repealed. (See chapter 200, Statutes of Nevada 1989, at page 438.)

§ 451.576. Coordination of procurement and use.

Each hospital in this state, after consultation with other hospitals and procurement organizations, shall establish agreements or affiliations for coordination of procurement and use of human bodies and parts.

§ 451.577. Identification of potential donors: Policies and procedures; search for and notification of information; administrative sanctions.

1. Every hospital shall establish policies and procedures to identify potential donors. The policies and procedures must require the administrator of the hospital or his representative:

(a) To determine whether a person is a donor.

(b) If the person is not a donor, to determine if the person is a potential donor including the consideration of:

(1) His religious and cultural beliefs; and

(2) The suitability of his organs and tissues for donation.

(c) At or near the time of death of a person identified as a potential donor, to request the person designated in subsection 1 of NRS 451.557, in the stated order of priority if persons in a prior class are not available, to consent to the gift of all or any part of the decedent's body as an anatomical gift.

(d) If he has actual knowledge of a contrary intent of the decedent or opposition by a person in the same class as or a prior class than a person who has consented to an anatomical gift, not to procure an anatomical gift.

(e) If an anatomical gift is made, to notify an organization which procures organs and tissues and cooperate in the procurement of the anatomical gift.

2. The following persons shall make a reasonable search for a document of gift or other information identifying the bearer as a donor or as a person who has refused to make an anatomical gift:

(a) A law enforcement officer, fireman, emergency medical technician or other emergency rescuer finding a person who the searcher believes is dead or near death; and

(b) A hospital, upon the admission of a person at or near the time of death, if there is not immediately available any other source of that information.

3. If a document of gift or evidence of refusal to make an anatomical gift is located by the search required by paragraph (a) of subsection 2, and the person or body to whom it relates is taken to a hospital, the hospital must be notified of the contents and the document or other evidence must be sent to the hospital.

4. If, at or near the time of death of a patient, a hospital knows that an anatomical gift has been made pursuant to subsection 1 of NRS 451.557 or that a patient or a person identified as in transit to the hospital is a donor, the hospital shall notify the donee if one is named and known to the hospital, or if not, it shall notify an appropriate procurement organization. The hospital shall cooperate in the implementation of the anatomical gift or release and removal of a part.

5. A person who fails to discharge the duties imposed by this section is not subject to criminal or civil liability but is subject to appropriate administrative sanctions.

§ 451.580. Rights and duties at death.

1. Rights of a donee created by an anatomical gift are superior to rights of others except with respect to autopsies under NRS 451.585. A donee may accept or reject an anatomical gift. If a donee accepts an anatomical gift of an entire body, the donee, subject to the terms of the gift, may allow embalming and use of the body in funeral services. If the gift is of a part of a body, the donee, upon the death of the donor and before embalming, shall cause the part to be removed without unnecessary mutilation. After removal of the part, custody of the remainder of the body vests in the person under obligation to dispose of the body.

2. The time of death must be determined by a physician who attends the donor at death, or, if none, the physician who certifies the death. Neither the physician who attends the donor at death nor the physician who determines the time of death may participate in the procedures for removing or transplanting a part unless the document of gift designates a particular physician pursuant to subsection 4 of NRS 451.555.

3. If there has been an anatomical gift, a technician may remove any donated parts and an enucleator may remove any donated eyes or parts of eyes, after determination of death by a physician.

§ 451.582. Examination of gifts; limitations on liability.

1. An anatomical gift authorizes any reasonable examination necessary to assure medical acceptability of the gift for the purposes intended.

2. A hospital, physician, coroner, local health officer, enucleator, technician or other person, who acts in accordance with the terms of NRS 451.500 to 451.590, inclusive, or with any other laws of the State of Nevada relating to anatomical gifts, or attempts in good faith to do so, is not liable for that act in a civil action or criminal proceeding.

3. A person who makes an anatomical gift pursuant to NRS 451.555 or 451.557 and his estate are not liable for any injury or damage that may result from the making or the use of the anatomical gift.

§ 451.583. Enucleation of eyes.

A licensed funeral director, a licensed embalmer, a medical technician or a licensed nurse may enucleate an eye of a dead person in order to carry out a gift made pursuant to the Uniform Anatomical Gift Act if the director, embalmer, technician or nurse has successfully completed a course, approved by the board of medical examiners, in the procedure for enucleation of eyes.

§ 451.585. Applicability of provisions governing autopsies.

The provisions of NRS 451.500 to 451.590, inclusive, are subject to the laws of this state governing autopsies.

§ 451.590. Sale or purchase of parts prohibited; penalties.

1. A person shall not knowingly, for valuable consideration, purchase or sell a part for transplantation or therapy.

2. Valuable consideration does not include reasonable payment for the removal, processing, disposal, preservation, quality control, storage, transportation or implantation of a part.

3. A person who violates this section is guilty of a felony and upon conviction is subject to a fine not exceeding $50,000 or imprisonment not exceeding 5 years, or both.

NEW HAMPSHIRE

ANATOMICAL GIFTS

291-A:1 Definitions.

As used in this chapter the following words shall have the following meanings:

I. "Bank or storage facility" means a facility licensed, accredited, or approved under the laws of any state for storage of human bodies or parts thereof.

II. "Decedent" means a deceased individual and includes a stillborn infant or fetus.

III. "Donor" means an individual who makes a gift of all or part of his body.

IV. "Hospital" means a hospital licensed, accredited, or approved under the laws of any state, and includes a hospital operated by the United States government although not required to be licensed under state law.

V. "Part" means organs, tissues, eyes, bones, arteries, blood, other fluids and any other portions of a human body.

VI. "Person" means an individual, corporation, government or governmental subdivision or agency, business trust, estate, trust, partnership or association, or any other legal entity.

VII. "Physician" or "surgeon" means a physician or surgeon licensed or authorized to practice under the laws of any state.

291-A:2 Persons Who May Execute Gift.

I. Any individual of sound mind and 18 years of age or more may give all or any part of his body for any purpose specified in RSA 291-A:3, the gift to take effect upon death.

II. Any of the following persons, in order of priority stated, when persons in prior classes are not available at the time of death, and in the absence of actual notice of contrary indications by the decedent or actual notice of opposition by a member of the same or a prior class, may give all or any part of the decedent's body for any purpose specified in RSA 291-A:3:

(a) The spouse, an adult son or daughter,

(b) Either parent,

(c) An adult brother or sister,

(d) A guardian of the person of the decedent at the time of his death,

(e) Any other person authorized or under obligation to dispose of the body,

III. If the donee has actual notice of contrary indications by the decedent or that a gift by a member of a class is opposed by a member of the same or a prior class, the donee shall not accept the gift. The persons authorized by paragraph II may make the gift after or immediately before death.

IV. A gift of all or part of a body authorizes any examination necessary to assure medical acceptability of the gift for the purposes intended.

V. The rights of the donee created by the gift are paramount to the rights of others except as provided by RSA 291-A:7, IV.

291-A:2a Request for Consent to an Anatomical Gift.

I. When, based on accepted medical standards, a patient in a hospital is a suitable candidate to donate an anatomical gift, any hospital licensed under RSA 151 shall request the gift of all or any part of the decedent's body for any purpose specified in RSA 291-A:3.

II. Each hospital licensed under RSA 151 shall develop a plan to be followed in requesting an anatomical gift. Such plan shall be filed with the director, division of public health services, department of health and human services, and shall be available for inspection by other hospitals during regular business hours.

291-A:3 Persons Who May Become Donees; Purposes for Which Gifts May Be Made.

The following persons may become donees of gifts or bodies or parts thereof for the purposes stated:

I. Any hospital, surgeon, or physician, for medical or dental education, research, advancement of medical or dental science, therapy, or transplantation; or

II. Any accredited medical or dental school, college or university for education, research, advancement of medical or dental science, or therapy; or

III. Any bank or storage facility, for medical or dental education, research, advancement of medical or dental science, therapy, or transplantation; or

IV. Any specified individual for therapy or transplantation needed by him.

291-A:4 Manner of Executing Gifts.

I. A gift of all or part of the body under RSA 291-A:2, I, may be made by will. The gift becomes effective upon the death of the testator without waiting for probate. If the will is not probated, or if it is declared invalid for testamentary purposes, the gift, to the extent that it has been acted upon in good faith, is nevertheless valid and effective.

II. A gift of all or part of the body under RSA 291-A:2, I may also be made by document other than a will. The gift becomes effective upon the death of the donor. The document, which may be a card designed to be carried on the person, must be signed by the donor in the presence of 2 witnesses who must sign the document in his presence. If the donor cannot sign, the document may be signed for him at his direction and in his presence in the presence of 2 witnesses who must sign the document in his presence. Delivery of the document of gift during the donor's lifetime is not necessary to make the gift valid.

III. The gift may be made to a specified donee or without specifying a donee. If the latter, the gift may be accepted by the attending physician as donee upon or following death. If the gift is made to a specified donee who is not available at the time and place of death, the attending physician upon or following death, in the absence of any expressed indication that the donor desired otherwise, may accept the gift as donee.

IV. Notwithstanding RSA 291-A:7, II, the donor may designate in his will, card, or other document of gift, the surgeon or physician to carry out the appropriate procedures. In the absence of a designation or if the designee is not available, the donee or other person authorized to accept the gift may employ or authorize any surgeon or physician for the purpose. Eye enucleations may also be performed by persons who have successfully completed a course of training acceptable to the eye bank of Massachusetts eye and ear infirmary and who have been licensed to perform such eye enucleations by the board of registration of funeral directors and embalmers.

V. Any gift by a person designated in RSA 291-A:2, II shall be made by a document signed by him or made by his telegraphic, recorded telephonic, or other recorded message.

291-A:5 Delivery of Document of gift.

If the gift is made by the donor to a specified donee, the will, card, or other document, or an executed copy thereof, may be delivered to the donee to expedite the appropriate procedures immediately after death. Delivery is not necessary to the validity of the gift. The will, card, or other document, or an executed copy thereof, may be deposited in any hospital, bank or storage facility, or registry office that accepts it for safekeeping or for facilitation of procedures after death. On request of any interested party upon or after the donor's death, the person in possession shall produce the document for examination.

291-A:6 Amendment or Revocation of Gift.

I. If the will, card, or other document or executed copy thereof, has been delivered to a specified donee, the donor may amend or revoke the gift by:

    (a) The execution and delivery to the donee of a signed statement, or

    (b) An oral statement made in the presence of 2 witnesses and communicated to the donee, or

    (c) A statement during a terminal illness or injury addressed to an attending physician or communicated to the donee, or

    (d) A signed card or document found on his person or in his effects.

II. Any document of gift which has not been delivered to the donee may be revoked by the donor in the manner set out in paragraph I, or by destruction, cancellation, or mutilation of the document and all executed copies thereof.

III. Any gift made by a will may be revoked in the manner provided for in RSA 551:13 for revocation of wills, or as provided in paragraph I.

291-A:7 Rights and Duties at Death.

I. The donee may accept or reject the gift. If the donee accepts a gift of the entire body, he may, subject to the terms of the gift, authorize embalming and the use of the body in funeral services. If the gift is of a part of the body, the donee, upon the death of the donor and prior to embalming, shall cause the part to be removed without unnecessary mutilation. After removal of the part, custody of the remainder of the body vests in the surviving spouse, next of kin, or other persons under obligation to dispose of the body.

II. The time of death shall be determined by a physician who attends the donor at his death, or; if none, the physician who certifies the death. The physician shall not participate in the procedures for removing or transplanting a part.

III. A person who acts in good faith in accord with the terms of this chapter is not liable for damages in any civil action or subject to prosecution in any criminal proceeding for his act.

IV. The provisions of this chapter are subject to RSA 611:10 through 611:15 prescribing powers and duties with respect to autopsies.

291-A:7-a Transportation and Preservation.

Notwithstanding any law or rule to the contrary, if a donee is an accredited medical or dental school and it accepts a gift of the entire body for the purposes of medical research and education, the school shall be responsible for all transportation arrangements and for all preservation procedures for such body. The preservation procedures shall be the responsibility of the donee institution and shall be conducted according to procedures in common use among American medical and dental schools. The provisions of RSA 325 shall not apply to this section.

291-A:8 Uniformity of Interpretation.

This chapter shall be so construed as to effectuate its general purpose to make uniform the law of those states which enact it.

291-A:9 Short Title.

This chapter may be cited as the Uniform Anatomical Gift Act.

NEW JERSEY

UNIFORM ANATOMICAL GIFT ACT

§ 26:6-57. Definitions.

As used in this act:

(a) "Bank or storage facility" means a facility licensed, accredited, or approved under the laws of any State for storage of human bodies or parts thereof.

(b) "Decedent" means a deceased individual and includes a stillborn infant or fetus.

(c) "Donor" means an individual who makes a gift of all or part of his body.

(d) "Hospital" means a hospital licensed, accredited, or approved under the laws of any State; includes a hospital operated by the United States Government, a State, or a subdivision thereof, although not required to be licensed under State laws.

(e) "Part" means organs, tissues, eyes, bones, arteries, blood, other fluids and any other portions of a human body.

(f) "Person" means an individual, corporation, government or governmental subdivision or agency, business trust, estate, trust, partnership or association, or any other legal entity.

(g) "Physician" or "surgeon" means a physician or surgeon licensed or authorized to practice under the laws of any State.

(h) "State" includes any State, district, commonwealth, territory, insular possession, and any other area subject to the legislative authority of the United States of America.

§ 26:6-58. Gift of all or part of body; consent; examination; rights of donee.

(a) Any individual of sound mind and 18 years of age or more may give all or any part of his body for any purpose specified in section 3, the gift to take effect upon death.

(b) Any of the following persons, in order of priority stated, when persons in prior classes are not available at the time of death, and in the absence of actual notice of contrary indications by the decedent or actual notice of opposition by a member of the same or a prior class, may give all or any part of the decedent's body for any purpose specified in section 3:

(1) The spouse,

(2) An adult son or daughter,

(3) Either parent,

(4) An adult brother or sister,

(5) A guardian of the person of the decedent at the time of his death,

(6) Any other person authorized or under obligation to dispose of the body.

(c) If the donee has actual notice of contrary indications by the decedent or that a gift by a member of a class is opposed by a member of the same or a prior class, the donee shall not accept the gift. The persons authorized by subsection (b) may make the gift after or immediately before death.

(d) A gift of all or part of a body authorizes any examination necessary to assure medical acceptability of the gift for the purposes intended.

(e) The rights of the donee created by the gift are paramount to the rights of others except as provided by section 7(d).

§ 26:6-58.1. Next-of-kin option to consent to anatomical gifts; procedures for informing; certificate of organ donation; good faith exemption from liability or prosecution.

a. When the decision has been made in a hospital to pronounce the death of a person who, based on accepted medical standards, is a suitable candidate for organ donation, the person in charge of the hospital, or that person's designated representative, other than a person connected with the determination of death, shall make known to any of the following persons, in order of priority stated, when persons in prior classes are not available at the time of death and in the absence of actual notice of contrary indications by the decedent or actual notice of opposition by a member of the same or a prior class specified in paragraph (1), (2), (3), (4), (5) or (6) or this subsection, or when there is any other reason to believe that an anatomical gift is contrary to the decedent's religious beliefs, that the person has the option to consent to the gift of all or any part of the decedent's body for any purpose specified in section 3 of P.L. 1969, c. 161 (C. 26:6-59):

(1) the spouse,

(2) an adult son or daughter,

(3) either parent,

(4) an adult brother or sister,

(5) a guardian of the person of the decedent at the time of the decedent's death, or

(6) any other person authorized or under the obligation to dispose of the body.

Consent or refusal need only be obtained from a person in the highest priority class available.

b. The person in charge of the hospital or that person's designated representative shall complete a certificate of organ donation option for an anatomical gift, on a form supplied by the Commissioner of Health. The certificate shall include a statement that the option for consent to an anatomical gift has been made known, and shall further indicate thereupon whether or not consent was granted, the name of the person granting or refusing the consent, and that person's relationship to the decedent. The death certificate required by R.S. 26:6-5.1 shall not be deemed complete unless a completed organ donation option certificate is attached thereto.

c. A gift made pursuant to the request required by this act shall be executed pursuant to the applicable provisions of P.L. 1969, c. 161 (C. 26:6-57 et seq.).

d. A person who acts in good faith in accordance with the provisions of this act is not liable for any damages in any civil action or subject to prosecution in any criminal proceeding for any act or omission of the person.

§ 26:6-58.2. Program to increase public awareness of act; investigation of methods of acquisition and distribution of human tissue and organs.

The Commissioner of Health shall establish a program to be administered by hospitals and other public and private agencies that are involved in the acquisition and distribution of human tissue and human organs to:

a. Increase public awareness of the provisions of this act regarding the acquisition and distribution of human tissue and human organs; and

b. Investigate the methods used by other states for the acquisition and distribution of human tissue and human organs, reciprocity agreements established between other states, and the development of similar agreements between New Jersey and other states.

§ 26:6-58.3. Rules and regulations.

In accordance with the "Administrative Procedure Act," P.L. 1968, c. 410 (C. 52:14B-1 et seq.) the commissioner, in consultation with professionals involved in organ transplants, shall adopt such rules and regulations as are necessary to effectuate the purposes of this act including, but not limited to, regulations concerning the training of hospital employees who may be designated to perform the request, the procedure to be employed in making the request, and where, based on medical criteria, the request would not yield a donation which would be suitable for use, the commissioner may, by regulation, authorize an exception to the request required by section 1 of this act.

§ 26:6-59. Donees; purposes.

The following persons may become donees of gifts of bodies or parts thereof for the purposes stated:

(1) Any hospital, surgeon, or physician, for medical or dental education, research, advancement of medical or dental science, therapy, or transplantation; or

(2) Any accredited medical or dental school, college or university for education, research, advancement of medical or dental science, or therapy; or

(3) Any bank or storage facility, for medical or dental education, research, advancement of medical or dental science, therapy, or transplantation; or

(4) Any specified individual for therapy or transplantation needed by him.

§ 26:6-60. Gift by will or other document or recorded message.

(a) A gift of all or part of the body under section 2(a) may be made by will. The gift becomes effective upon the death of the testator without waiting for probate. If the will is not probated, or if it is declared invalid for testamentary purposes, the gift, to the extent that it has been acted upon in good faith, is nevertheless valid and effective.

(b) A gift of all or part of the body under section 2(a) may also be made by document other than a will. The gift becomes effective upon the death of the donor. The document, which may be a card designed to be carried on the person, must be signed by the donor in the presence of two witnesses who must sign the document in his presence. If the donor cannot sign, the document may be signed for him at his direction and in his presence in the presence of two witnesses who must sign the document in his presence. Delivery of the document of gift during the donor's lifetime is not necessary to make the gift valid.

(c) The gift may be made to a specified donee or without specifying a donee. If the latter, the gift may be accepted by the attending physician as donee upon or following death. If the gift is made to a specified donee who is not available at the time and place of death, the attending physician upon or following death, in the absence of any expressed indication that the donor desired otherwise, may accept the gift as donee. The physician who becomes a donee under this subsection shall not participate in the procedures for removing or transplanting a part.

(d) Notwithstanding section 7(b), the donor may designate in his will, card, or other document of gift the surgeon or physician to carry out the appropriate procedures. In the absence of a designation or if the designee is not available, the donee or other person authorized to accept the gift may employ or authorize any surgeon or physician for the purpose or, in the case of a gift of eyes, he may employ or authorize a practitioner of mortuary science licensed by the State Board of Mortuary Science of New Jersey who has successfully completed a course in eye enucleation approved by the State Board of Medical Examiners to enucleate eyes for the gift after certification of death by a physician. A practitioner of mortuary science acting in accordance with the provisions of this subsection shall not have any liability, civil or criminal, for the eye enucleation.

(e) Any gift by a person designated in section 2(b), shall be made by a document signed by him or made by his telegraphic, recorded telephonic, or other recorded message.

§ 26:6-60.1. Anatomical gifts by hospital patients; ascertainment of existence of gift and identification of donee.

A hospital shall, if possible, ascertain from a patient upon admission whether or not the patient has made a gift of all or part of the patient's body pursuant to section 4 of P.L. 1969, c. 161 (C. 26:6-60), and the donee, if any, to whom the gift has been made.

§ 26:6-60.2. Anatomical gift records; contacting donee upon death of hospital patient donor.

A hospital shall maintain, as part of a patient's permanent record, the information required under this act and any other pertinent information concerning the anatomical gift which will facilitate the discharge of the patient's wishes in the event of the patient's death. Upon the death of a patient who has made an anatomical gift, a hospital shall make every good faith effort to contact, without delay, the donee, if any, to whom the gift has been made.

§ 26:6-61. Delivery of will, card, or other document to donee.

If the gift is made by the donor to a specified donee, the will, card, or other document, or an executed copy thereof, may be delivered to the donee to expedite the appropriate procedures immediately after death. Delivery is not necessary to the validity of the gift. The will, card, or other document, or an executed copy thereof, may be deposited in any hospital, bank, or storage facility, or registry office that accepts it for safekeeping or for facilitation of procedures after death. On request of any interested party upon or after the donor's death, the person in possession shall produce the document for examination.

§ 26:6-62. Amendment or revocation of gift by donor.

(a) If the will, card, or other document or executed copy thereof, has been delivered to a specified donee, the donor may amend or revoke the gift by:

    (1) The execution and delivery to the donee of a signed statement, or

    (2) An oral statement made in the presence of 2 persons and communicated to the donee, or

    (3) A statement during a terminal illness or injury addressed to an attending physician and communicated to the donee, or

    (4) A signed card or document found on his person or in his effects.

(b) Any document of gift which has not been delivered to the donee may be revoked by the donor in the manner set out in subsection (a) or by destruction, cancellation, or mutilation of the document and all executed copies thereof.

(c) Any gift made by a will may also be amended or revoked in the manner provided for amendment or revocation of wills or as provided in subsection (a).

§ 26:6-63. Acceptance or rejection of gift; determination of time of death; civil liability; application of autopsy laws.

(a) The donee may accept or reject the gift. If the donee accepts a gift of the entire body, he may, subject to the terms of the gift, authorize embalming and the use of the body in funeral services, and after it has served its scientific purposes, provide for its disposal by burial or cremation. If the gift is of a part of the body, the donee, upon the death of the donor and prior to embalming, shall cause the part to be removed without unnecessary mutilation. After removal of the part, custody of the remainder of the body vests in the surviving spouse, next of kin, or other persons under obligation to dispose of the body.

(b) The time of death shall be determined by a physician who attends the donor at his death, or, if none, the physician who certifies the death. The physician shall not participate in the procedures for removing or transplanting a part.

(c) A person who acts in good faith in accord with the terms of this act or the anatomical gift laws of another State or foreign country is not liable for damages in any civil action or subject to prosecution in any criminal proceeding for his act.

(d) The provisions of this act are subject to the laws of this State prescribing powers and duties with respect to autopsies.

§ 26:6-64. Construction of act.

This act shall be so construed as to effectuate its general purpose to make uniform the law of those States which enact it.

§ 26:6-65. Short title.

This act may be cited as the "Uniform Anatomical Gift Act."

NEW MEXICO

ANATOMICAL GIFTS

§ 24-6-1. Definitions.

As used in the Uniform Anatomical Gift Act [this article]:

A. "bank or storage facility" means a facility licensed, accredited or approved under the laws of any state for storage of human bodies or parts thereof;

B. "decedent" means a deceased individual and includes a stillborn infant or fetus;

C. "donor" means an individual who makes a gift of all or part of his body;

D. "eye bank" means any nonprofit agency which is organized to procure eye tissue for the purpose of transplantation or research and which meets the medical standards set by the eye bank association of America;

E. "hospital" means a hospital licensed, accredited or approved under the laws of any state and includes a hospital operated by the United States government, a state or a subdivision thereof, although not required to be licensed under state laws;

F. "organ procurement agency" means any nonprofit agency designated by the health care financing administration to procure and place human organs and tissues for transplantation, therapy or research;

G. "part" includes organs, tissues, eyes, bones, arteries, blood, other fluids and other portions of a human body, and includes parts;

H. "person" means an individual, corporation, government or governmental subdivision or agency, business trust, estate, trust, partnership or association or any other legal entity;

I. "physician" or "surgeon" means a physician or surgeon licensed or authorized to practice under the laws of any state; and

J. "state" includes any state, district, commonwealth, territory, insular possession and any other area subject to the legislative authority of the United States of America.

§ 24-6-2. Persons who may execute an anatomical gift.

A. Any individual of sound mind and eighteen years of age or more may give all or any part of his body for any purposes specified in Section 24-6-3 NMSA 1978, the gift to take effect upon death.

B. Any of the following persons in order of priority stated, when persons in prior classes are not available at the time of death and in the absence of actual notice of contrary indications by the decedent, may give all or any part of the decedent's body for any purposes specified in Section 24-6-3 NMSA 1978:

(1) the spouse;

(2) an adult son or daughter;

(3) either parent;

(4) an adult brother or sister;

(5) a guardian of the person of the decedent at the time of his death; or

(6) any other person authorized or under obligation to dispose of the body.

C. If the donee has actual notice of contrary indications by the decedent, the donee shall not accept the gift. The persons authorized by Subsection B of this section may make the gift after death or immediately before death.

D. A gift of all or part of a body authorizes any examination necessary to assure medical acceptability of the gift for the purposes intended.

E. The rights of the donee created by the gift are paramount to the rights of others except as provided by Subsection D of Section 24-6-7 NMSA 1978.

F. If a decedent is a donor who has executed an anatomical gift as provided in Section 24-6-4 NMSA 1978 and has not revoked that gift as provided in Section 24-6-6 NMSA 1978, his gift of all or a part of his body, as amended if applicable, shall be valid and effective and shall not be revoked by any other person listed in Paragraphs (1) through (6) of Subsection B of this section.

§ 24-6-3. Persons who may become donees, and purposes for which anatomical gifts may be made.

The following persons may become donees of gifts of bodies or parts thereof for the purposes stated:

A. any hospital, surgeon or physician, for medical or dental education, research, advancement of medical or dental science, therapy or transplantation; or

B. any accredited medical or dental school, college or university, for education, research, advancement of medical or dental science, therapy or transplantation; or

C. any bank or storage facility, for medical or dental education, research, advancement of medical or dental science, therapy or transplantation; or

D. any specified individual for therapy or transplantation needed by him.

§ 24-6-4. Manner of executing anatomical gifts.

A. A gift of all or part of the body under Subsection A of Section 24-6-2 NMSA 1978 may be made by will. The gift becomes effective upon the death of the testator without waiting for probate. If the will is not probated or if it is declared invalid for testamentary purposes, the gift, to the extent that it has been acted upon in good faith, is nevertheless valid and effective.

B. A gift of all or part of the body under Subsection A of Section 24-6-2 NMSA 1978 may also be made by a document other than a will. The gift becomes effective upon the death of the donor. The document, which may be a card designed to be carried on the person, must be signed by the donor in the presence of two witnesses who must sign the document in his presence, unless the document is a driver's license application or renewal form or a driver's license, in which case, the presence and signature of only one witness is necessary. If the donor cannot sign, the document may be signed for him at his direction and in his presence and in the presence of two witnesses who must sign the document in his presence. Delivery of the document of gift during the donor's lifetime is not necessary to make the gift valid.

C. The gift may be made to a specified donee or without specifying a donee. If the latter, the gift may be accepted by the attending physician as donee upon or following death. If the gift is made to a specified donee who is not available at the time and place of death, the attending physician upon or following death, in the absence of any expressed indication that the donor desired otherwise, may accept the gift as donee. The physician who becomes a donee under this subsection shall not participate in the procedures for removing or transplanting a part.

D. Notwithstanding Subsection B of Section 24-6-7 NMSA 1978, the donor may designate in his will, card or other document of gift the surgeon or physician to carry out the appropriate procedures. In the absence of a designation or if the designee is not available, the donee or other person authorized to accept the gift may employ or authorize any surgeon or physician for the purpose.

E. Any gift by a person designated in Subsection B of Section 24-6-2 NMSA 1978 shall be made by a document signed by him or made by his telegraphic, recorded telephonic or other recorded message.

§ 24-6-5. Delivery of document of gift.

If the gift is made by the donor to a specified donee, the will, card or other document or an executed copy thereof may be delivered to the donee to expedite the appropriate procedures immediately after death, but delivery is not necessary to the validity of the gift. The will, card or other document or an executed copy thereof may be deposited in any hospital, bank or storage facility or registry office that accepts them for safekeeping or for facilitation of procedures after death. On request of any interested party upon or after the donor's death, the person in possession shall produce the document for examination. If the document is executed pursuant to a driver's license application or renewal, it shall be microfilmed and filed in the statewide organ and tissue donor registry provided pursuant to Section 66-5-10 NMSA 1978. Upon request of authorized hospital, and/or organ and tissue donor program personnel, immediately prior to or after the donor's death, the New Mexico state police shall verify the donor information on the microfilmed document. The motor vehicle division of the transportation department shall produce a copy of the document upon request to authorized hospital personnel or any other interested party immediately prior to or after the donor's death.

§ 24-6-6. Amendment or revocation of the gift.

A. If the will, card or other document or executed copy thereof has been delivered to a specified donee, the donor may amend or revoke the gift by:

    (1) the execution and delivery to the donee of a signed statement;

    (2) an oral statement made in the presence of two persons and communicated to the donee;

    (3) a statement during a terminal illness or injury addressed to an attending physician and communicated to the donee; or

    (4) a signed card or document found on his person or in his effects.

B. Any document of gift which has not been delivered to the donee may be revoked by the donor in the manner set out in Subsection A of this section, by destruction, cancellation or mutilation of the document and all executed copies thereof or in the case of a driver's license and the document executed pursuant to application for or renewal of such driver's license, by written notice to the motor vehicle division of the transportation department revoking the gift or by signing a donor revocation statement in person at any motor vehicle field office in the presence and with the signature of one witness.

C. Any gift made by a will may also be amended or revoked in the manner provided for amendment or revocation of wills or as provided in Subsection A of this section.

§ 24-6-7. Rights and duties at death.

A. The donee may accept or reject the gift. If the donee accepts a gift of the entire body, he may, subject to the terms of the gift, authorize embalming and the use of the body in funeral services. If the gift is a part of the body, the donee, upon the death of the donor and prior to embalming, shall cause the part to be removed without unnecessary mutilation. After removal of the part, custody of the remainder of the body vests in the surviving spouse, next of kin or some other persons under obligation to dispose of the body.

B. The time of death shall be determined by a physician who attends the donor at his death, or if none, the physician who certifies the death. This physician shall not participate in the procedures for removing or transplanting a part.

C. A person who acts in good faith in accord with the terms of the Uniform Anatomical Gift Act [24-6-1 to 24-6-9 NMSA 1978], or under the anatomical gift laws of another state is not liable for damages in any civil action or subject to prosecution in any criminal proceeding for such action.

D. The provisions of the Uniform Anatomical Gift Act are subject to the laws of this state prescribing powers and duties with respect to autopsies.

E. In respect to a gift of an eye, a licensed funeral service practitioner who has completed a course in eye enucleation conducted and certified by an accredited school of medicine and who holds a certificate of competence for completing such course may enucleate eyes for a gift after the death of a donor. A written release authorizing the enucleation shall be obtained prior to the performance of the eye enucleation from a relative or other person in order of priority stated in Subsection B of Section 24-6-2 NMSA 1978. A licensed funeral service practitioner acting in accordance with this subsection is not liable for damages in any civil act or subject to prosecution in any criminal proceeding for performing the eye enucleation.

§ 24-6-8. Uniformity of interpretation.

This act [24-6-1 to 24-6-9 NMSA 1978] shall be so construed as to effectuate its general purpose to make uniform the law of those states which enact it.

§ 24-6-9. Short title.

This act [24-6-1 to 24-6-9 NMSA 1978] may be cited as the "Uniform Anatomical Gift Act".

§ 24-6-10. Organ and tissue donation policy and procedure; duties; immunity from liability.

A. Every hospital in New Mexico shall adopt and implement an organ and tissue donation policy and procedure to assist the medical, surgical and nursing staff in identifying and evaluating potential organ or tissue donors.

B. The organ and tissue donation policy and procedure shall contain information on acceptable donor criteria, methods for routine education of the hospital staff about the policy and procedure, the name and telephone number of the local organ procurement agency and eye bank which will provide a standard organ and tissue donation consent form, mechanisms for informing the next of kin of a potential donor about organ and tissue donation options and provisions for the maintenance and procurement of donated organs and tissues.

C. Every hospital's written policy and procedure for the identification of potential organ and tissue donors shall:

(1) assure that families of potential organ or tissue donors are made aware of the option of organ or tissue donation and the option to decline;

(2) encourage discretion and sensitivity with respect to the circumstances, views and beliefs of those families; and

(3) require that the appropriate organ procurement agency or eye bank be notified when a potential organ or tissue donor is identified.

D. All physicians and hospital personnel shall make every reasonable effort to carry out the organ and tissue donation policy and procedure adopted by the hospital so that the wishes of a donor may be conveyed to an appropriate local organ procurement agency or eye bank and the necessary donation documents may be properly executed.

E. Every hospital shall develop and implement a policy and procedure for the determination of brain death pursuant to Section 12-2-4 NMSA 1978.

F. The health and environment department shall issue an annual report summarizing the data pertaining to the implementation of this section and its impact on organ and tissue procurement activity.

G. Laws pertaining to notification of the office of the medical investigator should be complied with in all cases of reportable deaths.

H. Failure to comply with any provision of this section shall not subject any physician, hospital, hospital employee or other person to civil or criminal liability for such failure.

I. As used in this section, "hospital" means any general acute care hospital in New Mexico.

§ 24-6-11. Human organ or tissue transfers; prohibited actions; penalty.

A. No person may acquire, receive or otherwise transfer for valuable consideration any human organ or tissue.

B. All costs which are incurred at the request of an organ procurement agency or eye bank and which are related to the evaluation of a potential organ or tissue donor, maintenance of organ or tissue viability following a brain death declaration or removal of donated organs and tissues shall be paid by the receiving organ procurement agency or eye bank. The next of kin or the estate of the donor shall not be responsible for payment of any of these costs.

C. Any person who violates any provision of this section is guilty of a misdemeanor and upon conviction shall be punished in accordance with the provisions of Section 31-19-1 NMSA 1978.

NEW YORK

UNIFORM ANATOMICAL GIFT ACT

§ 4300. Definitions.

As used in this section, the following terms shall have the following meanings:

1. "Bank or storage facility" means a hospital, laboratory or other facility licensed or approved under the laws of any state for storage of human bodies or parts thereof, for use in medical education, research, therapy, or transplantation to individuals.

2. "Decedent" means a deceased individual of any age and includes a stillborn infant or fetus.

3. "Donor" means an individual who makes a gift of all or part of his body.

4. "Hospital" means a hospital licensed, accredited, or approved under the laws of any state and includes a hospital operated by the United States Government, a state, or a subdivision thereof, although not required to be licensed under state laws.

5. "Part" of a body includes organs, tissues, eyes, bones, arteries, blood, other fluids and other portions of a human body, and "part" includes "parts".

6. "Person" means an individual, corporation, government or governmental subdivision or agency, business trust, estate, trust, partnership or association, or any other legal entity.

7. "Physician" or "surgeon" means a physician or surgeon licensed or authorized to practice under the laws of any state.

8. "State" includes any state, district, commonwealth, territory, insular possession, and any other are subject to the legislative authority of the United States of America.

§ 4301. Persons who may execute an anatomical gift.

1. Any individual of sound mind and eighteen years of age or more may give all or any part of his body for any purpose specified in section four thousand three hundred two of this article, the gift to take effect upon death.

2. Any of the following persons, in the order of priority stated, may, when persons in prior classes are not available at the time of death, and in the absence of actual notice of contrary indications by the decedent, or actual notice of opposition by a member of any of the classes specified in paragraph (a), (b), (c), (d) or (e), or other reasons to believe that an anatomical gift is contrary to the decedent's religious or moral beliefs, give all or any part of the decedent's body for any purpose specified in section four thousand three hundred two of this article:

   (a) the spouse,
   (b) a son or daughter twenty-one years of age or older,
   (c) either parent,
   (d) a brother or sister twenty-one years of age or older,
   (e) a guardian of the person of the decedent at the time of his death,
   (f) any other person authorized or under the obligation to dispose of the body.

3. If the donee has actual notice of contrary indication by the decedent or that the gift is opposed by a member of any of the classes specified in paragraph (a), (b), (c), (d) or (e), or other reasons to believe that an anatomical gift is contrary to the decedent's religious or moral beliefs, the donee shall not accept the gift.

4. A gift of all or part of a body authorizes any examination necessary to assure medical acceptability of gift for the purposes intended.

5. The rights of the donee created by the gift are paramount to the rights of others except as provided by section four thousand three hundred seven of this article.

§ 4302. Persons who may become donees and purposes for which anatomical gifts may be made.

The following persons may become donees of gifts or bodies or parts thereof for the purposes stated:

1. any hospital, surgeon, or physician, for medical or dental education, research, advancement of medical or dental science, therapy, or transplantation; or

2. any accredited medical or dental school, college or university for education, research, advancement of medical or dental science, or therapy; or

3. any bank or storage facility, for medical or dental education, research, advancement of medical or dental science, therapy or transplantation; or

4. any specific donee, for therapy or transplantation needed by him.

§ 4303. Manner of executing anatomical gifts.

1. A gift of all or part of the body under this article may be made by will. The gift becomes effective upon the death of the testator without waiting for probate. If the will is not probated, or if it is declared invalid for testamentary purposes, the gift, to the extent that it has been acted upon in good faith, is nevertheless valid and effective.

2. A gift of all or part of the body under this article may also be made by document other than a will. The gift becomes effective upon the death of the donor. The document, which may be a card designed to be carried on the person, must be signed by the donor

in the presence of two witnesses who must sign the document in the donor's presence. Delivery of the document of gift during the donor's lifetime is not necessary to make the gift valid.

3. The gift may be made either to a specified donee or without specifying a donee. If the latter, the gift may be accepted by and utilized under the direction of the attending physician upon or following death. If the gift is made to a specified donee who is not available at the time and place of death, the attending physician upon or following death, in the absence of any expressed indication that the donor desired otherwise, may accept the gift as donee. The physician who becomes a donee under this subdivision shall not participate in the procedures for removing or transplanting a part.

4. Subject to the prohibitions in subdivision two of section four thousand three hundred six the donor may designate in his will, card or other document of gift the surgeon or physician to carry out the appropriate procedures. In the absence of a designation, or if the designee is not available, the donee or other person authorized to accept the gift may employ or authorize any surgeon or physician for the purpose.

5. Any gift by a person designated in subdivision two of section four thousand three hundred one of this article shall be by a document signed by him or made by his telegraphic, recorded telephonic, or other recorded message.

§ 4304. Delivery of document of gift.

If the gift is made by the donor to a specified donee, the will, card or other document or an executed copy thereof, may be delivered to him to expedite the appropriate procedures immediately after death delivery is not necessary to validity of the gift. The will, card or other document, or an executed copy thereof, may be deposited in any hospital, bank, storage facility or registry office that accepts it for safekeeping or for facilitation of procedures after death. On request of an interested party upon or after the donor's death, the person in possession shall produce the document for examination.

§ 4305. Revocation of the gift.

1. If the will, card, or other document or executed copy thereof has been delivered to a specified donee, the donor may amend or revoke the gift by:

(a) the execution and delivery to the donee of a signed statement, or

(b) an oral statement of revocation made in the presence of two persons, communicated to the donee, or

(c) a statement during a terminal illness or injury addressed to an attending physician and communicated to the donee, or

(d) a signed card or document, found on his person or in his effects.

2. Any document of gift which has not been delivered to the donee may be revoked in the manner set out in subdivision one of this section or by destruction, cancellation, or mutilation of the document and all executed copies thereof.

3. Any gift made by a will may be revoked or amended in the manner provided for revocation or amendment of wills or as provided in subdivision one of this section.

§ 4306. Rights and duties at death.

1. The donee may accept or reject the gift. If the donee accepts a gift of the entire body, he may, subject to the terms of the gift, authorize embalming and the use of the body in funeral services. If the gift is of a part of the body, the donee upon the death of the donor and prior to embalming, may cause the part to be removed without unnecessary mutilation. After removal of the part, custody of the remainder of the body vests in the surviving spouse, next of kin, or other persons under obligation to dispose of the body.

2. The time of death shall be certified by the physician who attends the donor at his death and one other physician, neither of whom shall participate in the procedure for removing or transplanting the part.

3. A person who acts in good faith in accord with the terms of this article or with the anatomical gift laws of another state is not liable for damages in any civil action or subject to prosecution in any criminal proceeding for his act.

§ 4307. Prohibition of sales and purchases of human organs.

It shall be unlawful for any person to knowingly acquire, receive, or otherwise transfer for valuable consideration any human organ for use in human transplantation. The term human organ means the human kidney, liver, heart, lung, bone marrow, and any other human organ or tissue as may be designated by the commissioner but shall exclude blood. The term "valuable consideration" does not include the reasonable payments associated with the removal, transportation, implantation, processing, preservation, quality control, and storage of a human organ or the expenses of travel, housing, and lost wages incurred by the donor of a human organ in connection with the donation of the organ. Any person who violates this section shall be guilty of a misdemeanor.

§ 4308. Application.

The provisions of this article shall not be deemed to supersede or affect the provisions of the public health law relating to the functions, powers and duties of coroners, coroner's physicians or medical examiners.

NORTH CAROLINA

UNIFORM ANATOMICAL GIFT ACT

§ 130A-402. Short title.

This Part may be cited as the Uniform Anatomical Gift Act.

§ 130A-403. Definitions.

The following definitions shall apply throughout this Part:

(1) "Bank or storage facility" means a facility licensed, accredited or approved under the laws of any state for storage or distribution of a human body or its parts.

(2) "Decedent" means a deceased individual and includes a stillborn infant or fetus.

(3) "Donor" means an individual who makes a gift of all or part of the individual's body.

(4) "Hospital" means a hospital licensed, accredited or approved under the laws of any state and a hospital operated by the United States government, a state or its subdivision, although not required to be licensed under state laws.

(5) "Part" means organs, tissues, eyes, bones, arteries, blood, other fluids and any other portions of a human body.

(6) "Physician" or "surgeon" means a physician or surgeon licensed to practice medicine under the laws of any state.

(7) "State" includes any state, district, commonwealth, territory, insular possession and any other area subject to the legislative authority of the United States of America.

(8) "Qualified individual" means any of the following individuals who has completed a course in eye enucleation and has been certified as competent to enucleate eyes by an accredited school of medicine in this State:

a. An embalmer licensed to practice in this State;

b. A physician's assistance approved by the Board of Medical Examiners pursuant to G.S. 90-18(13);

c. A registered or a licensed practical nurse licensed by the Board of Nursing pursuant to Article 9A of Chapter 90 of the General Statutes;

d. A student who is enrolled in an accredited school of medicine operating within this State and who has completed two or more years of a course of study leading to the awarding of a degree of doctor of medicine;

e. A technician who has successfully completed a written examination by the North Carolina Eye and Human Tissue Bank, Inc., certified by the eye Bank Association of America.

§ 130A-404. Persons who may make an anatomical gift.

(a) An individual of sound mind and 18 years of age or more may give all or any part of that individual's body for any purpose specified in G.S. 130A-405. The gift shall take effect upon death.

(b) Any of the following persons, in order of priority stated, when persons in prior classes are not available at the time of death, and in the absence of actual notice of contrary indications by the decedent or actual notice of opposition by a member of the same or a prior class, may give all or any part of the decedent's body for any purpose specified in G.S. 130A-405.

(1) The spouse;

(2) An adult child;

(3) Either parent;

(4) An adult sibling;

(5) A guardian of the person of the decedent at the time of decedent's death;

(6) Any other person authorized or under obligation to dispose of the body.

(c) The persons authorized by subsection (b) may make the gift after or immediately before death. However, the guardian of the person of a ward may make the gift at any time during the guardianship and the gift shall become effective upon the death of the ward unless the guardianship terminated before death.

(d) If the donee has actual notice of contrary indications by the decedent or that a gift by a member of a class is opposed by a member of the same or a prior class, the donee shall not accept the gift.

(e) A gift of all or part of a body authorizes any examination necessary to assure medical acceptability of the gift for the purposes intended.

(f) The rights of the donee created by the gift are paramount to the rights of others except as provided by G.S. 130A-409(d).

§ 130A-405. Persons who may become donees; purposes for which anatomical gifts may be made.

The following persons may become donees of gifts of a human body or its parts for the purposes stated:

(1) A hospital, surgeon or physician for medical or dental education, research, advancement of medical or dental science, therapy or transplantation;

(2) An accredited medical or dental school, college or university for education, research, advancement of medical or dental science or therapy;

(3) A bank or storage facility, for medical or dental education, research, advancement of medical or dental science, therapy or

transplantation;

(4) A specified individual for therapy or transplantation needed by that individual; or

(5) The Commission of Anatomy for the distribution of a human body or its parts for the purpose of promoting the study of anatomy in this State.

§ 130A-406. Manner of making anatomical gifts.

(a) A gift of all or part of the body under G.S. 130A-404(a) may be made by will. The gift becomes effective upon the death of the testator without waiting for probate. If the will is not probated, or if it is declared invalid for testamentary purposes, the gift, to the extent that it has been acted upon in good faith, is valid and effective.

(b) A gift of all or part of the body under G.S. 130A-404(a) may also be made by a document other than a will. The gift becomes effective upon the death of the donor. The document, which may be a card designed to be carried on the individual, must be signed by the donor in the presence of two witnesses who must sign the document in the donor's presence. If the donor cannot sign, the document may be signed for the donor at the direction and in the presence of the donor and in the presence of two witnesses who must sign the document in the donor's presence. Delivery of the document of gift during the donor's lifetime is not necessary to make the gift valid.

(c) The gift may be made to a specified donee or without specifying a donee. If the latter, the gift may be accepted by the attending physician as donee upon or following death. If the gift is made to a specified donee who is not available at the time and place of death, the attending physician upon or following death, in the absence of any expressed indication that the donor desired otherwise, may accept the gift as donee.

(d) The donor may designate by will, card or other document of gift the surgeon or physician to carry out the appropriate procedures, subject to the provisions of G.S. 130A-409(b). In the absence of a designation or if the designee is not available, the donee or other person authorized to accept the gift may employ or authorize any surgeon or physician for that purpose.

(e) In respect to a gift of an eye, a qualified individual may enucleate eyes for the gift after proper certification of death by a physician and upon the express direction of a physician other than the one who certified the death of the donor.

(f) A gift by a person designated in G.S. 130A-404(b) shall be made by a document signed by the donor or made by the donor's telegraphic, recorded telephonic, or other recorded message. However, a guardian of the person of a ward who makes a gift of all or any part of the ward's body prior to the ward's death shall make the gift by a document signed by the guardian and filed with the clerk of court having jurisdiction over the guardian.

(g) The making of a gift shall be deemed to include an authorization to the donee to review any medical records of the donor after the death of the donor.

§ 130A-407. Delivery of document of gift.

If the gift is made by the donor or the guardian to a specified donee, the will, card or other document or executed copy may be delivered to the donee at any time to expedite the appropriate procedures immediately after death. Delivery is not necessary to the validity of the gift. The will, card or other document or executed copy may be deposited in a hospital, bank or storage facility, or registry office that accepts it for safekeeping or for facilitation of procedures after death. On request of any interested party upon or after the donor's or ward's death, the person in possession shall produce the document for examination.

§ 130A-408. Amendment or revocation of the gift.

(a) If the will, card or other document or executed copy has been delivered to a specified donee, the donor may amend or revoke the gift by:

(1) The execution and delivery to the donee of a signed statement;

(2) An oral statement made in the presence of two persons and communicated to the donee;

(3) A statement during a terminal illness or injury addressed to an attending physician and communicated to the donee; or

(4) A signed card or document found on the individual or in the individual's effects, and made known to the donee.

(b) A guardian may amend or revoke the gift by the execution and delivery to the donee of a signed statement.

(c) Any document of gift which has not been delivered to the donee may be revoked by the donor or guardian in the manner set out in subsection (a) or by destruction, cancellation or mutilation of the document and all executed copies.

(d) Any gift made by a will may also be amended or revoked in the manner provided for amendment or revocation of wills or as provided in subsection (a).

§ 130A-409. Rights and duties at death.

(a) The donee may accept or reject the gift. If the donee accepts a gift of the entire body, the donee shall, subject to the terms of the gift, authorize embalming and the use of the body in funeral services, upon request of the surviving spouse or other person listed in the order stated in G.S. 130A-404(b). If the gift is of a part of the body, the donee, upon the death of the donor or ward and prior to embalming, shall, within 24 hours, cause the part to be removed without unnecessary mutilation. After removal of the part, custody of the remainder of the body vests in the surviving spouse, next-of-kin or other persons under obligation to dispose of the body.

(b) The time of death shall be determined by a physician who attends the donor or ward at death, or, if none, the physician who certifies the death. The physician shall not participate in the procedures for removing or transplanting a part.

(c) A person who acts with due care in accord with the terms of this Part or the anatomical gift laws of another state is not liable for damages in any civil action or subject to prosecution in any criminal proceeding for the act.

(d) The provisions of this Part are subject to the laws of this State prescribing powers and duties with respect to autopsies.

§ 130A-410. Use of tissue declared a service; standard of care; burden of proof.

The procurement, processing, distribution or use of whole blood, plasma, blood products, blood derivatives and other human tissues such as corneas, bones or organs for the purpose of injecting, transfusing or transplanting any of them into the human body is declared to be, for all purposes, the rendition of a service by every participating person or institution. Whether or not any remuneration is paid, the service is declared not to be a sale of whole blood, plasma, blood products, blood derivatives or other human tissues, for any purpose. No person or institution shall be liable in warranty, express or implied, for the procurement, processing, distribution or use of these items but nothing in this section shall alter or restrict the liability of a person or institution in negligence or tort in consequence of these services.

§ 130A-411. Giving of blood by persons 17 years of age or more.

A person who is 17 years of age or more may give or donate blood to an individual, hospital blood bank or blood collection center without the consent of the parent or parents or guardian of the donor. It shall be unlawful for a person under the age of 18 years to sell blood.

§ 130A-412. Uniformity of interpretation.

This Part shall be so construed to effectuate its general purpose to make uniform the law of those states which enact it.

§ 130A-412.1. Duty of hospitals to establish organ procurement protocols.

(a) In order to facilitate the goals of this Part, each hospital shall be required to establish written protocols for the identification of potential organ and tissue donors that:

(1) Assure that the families of potential organ and tissue donors are made aware of the option of organ or tissue donation and their option to decline;

(2) Encourage discretion and sensitivity with respect to the circumstances, views and beliefs of such families;

(3) Require that only the organ procurement agency designated by the Secretary of Health and Human Services be notified of potential organ and tissue donors; and

(4) Assure that procedures are established for identifying and consulting with holders of properly executed donor cards.

(b) The family of any person whose organ or tissue is donated for transplantation shall not be financially liable for any costs related to the evaluation of the suitability of the donor's organ or tissue for transplantation or any costs of retrieval of the organ or tissue.

(c) The requirements of this section, or of any hospital organ procurement protocols established pursuant to this section shall not exceed those provided for by the hospital organ protocol provisions of Title XI of the Social Security Act, except for the purposes of this section the term "organ and tissue donors" shall include cornea and tissue donors for transplantation.

NORTH DAKOTA

UNIFORM ANATOMICAL GIFT ACT

§ 23-06.2-01. Definitions.

As used in this chapter, unless the context or subject matter otherwise requires:

1. "Anatomical gift" means a donation of all or part of a human body to take effect upon or after death.

2. "Decedent" means a deceased individual and includes a stillborn infant or fetus.

3. "Document of gift" means a card, a statement attached to or imprinted upon a motor vehicle operator's license, a will, or any other writing used to make an anatomical gift.

4. "Donor" means an individual who makes an anatomical gift of all or part of the individual's body.

5. "Enucleator" means an individual who has successfully completed a course in eye enucleation conducted by the department of ophthalmology of an accredited college of medicine that has been approved by the state board of medical examiners.

6. "Hospital" means a facility licensed, accredited, or approved as a hospital under the laws of any state and includes a hospital operated by the United States government, a state, or a subdivision thereof, although not required to be licensed under state law.

7. "Part" means an organ, tissue, eye, bone, artery, blood, fluid, and any other portion of a human body.

8. "Physician" or "surgeon" means an individual licensed or authorized to practice medicine and surgery or osteopathy and surgery under the laws of any state.

9. "Procurement organization" means a person licensed, accredited, or approved under the laws of any state for procurement, distribution, or storage of human bodies or parts thereof.

10. "State" means any state, district, commonwealth, territory, insular possession, or other area subject to the legislative authority of the United States of America.

11. "Technician" means an individual who is licensed or certified by the state board of medical examiners to remove or process a part.

§ 23-06.2-02. Making, amending, revoking, and refusing to make anatomical gifts by individual.

1. An individual who has attained eighteen years of age may make an anatomical gift for any of the purposes specified in subsection 1 of section 23-06.2-06 or may refuse to make an anatomical gift. An individual may limit an anatomical gift to one or more of the purposes specified in subsection 1 of section 23-06.2-06.

2. An anatomical gift may be made by a document of gift.

a. A document of gift must be signed by the donor. If the donor cannot sign, the document of gift must state that it has been signed by another individual and by two witnesses, all of whom have signed at the direction and in the presence of the donor and in the presence of each other.

b. A document of gift may be a statement attached to or imprinted upon a donor's motor vehicle operator's license, subject to subdivision a. Revocation, suspension, expiration, or cancellation of the license does not invalidate the anatomical gift.

c. Notwithstanding subsection 2 of section 23-06.2-08, a document of gift may designate a particular physician or surgeon to carry out the appropriate procedures. In the absence of a designation or if the designee is not available, the donee or other person authorized to accept the anatomical gift may employ or authorize any physician, surgeon, technician, or enucleator for the purpose.

3. An anatomical gift by will becomes effective upon death of the testator without waiting for probate. If the will is not probated, or if, after death, it is declared invalid for testamentary purposes, the gift is nevertheless valid.

4. The donor may amend or revoke an anatomical gift, not made by will, only by:

a. A signed statement;

b. An oral statement made in the presence of two individuals;

c. Any form of communication during a terminal illness or injury addressed to a physician or surgeon; or

d. The delivery of a signed statement to a specified donee to whom a document of gift had been delivered.

5. An anatomical gift made by a will may be amended or revoked in the manner provided for amendment or revocation of wills, or as provided in subsection 4.

6. An anatomical gift that is not revoked by the donor is irrevocable and does not require the consent or concurrence of any other person after the death of the donor but is subject to subsection 2 of section 23-06.2-11.

7. A potential donor may refuse to make an anatomical gift by a writing executed in the same manner as an anatomical gift is made or any other instrument used to identify the individual as refusing to make an anatomical gift. It may be an oral statement or other form of communication during a terminal illness or injury.

8. An anatomical gift of a part by a donor pursuant to subsection 1 is not a refusal to give other parts in the absence of contrary indications by the donor and is not a limitation on a gift or release of other parts pursuant to sections 23-06.2-03 and 23-06.2-04.

9. A revocation or amendment of an anatomical gift by a donor is not a refusal to make another anatomical gift in the absence of contrary indications by the donor. If the donor intends a revocation to be a refusal to make an anatomical gift, the donor must make a refusal pursuant to subsection 7.

§ 23-06.2-03. Making revoking, and objecting to anatomical gifts by others.

1. Unless an individual at the time of death has refused to make any anatomical gift, then any member of the following classes of persons, in the order of priority stated, may make an anatomical gift of all or any part of the decedent's body for any purpose specified in section 23-06.2-06:

    a. The spouse of the decedent.

    b. An adult son or daughter of the decedent.

    c. Either parent of the decedent.

    d. An adult brother or sister of the decedent.

    e. A grandparent of the decedent.

    f. A guardian of the person of the decedent at the time of death.

2. A gift may not be made by a person specified in subsection 1 if:

    a. A person in a prior class is available at the time of death to make an anatomical gift;

    b. The person has knowledge of contrary indications by the decedent; or

    c. The person has knowledge of an objection by a member of the person's class or a prior class.

3. An anatomical gift by a person under subsection 1 must be made by a document of gift signed by the person, or by the person's telegraphic, recorded telephonic, or other recorded message, or other type of communication from the person that is contemporaneously reduced to writing and signed by the recipient.

4. An anatomical gift by a person under subsection 1 may be revoked by any member of the same or a prior class if, before commencement of procedures for the removal of any part from the body of the decedent, the physician, surgeon, technician, or enucleator taking the part knows of the revocation.

5. A failure to make an anatomical gift under subsection 1 is not an objection to the making of an anatomical gift.

§ 23-06.2-04. Authorization by coroner or local public health official.

1. The coroner may permit the removal and release of any part from a body within the coroner's custody, for transplant or therapeutic purposes, if the following requirements are met:

    a. A request has been received from a person specified in subsection 1 of section 23-06.2-06;

    b. A reasonable effort has been made, taking into account the useful life of the part, to locate and examine the decedent's medical records, and to inform persons specified in subsection 1 of section 23-06.2-03 of the option to make or object to the making of an anatomical gift;

    c. That official does not know of a contrary indication by the decedent or objection by a person having priority to act as specified in subsection 1 of section 23-06.2-03;

    d. The removal will be by a physician, surgeon, or technician; but in the case of eyes, removal may be by an enucleator;

    e. The removal will not interfere with any autopsy or investigation; and

    f. The removal will be in accordance with accepted medical standards and cosmetic restoration will be done if appropriate.

2. If the body is not within the custody of the coroner, the local public health officer may permit the removal and release of any part from a body within the local public health officer's custody for transplant or therapeutic purposes if the enumerated requirements of subsection 1 are met.

3. An official permitting the removal and release of any part shall maintain a permanent record of the name of the decedent, the person making the request, the date and purpose of the request, the part requested, and the person to whom it is released.

§ 23-06.2-05. Request for consent to an anatomical gift — Protocol — Exceptions.

1. When death occurs, or is deemed to be imminent, in a hospital to a patient who has not made an anatomical gift, the hospital administrator or a designated representative, other than a person connected with the determination of death, shall request the person described in subsection 1 of section 23-06.2-03, in the order of priority stated, when persons in prior classes are not available at the time of death, and in the absence of actual notice of contrary indication by the decedent or one in a prior class, to consent to the gift of organs of the decedent's body as an anatomical gift. The hospital must develop a protocol that includes the training of employees or other persons designated to make the request, the procedure to be followed in making the request, and a form of record identifying the person making the request and the response and relationship to the decedent. The protocol must encourage reasonable discretion and sensitivity to the family circumstances in all discussions regarding anatomical gifts.

2. If, based upon medical criteria, a request would not yield an anatomical gift that would be suitable for use, there is authorized an exception to the request required by this section.

3. If, based upon the attending physician's special and peculiar knowledge of the decedent or the circumstances surrounding the death of the patient, the attending physician determines that a request will not be made for an anatomical gift, that determination must be noted in the patient's medical record. The determination is an exception to the request required by this section.

4. A reasonable search for a document of gift or other information identifying the bearer as an anatomical gift donor or as an individual who has refused to make an anatomical gift must be made by:

    a. A law enforcement officer, fireman, paramedic, or other emergency rescuer finding an individual whom the searcher believes to be dead or near death; and

    b. A hospital representative upon the admission of an individual at or near the time of death, if there is no other source of that information immediately available.

5. If a document of gift or evidence of refusal to make a gift is located by the search required by subdivision a of subsection 3, a hospital must be notified of the contents and the document must be sent to the hospital with the individual to whom it applies.

6. If, at or near the time of death, a hospital knows that an anatomical gift has been made pursuant to subsection 1 of section 23-06.2-03 or has been authorized pursuant to section 23-06.2-04, or that a patient or an individual identified as in transit to the hospital is a donor, the hospital shall notify the donee if one is specified; if not, the hospital shall notify an appropriate procurement organization. The hospital shall cooperate in the implementation of the anatomical gift.

7. Any person who fails to discharge the duties imposed by this section is not subject to criminal or civil liability but is subject to appropriate administrative sanctions.

§ 23-06.2-06. Persons who may become donees — Purposes for which anatomical gifts may be made.

1. The following persons may become donees of anatomical gifts for the purposes stated:

a. Any hospital, physician, surgeon, or procurement organization, for transplantation, therapy, medical or dental education, research, or advancement of medical or dental science.

b. Any accredited medical or dental school, college or university for education, research, advancement of medical or dental science, or therapy.

c. Any specified individual for transplantation or therapy needed by that individual.

2. An anatomical gift may be made to a specified donee or without specifying a donee. If a donee is not specified or if the donee is not available or rejects the anatomical gift, the anatomical gift may be accepted by any hospital.

3. If the donee has knowledge of contrary indications by the decedent or that a gift by a member of a class is opposed by a member of the same or a prior class under subsection 1 of section 23-06.2-03, the donee may not accept the gift.

§ 23-06.2-07. Delivery of document of gift.

1. Delivery of a document of gift during the donor's lifetime is not necessary to the validity of an anatomical gift.

2. If an anatomical gift is made to a specified donee, the document of gift, or a copy, may be delivered to the donee to expedite the appropriate procedures immediately after death. The document of gift, or a copy, may be deposited in any hospital, procurement organization, or registry office that accepts it for safekeeping or for facilitation of procedures after death. On request of any interested person, upon or after the donor's death, the person in possession shall provide the document of gift or a copy for examination.

§ 23-06.2-08. Rights and duties at death.

1. Rights of a donee created by an anatomical gift are paramount to rights of others except as provided by subsection 2 of section 23-06.2-11. A donee may accept or reject an anatomical gift. If a donee accepts a gift of the entire body, the donee, subject to the terms of the gift, may authorize embalming and the use of the body in funeral services. If the gift is of a part of the body, the donee, upon the death of the donor and before embalming, shall cause the part to be removed without unnecessary mutilation. After removal of the part, custody of the remainder of the body vests in the surviving spouse, next of kin, or other persons under obligation to dispose of the body.

2. The time of death shall be determined by a physician or surgeon who attends the donor at death or, if none, the physician or surgeon who certifies the death. Neither the attending physician or surgeon nor the physician or surgeon who determines the time of death may participate in the procedures for removing or transplanting a part, except as provided in subdivision c of subsection 2 of section 23-06.2-02.

3. If there has been an anatomical gift, a technician may remove any donated parts and an enucleator may remove any donated eyes or parts of eyes, after determination of death by a physician or surgeon.

§ 23-06.2-09. Coordination of procurement and utilization.

Each hospital, after consultation with other hospitals and procurement organizations in the region, shall establish agreements or affiliations for coordination of procurement and utilization of anatomical gifts.

§ 23-06.2-10. Sale or purchase prohibited — Penalty.

1. A person may not knowingly, for valuable consideration, purchase or sell any part for transplantation or therapy, if removal of the part is intended to occur after the death of the decedent.

2. Valuable consideration does not include reasonable payments for removal, processing, disposal, preservation, quality control, storage, transportation, and implantation of a part.

3. Any person who violates this section is guilty of a class B misdemeanor.

§ 23-06.2-11. Examination — Autopsy — Liability.

1. An anatomical gift authorizes any reasonable examination necessary to assure medical acceptability of the gift for the purposes intended.

2. This chapter is subject to the laws of this state prescribing powers and duties with respect to autopsies.

3. Except as provided in section 23-06.2-10, a hospital, physician, surgeon, coroner, local public health officer, enucleator, technician, or any other person who acts in accordance with this chapter or with the applicable anatomical gift law of another state or a foreign country or attempts in good faith to do so is not liable for that activity in any civil action or criminal proceeding.

4. An individual who makes an anatomical gift and the individual's estate are not liable for any injury or damage that may result from the use of the anatomical gift.

§ 23-06.2-11.1. Anatomical parts testing — Exception.

No anatomical parts of human bodies, including whole blood, plasma, blood products, blood derivatives, semen, body tissue, organs, and parts of organs or products derived from parts of organs may be used for injection, transfusion, or transplantation into a human body unless the anatomical parts or the donor have been examined for the presence of antibodies to or antigens of the human immunodeficiency virus and the test is negative for the presence of such antibodies or antigens. The testing requirement of this section does not apply if, in a medical emergency constituting a serious threat to the life of a potential anatomical part recipient, a required anatomical part that has been subjected to the testing required under this section is not available. The state department of health and consolidated laboratories may adopt rules to implement the requirements of this section.

§ 23-06.2-12. Application.

This chapter applies to a document of gift or refusal to make a gift signed by the donor before, on, or after July 12, 1989.

OHIO

ANATOMICAL GIFTS

§ 2108.02. Gift of body or part; rights of next of kin to donate; when donee shall not accept; examination; rights of donee and of coroner conducting autopsy.

(A) Any individual of sound mind may give all or any part of his body for any purpose specified in section 2108.03 of the Revised Code, the gift to take effect upon his death, if either of the following conditions applies:

(1) The individual is eighteen years of age or more;

(2) The individual is less than eighteen years of age and a parent or guardian of the individual signs a document pursuant to division (B)(2) or a statement pursuant to division (C) of section 2108.04 of the Revised Code.

(B) Any of the following persons, in the order of priority stated, when persons in prior classes are not available at the time of death, and in the absence of actual notice of contrary indications by the decedent or actual notice of opposition by a member of the same or a prior class, may give any part of the decedent's body for any purpose specified in section 2108.03 of the Revised Code:

(1) The spouse;

(2) An adult son or daughter;

(3) Either parent;

(4) An adult brother or sister;

(5) A guardian of the person of the decedent at the time of his death;

(6) Any other person authorized or under obligation to dispose of the body.

(C) The donee shall not accept the gift if he has actual notice of contrary indications by the decedent or that a gift by a member of a class is opposed by a member of the same or a prior class. The persons authorized in division (B) of this section may make the gift after or immediately before death.

(D) A gift of all or part of a body authorizes any examination necessary to ensure medical acceptability of the gift for the purpose intended.

(E) The rights of the donee created by the gift are paramount to the rights of others except that a coroner or, in his absence, a deputy coroner, who has, under section 313.13 of the Revised Code, taken charge of the decedent's dead body and decided that an autopsy is necessary, has a right to the dead body and any part that is paramount to the rights of the donee. The coroner, or in his absence, the deputy coroner, may waive this paramount right and permit the donee to take a donated part if the donated part is or will be unnecessary for successful completion of the autopsy or for evidence. If the coroner or deputy coroner does not waive his paramount right and later determines, while performing the autopsy, that the donated part is or will be unnecessary for successful completion of the autopsy or for evidence, he may thereupon waive his paramount right and permit the donee to take the donated part, either during the autopsy or after it is completed.

§ 2108.021. Protocol for requests by hospital for certificate of request.

(A) As used in this section, "certified organ and tissue procurement organization" means a nonprofit organ or tissue procurement organization that has its principal place of business in this state and is certified under Title XVIII of the "Social Security Act," 49 Stat. 620 (1935), 42 U.S.C. 301, as amended, or by the eye bank association of America.

(B) Every hospital shall develop an organ and tissue procurement protocol in consultation with a certified organ and tissue procurement organization. The protocol shall encourage reasonable discretion and sensitivity to the family circumstances in all discussions regarding donations of tissue or organs. The protocol shall identify the appropriate circumstances under which a request for organ or tissue donation is made or not made and shall require that families of potential organ donors be informed of the option to donate tissue or organs. Such notification shall be the responsibility of the certified organ and tissue procurement organization unless otherwise designated. In any case in which a hospital patient is suitable as an organ or tissue donor based on the hospital's protocol, the certified organ and tissue procurement organization, the hospital administrator, or his designated representative shall request one or more of the persons described in division (B) of section 2108.02 of the Revised Code to make a gift of appropriate parts of the patient's body, except that the certified organ and tissue procurement organization, the hospital administrator, or his designated representative shall not make such a request if he has actual notice of contrary intentions by the patient, actual notice of opposition by any of the persons described in division (B) of section 2108.02 of the Revised Code, or reason to believe that a gift for purposes described in section 2108.03 of the Revised Code is contrary to the patient's religious beliefs.

When a gift is requested under this section, the certified procurement organization, the hospital administrator, or his designated representative shall complete a certificate of request for an anatomical gift, on a form prescribed by the director of health. The certificate shall state whether or not a request for an anatomical gift was made, shall state the name of the person or persons to whom the request was made and his or their relationship to the patient, and shall state whether or not the gift was granted. Upon completion of the certificate, the certified organ and tissue procurement organization, the hospital administrator, or his designated representative shall retain the certificate in a central location for no less than three years after the date of the patient's death. Upon the request of the director of health, the certified organ and tissue organization, hospital administrator, or his designated representative shall permit the director or his authorized representative to inspect or copy the certificates or shall provide a summary of the information contained in the certificates to the director on a form prescribed by the director. All copies of such certificates or summaries in the possession of the director, except for any patient-identifying information contained in them, are public records as defined in section 149.43 of the Revised Code.

(C) The director of health shall issue guidelines establishing:

(1) Recommendations for the training of persons representing certified organ and tissue procurement organizations, hospital administrators, and representatives designated to make requests for anatomical gifts under this section;

(2) Communication and coordination procedures to improve the efficiency of making donated organs available. The guidelines shall include procedures for communicating with the appropriate certified organ and tissue procurement organization.

§ 2108.03. Permissible donees.

Any of the following persons may become donees of gifts of bodies or parts thereof for the purposes stated:

(A) A hospital, surgeon, or physician, for medical or dental education, research, advancement of medical or dental science, therapy, or transplantation;

(B) An accredited medical or dental school, college, or university, for education, research, advancement of medical or dental science, or therapy;

(C) A bank or storage facility, for medical or dental education, research advancement of medical or dental science, therapy, or transplantation;

(D) A specified individual for therapy or transplantation, needed by him.

§ 2108.04. Instrument of gift; acceptance by physician.

(A) A gift of all or part of the body under division (A) of section 2108.02 of the Revised Code may be made by will when the individual is eighteen years of age or more. The gift becomes effective upon the death of the testator without waiting for probate. If the will is not probated or if it is declared invalid for testamentary purposes, the gift, to the extent that it has been acted upon in good faith, is nevertheless valid and effective.

(B)(1) A gift of all or part of the body under division (A) of section 2108.02 of the Revised Code may also be made by any document other than a will. The gift becomes effective upon the death of the donor. The document, which may be a card designed to be carried on the person, shall be signed by the donor in the presence of two witnesses who shall sign the document in his presence. If the donor cannot sign, the document may be signed for him at his direction and in the presence of two witnesses, having no affiliation with the donee, who shall sign the document in his presence. Delivery of the document of gift during the donor's lifetime is not necessary to make the gift valid.

(2) If a person less than eighteen years of age wishes to make a gift under division (B)(1) of this section, one of the witnesses who signs the document shall be a parent or guardian of that person.

(C) A gift of parts of the body under division (A) of section 2108.02 of the Revised Code may also be made by a designation, to be provided for on all Ohio driver's or commercial driver's licenses and motorcycle operator's licenses or endorsements, and on all identification cards. The gift becomes effective upon the death of the donor. The holder of the driver's or commercial driver's license or endorsement, or the holder of the identification card must sign a statement at the time of application or renewal of the license, endorsement, or identification card in the presence of two witnesses, who must sign the statement in the presence of the donor; except that when the holder of the license or card is less than eighteen years of age, one of the witnesses who signs shall be a parent or guardian of the holder. Delivery of the license or identification card during the donor's lifetime is not necessary to make the gift valid. The gift shall become invalidated upon expiration or cancellation of the license, endorsement, or identification card. Revocation or suspension of the license or endorsement will not invalidate the gift. The gift must be renewed upon renewal of each license, endorsement, or identification card. If the statement is ambiguous as to whether a general or specific gift is intended by the donor, the statement shall be construed as evidencing the specific gift only. As used in this division, "identification card" means an identification card issued under section 4507.50 of the Revised Code.

(D) The gift may be made to a specified donee or without specifying a donee. If the latter, the gift may be accepted by the attending physician as donee upon or following death. If the gift is made to a specified donee who is not available at the time and place of death, the attending physician may accept the gift as donee upon or following death, in the absence of any expressed indication that the donor desired otherwise. The physician who accepts the gift as donee under this division shall not participate in the procedures for removing or transplanting a part.

(E) Notwithstanding division (B) of section 2108.07 of the Revised Code, the donor may designate in his will, card, or other document of gift the surgeon or physician to carry out the appropriate procedures. In the absence of a designation or if the designee is not available, the donee or other person authorized to accept the gift may employ or authorize any surgeon or physician to carry out the appropriate procedures.

(F) Any gift by a person specified in division (B) of section 2108.02 of the Revised Code shall be made by a document signed by him or made by his telegraphic, recorded telephonic, or other recorded message.

§ 2108.05. Delivery or deposit of instrument.

If the gift is made by the donor to a specified donee, the will, card, or other document, or an executed copy thereof, may be delivered to the donee to expedite the appropriate procedures immediately after death. Delivery is not necessary to the validity of the gift. The will, card, or other document, or an executed copy thereof, may be deposited in any hospital, bank or storage facility, or registry office that accepts it for safekeeping or for facilitation of procedures after death. On request of any interested party upon or after the donor's death, the person in possession shall produce the document for examination.

§ 2108.06. Manner of amendment or revocation.

(A) If the will, card, or other document, or an executed copy thereof, has been delivered to a specified donee, the donor may amend or revoke the gift by any of the following means:

(1) The execution and delivery to the donee of a signed statement;

(2) An oral statement made in the presence of two persons and communicated to the donee;

(3) A statement during a terminal illness or injury addressed to an attending physician and communicated to the donee;

(4) A signed card or document found on his person or in his effects.

(B) The donor may revoke any document of gift which has not been delivered to the donee, in any manner specified in division (A) of this section or by destruction, cancellation, or mutilation of the document and all executed copies thereof.

(C) Any gift made by a will may also be amended or revoked in the manner provided for amendment or revocation of wills or as provided in division (A) of this section.

§ 2108.07. Acceptance and use of body; time of death.

(A) The donee may accept or reject the gift. If the donee accepts a gift of the entire body, the surviving spouse or next of kin may, subject to the terms of the gift, authorize embalming and the use of the body in funeral services. If the gift is of a part of the body, the donee, upon the death of the donor and prior to embalming, shall cause the part to be removed without unnecessary mutilation. After removal of the part, custody of the remainder of the body vests in the surviving spouse, next of kin, or other persons under obligation to dispose of the body.

(B) The attending physician or a physician selected by the donor shall determine the time of death. If it is not possible for such physician to attend the donor at his death or to certify the death within a period of time which would make it possible to carry out the terms of the gift, the time of death shall be determined by two physicians having no affiliation with the donee. The physician or physicians determining the time of death or certifying the death shall not participate in the procedure for removing or transplanting a part.

§ 2108.071. Enucleation of eyes; definition.

(A) With respect to the gift of an eye, an embalmer licensed pursuant to Chapter 4717, of the Revised Code who has completed a course in eye enucleation and has received a certificate of competency to that effect from a school of medicine recognized by the state medical board may enucleate eyes for the gift after proper certification of death by a physician and compliance with the intent of the gift as defined by sections 2108.01 to 2108.10 of the Revised Code.

(B) As used in this section, "eye enucleation" means the removal of the eyeball in such a way that it comes out clean and whole.

§ 2108.08. Person who acts in good faith not liable.

A person who acts in good faith in accordance with sections 2108.01 to 2108.10, inclusive, of the Revised Code, or the anatomical gift laws of another state, is not liable for damages in any civil action or subject to prosecution in any criminal proceeding for his act.

§ 2108.09. Adoption of Uniform Anatomical Gift Act; uniform construction.

Sections 2108.01 to 2108.09, inclusive, of the Revised Code, are enacted to adopt the Uniform Anatomical Gift Act (1968), national conference of commissioners on uniform state laws, and shall be construed so as to effectuate its general purpose to make uniform the law of those states which enact it.

§ 2108.10. Forms of document of gift.

(A) The document of gift provided for in division (B) of section 2108.04 of the Revised Code shall conform substantially to the following forms:

UNIFORM DONOR CARD

OF

_____

Print or type name of donor

In the hope that I may help others, I hereby make this anatomical gift, if medically acceptable, to take effect upon my death. The words and marks below indicate my desire.

I give: (A) ___ any needed organs or parts
      (B) ___ only the following organs or parts
_____
                         Specify the organ(s) or part(s)

for the purpose of transplantation, therapy, or medical research or education.
      (C) ___ my body for anatomical study, if needed. Limitations or special wishes, if any:
_____

Signed by the donor and the following two witnesses in the presence of each other:

_____
                    Signature of Donor

_____
                  Date of Birth of Donor

_____
                      Date Signed

_____
                        Witness

_____
                        Witness

This is a legal document under the Uniform Anatomical Gift Act or similar laws.

ANATOMICAL GIFT BY NEXT OF KIN
OR OTHER AUTHORIZED PERSON

I hereby make this anatomical gift from the body of (name) who died on (date) in (city and state).

The marks in the appropriate squares and the words filled into the blanks below indicate my relationship to the deceased according to the following order of priority as presented by Ohio law, and indicate my desires respecting the gift.

    1. I am the surviving:
        1. ___ spouse;
        2. ___ adult son or daughter;
        3. ___ parent;
        4. ___ adult brother or sister;
        5. ___ guardian;
        6. ___ authorized to dispose of the body;
    2. I give:
        ___ any needed organs or parts;
        ___ the following organs or parts _____
_____;
    3. To the following person (or institution): _____
_____
                (insert the name of a physician, hospital, research or
                educational institution, storage banks, or individual);
    4. For the following purposes:
        ___ any purpose authorized by section 2108.03 of the Revised Code;
        ___ transplantation;
        ___ therapy;
        ___ medical research and education;
    5. After the donated organs or parts are removed, the remains of the body shall be disposed of in the following manner:
_____; at the expense of the following person: _____
Dated _____City and State _____

_____
                    Signature of Survivor

_____
                    Address of Survivor

    (B) The statement of gift provided for in division (C) of section 2108.04 of the Revised Code shall conform substantially to the following form:

I hereby make an anatomical gift, to be effective upon my death, of:

  (A) ___ Any needed organs or parts (if you mark this box, go to section (C) or

  (B) ___ Only the following organs or body part(s): (list)

_____

  (C) Donee _____

Date _____

Signature of donor _____

Witness _____

Witness _____

§ 2108.11. Transaction involving human tissue not a sale.

The procuring, furnishing, donating, processing, distributing, or using human whole blood, plasma, blood products, blood derivatives, and products, corneas, bones, organs, or other human tissue except hair, for the purpose of injecting, transfusing, or transplanting any of them in the human body, is declared for all purposes to be the rendition of a service by every person, firm, or corporation participating therein, whether or not any remuneration is paid therefor, is declared not to be a sale of any such items, and no warranties of any kind or description are applicable thereto.

§ 2108.21. Seventeen-year-olds may donate blood; publicity.

Any person seventeen years of age or older may donate blood in a voluntary blood program, which is not operated for profit, without consent of his parent or guardian. Before obtaining blood donations from students at high schools, joint vocational schools, or technical schools, a blood program shall arrange for the dissemination of written donation information to students to be shared with their parents or guardians. This information shall include a statement that the students will be requested to donate blood.

§ 2108.30. Determination that death has occurred; immunity of physician.

An individual is dead if he has sustained either irreversible cessation of circulatory and respiratory functions or irreversible cessation of all functions of the brain, including the brain stem, as determined in accordance with accepted medical standards. If the respiratory and circulatory functions of a person are being artificially sustained, under accepted medical standards a determination that death has occurred is made by a physician by observing and conducting a test to determine that the irreversible cessation of all functions of the brain has occurred.

A physician who makes a determination of death in accordance with this section and accepted medical standards is not liable for damages in any civil action or subject to prosecution in any criminal proceeding for his acts or the acts of others based on that determination.

Any person who acts in good faith in reliance on a determination of death made by a physician in accordance with this section and accepted medical standards is not liable for damages in any civil action or subject to prosecution in any criminal proceeding for his actions.

OKLAHOMA

ANATOMICAL GIFT ACT

§ 2201. Citation

This act shall be known and may be cited as the Uniform Anatomical Gift Act.

§ 2202. Definitions

(a) "Bank or storage facility" means a facility licensed, accredited, or approved under the laws of any state for storage of human bodies or parts thereof.

(b) "Decedent" means a deceased individual and includes a stillborn infant or fetus.

(c) "Donor" means an individual who makes a gift of all or part of his body.

(d) "Hospital" means a hospital licensed, accredited, or approved under the laws of any state; including a hospital operated by the United States government, a state, or a subdivision thereof, although not required to be licensed under state laws.

(e) "Part" means organs, tissues, eyes, bones, arteries, blood, other fluids and any other portions of a human body.

(f) "Person" means an individual, corporation, government or governmental subdivision or agency, business trust, estate, trust, partnership or association, or any other legal entity.

(g) "Physician" or "surgeon" means a physician or surgeon licensed or authorized to practice under the laws of any state.

(h) "State" includes any state, district, commonwealth, territory, insular possession, and any other area subject to the legislative authority of the United States of America.

§ 2203. Persons who may execute an anatomical gift

1. Any adult of sound mind may give all or any part of his body for any purpose specified in Section 2204 of this title, the gift to take effect upon death.

2. Any of the following persons, in order of priority stated, when persons in prior classes are not available at the time of death, and in the absence of actual notice of contrary indications by the decedent or actual notice of opposition by a member of the same or a prior class, may give all or any part of the decedent's body for any purpose specified in Section 2204 of this title:

     a. the spouse,

     b. an adult son or daughter,

     c. either parent,

     d. an adult brother or sister,

     e. a guardian of the person of the decedent at the time of his death, or

     f. any other person authorized or under obligation to dispose of the body.

3. If the donee has actual notice of contrary indications by the decedent or that a gift by a member of a class is opposed by a member of the same or a prior class, the donee shall not accept the gift. The persons authorized by subsection 2 may make the gift after or immediately before the decedent's death.

4. A gift of all or part of a body authorizes any examination necessary to assure medical acceptability of the gift for the purposes intended.

5. The rights of the donee created by the gift are paramount to the rights of others except as provided by Section 2208(d) of this title.

§ 2204. Persons who may become donees—Purposes for which anatomical gifts may be made—Anatomical Board approval to donees

A. The following persons may become donees of gifts of bodies or parts thereof for the purposes stated:

1. Any hospital, surgeon, or physician, for medical or dental education, research, advancement of medical or dental science, therapy or transplantation;

2. Any accredited medical or dental school, college or university for education, research, advancement of medical or dental science or therapy;

3. Any bank or storage facility, for medical or dental education, research, advancement of medical or dental science, therapy or transplantation;

4. Any specified individual for therapy or transplantation needed by him; or

5. The Anatomical Board of the State of Oklahoma.

B. Any donee receiving a whole body donation from any source shall have approval from the Anatomical Board of the State of Oklahoma prior to receiving such donation.

§ 2205. Manner of executing anatomical gifts

(a) A gift of all or part of the body under Section 3(a) may be made by will. The gift becomes effective upon the death of the testator without waiting for probate. If the will is not probated, or if it is declared invalid for testamentary purposes, the gift to the extent that it has been acted upon in good faith, is nevertheless valid and effective.

(b) A gift of all or part of the body under Section 3(a) may also be made by document other than a will. The gift becomes effective upon the death of the donor. The document, which may be a card designed to be carried on the person, must be signed by the donor in the presence of two witnesses who must sign the document in his presence. If the donor cannot sign, the document may be signed for him at his direction and in his presence in the presence of two witnesses who must sign the document in his presence. Delivery of the document of gift during the donor's lifetime is not necessary to make the gift valid.

(c) The gift may be made to a specified donee or without specifying a donee. If the latter, the gift may be accepted by the attending physician as donee upon or following death. If the gift is made to a specified donee who is not available at the time and place of death, the attending physician upon or following death, in the absence of any expressed indication that the donor desired otherwise, may accept the gift as donee. The physician who becomes a donee under this subsection shall not participate in the procedures for removing or transplanting a part.

(d) Notwithstanding Section 8(b), the donor may designate in his will, card, or other document of gift the surgeon or physician to carry out the appropriate procedures. In the absence of a designation or if the designee is not available, the donee or other person authorized to accept the gift may employ or authorize any surgeon or physician for the purpose.

(e) Any gift by a person designated in Section 3(b) shall be made by a document signed by him or made by his telegraphic, recorded telephonic, or other recorded message.

§ 2206. Delivery of document of gift

If the gift is made by the donor to a specified donee, the will, card, or other document, or an executed copy thereof, may be delivered to the donee to expedite the appropriate procedures immediately after death. Delivery is not necessary to the validity of the gift. The will, card, or other document, or an executed copy thereof, may be deposited in any hospital, bank or storage facility, or registry office that accepts it for safekeeping or for facilitation of procedures after death. On request of any interested party upon or after the donor's death, the person in possession shall produce the document for examination.

§ 2207. Revocation or amendment of gift

(a) If the will, card, or other document, or executed copy thereof, has been delivered to a specified donee, the donor may amend or revoke the gift by:

(1) the execution and delivery to the donee of a signed statement,

(2) an oral statement made in the presence of two persons and communicated to the donee,

(3) a statement during a terminal illness or injury addressed to an attending physician and communicated to the donee, or

(4) a signed card or document found on his person or in his effects.

(b) Any document of gift which has not been delivered to the donee may be revoked by the donor in the manner set out in subsection (a) or by destruction, cancellation, or mutilation of the original document.

(c) Any gift made by a will may also be amended or revoked in the manner provided for amendment or revocation of wills, or as provided in subsection (a).

§ 2208. Rights and duties at death

(a) The donee may accept or reject the gift. If the donee accepts a gift of the entire body, he may, subject to the terms of the gift, authorize embalming and the use of the body in funeral services. If the gift is of a part of the body, the donee, upon the death of the decedent and prior to embalming, shall cause the part to be removed without unnecessary mutilation. After removal of the part, custody of the remainder of the body vests in the surviving spouse, next of kin, or other persons under obligation to dispose of the body.

(b) The time of death shall be determined by a physician who attends the donor at his death, or, if none, the physician who certifies the death. The physician shall not participate in the procedures for removing or transplanting a part.

(c) A person who acts in good faith in accord with the terms of this act or the anatomical gift laws of another state or of a foreign country is not liable for damages in any civil action or subject to prosecution in any criminal proceeding for his act.

(d) The provisions of this act are subject to the laws of this state prescribing powers and duties with respect to autopsies.

§ 2209. Uniformity of interpretation

This act shall be so construed as to effectuate its general purpose to make uniform the law of those states which enact it.

§ 2210. Eye enucleation

In respect to a gift of an eye as provided for in this chapter, a licensed embalmer, as defined by Sections 396 et seq. of Title 59 of the Oklahoma Statutes, or other persons who have successfully completed a course in eye enucleation in the State of Oklahoma or elsewhere and have received a certificate of competence from the Department of Ophthalmology of the University of Oklahoma School of Medicine, may enucleate eyes for such gift after proper certification of death by a physician and compliance with the extent of such gift as defined by Sections 2201 et seq. of this title. No such properly-certified embalmer or other person acting in accordance with the terms of this chapter shall have any liability, civil or criminal, for such eye enucleation.

§ 2211. Donor cards

A. In order to provide an expeditious procedure for a person to make a gift of all or part of his body pursuant to the provisions of the Uniform Anatomical Gift Act, the Department of Public Safety and all motor license agents shall make space available on the reverse side of the driver's license and the identification license for an organ donor card to be signed by the donor and two witnesses. The donor card shall state that the person, upon death, is a donor of specified body organs or of his entire body or parts of said body for the purposes of transplantation, therapy, medical research, or education pursuant to the provisions of the Uniform Anatomical Gift Act.

B. Said signed donor card shall constitute sufficient legal authority for the removal of the designated organs or parts of the body upon the death of said person in accordance with the provisions of the Uniform Anatomical Gift Act. Except as provided by law, every surgeon, physician, hospital, or person or entity acting pursuant to the provisions of the Uniform Anatomical Gift Act may rely upon said donor card as sufficient legal authority to remove, process, store, and use the organs or parts of the body as designated on said card in accordance with accepted medical practice.

C. The carrying of said card on the person shall be prima facie evidence that the person carrying the card is the donor named on said card. No surgeon, physician, hospital, or person or entity acting pursuant to the provisions of this section or the Uniform Anatomical Gift Act shall be held civilly or criminally liable for relying in good faith upon said donor card or its contents, or for presuming that the person carrying the card is the donor named on said card.

D. The donor card authorized and issued pursuant to the provisions of this section shall be personal to the donor, who shall be solely responsible for the accuracy of its contents. It shall be unlawful and a misdemeanor for any person to carry said signed donor card except the donor named on said card. Upon the death of the donor, the donor card may be removed and retained in the files of any surgeon, physician, hospital, or person or entity participating pursuant to the provisions of the Uniform Anatomical Gift Act and copies of said card may be made for the record or file of any other participant.

E. The gift designated may be revoked by the donor at any time by destroying the donor card, and the following shall be printed above the donor's signature line on the donor card form:

"I declare that I am at least eighteen (18) years of age and hereby make a gift of my body, organs, or body parts as designated on this card. I understand that this donor card shall constitute sufficient legal authority for donation and acceptance of such designated gift pursuant to the provisions of the Uniform Anatomical Gift Act and that I may revoke such gift at any time only by destroying this donor card."

F. The donor card shall contain other information in a format to be prescribed by the Commissioner of Public Safety, which shall be approved by the Attorney General prior to issuance to the public.

G. Upon revocation of the gift and destruction of the organ donor card, the person shall be required to make application for a renewal or duplicate of the driver's license or identification license of said person.

H. Nothing in this section shall be construed to prevent persons under eighteen (18) years of age from being organ donors.

§ 2212. Removal or organs—Consent

In any death that the Office of the Chief Medical Examiner of the State of Oklahoma is required by law to investigate, a medical examiner may remove organs from the deceased for donation to a suitable donee pursuant to the provisions of the Uniform Anatomical Gift Act if the next of kin of the deceased has been consulted and consents to said removal. In such cases where the deceased has an organ donor card the consent from next of kin shall not be required.

§ 2213. Accidental deaths, homicides and suicides—Organ donors

Law enforcement and medical personnel involved with the investigation of accidental deaths, homicides, and suicides shall make reasonable efforts to ascertain if the victims are organ donors and, if so, to pass that information on to the proper officials. Said law enforcement and medical personnel shall not be subject to criminal or civil liability for complying with the provisions of this section.

§ 2214. Requests for consent to anatomical gift

A. When death occurs in a general hospital as defined by Section 1-701 of Title 63 of the Oklahoma Statutes, to a person determined to be a suitable candidate for organ or tissue donation based on accepted medical standards, the hospital administrator or designated representative shall request the appropriate person described in paragraph 2 of Section 2203 of Title 63 of the Oklahoma Statutes to consent to the gift of any part of the body of the decedent as an anatomical gift.

B. No request shall be required, pursuant to this section, when the hospital administrator or designated representative has actual notice of contrary intention by the decedent or those persons described in paragraph 2 of Section 220 of Title 63 of the Oklahoma Statutes according to the order of priority stated therein, or reason to believe that an anatomical gift is contrary to the religious beliefs of the decedent.

C. Upon consent of the appropriate person specified in paragraph 2 of Section 2203 of Title 63 of the Oklahoma Statutes, the hospital administrator or designated representative shall notify an appropriate organ or tissue bank, or retrieval organization and cooperate in the procurement of the anatomical gift pursuant to the Uniform Anatomical Gift Act.

D. The person consenting to the request for the anatomical gift may give such consent in person or by telephone, telegraph or other appropriate means pursuant to procedures established by rules and regulations of the State Board of Health.

§ 2215. Certificate of request for anatomical gift

A. When a request is made, pursuant to Section 1 of this act, the person making the request shall complete a certificate of request for an anatomical gift, on a form to be supplied by the State Board of Health. The certificate shall include the following:

1. A statement indicating that a request for an anatomical gift was made;
2. The name and affiliation of the person making the request;
3. An indication of whether consent was granted and, if so, what organs and tissues were donated;
4. The name of the person granting or refusing the request, and his relationship to the decedent; and
5. Whether the consent was given in person, by telephone, telegraph or other appropriate means.

B. A copy of the certificate required by subsection A of this section shall be included in the medical records of the decedent.

§ 2216. Rules and regulations

A. The State Board of Health shall promulgate rules and regulations, concerning but not limited to:

1. The training and qualification of hospital personnel or designated representatives who perform the request; and
2. The procedures to be employed in making the request.

B. The State Board of Health shall promulgate such rules and regulations as are necessary to implement appropriate procedures to facilitate proper coordination among hospitals, organ and tissue banks and retrieval organizations.

§ 2217. Civil liability—Limitations

No additional civil liability shall be created as a result of the duties imposed by this act.

§ 2218. Exemptions

All hospitals with a capacity of fewer than fifty (50) beds shall be exempt from the mandatory provisions of this act, but may elect to voluntary comply with the provisions of this act and the rules and regulations promulgated by the State Board of Health, and to participate in any training program established or required by the State Board of Health.

OREGON

ANATOMICAL GIFTS

§ 97.250. Short title for ORS 97.250 to 97.290.

ORS 97.250 to 97.290 may be cited as the Uniform Anatomical Gift Act.

§ 97.255. Definitions for ORS 97.250 to 97.290.

As used in ORS 97.250 to 97.290, unless the context requires otherwise:

(1) "Bank or storage facility" means a facility licensed, accredited or approved under the laws of any state for storage of human bodies or parts thereof.

(2) "Decedent" includes a deceased individual, stillborn infant or fetus.

(3) "Donor" means an individual who makes a gift of all or part of the body of the donor.

(4) "Hospital" includes a hospital licensed, accredited or approved under the laws of any state or a hospital operated by the United States Government, a state or a subdivision thereof, although not required to be licensed under state laws.

(5) "Part" means organs, tissues, eyes, bones, arteries, blood, other fluids and any other portions of a human body.

(6) "Person" includes an individual, corporation, government or governmental subdivision or agency, business trust, estate, trust, partnership or association or any other legal entity.

(7) "Physician" or "surgeon" includes a physician or surgeon licensed or authorized to practice under the laws of any state.

(8) "State" includes any state, district, commonwealth, territory, insular possession and any other area subject to the legislative authority of the United States of America.

§ 97.260. Construction of ORS 97.250 to 97.290.

ORS 97.250 to 97.290 shall be so construed as to effectuate their general purpose to make uniform the law of those states which enact the Uniform Anatomical Gift Act.

§ 97.265. Authority to make anatomical gift; rights of donee.

(1) Any individual of sound mind and 18 years of age or older may give all or any part of the body of the individual for any purpose specified in ORS 97.270, the gift to take effect upon death.

(2) Any of the following persons, in order of priority stated, when persons in prior classes are not available at the time of death, and in the absence of actual notice of contrary indications by the decedent or actual notice of opposition by a member of the same or a prior class, may give all or any part of a decedent's body for any purpose specified in ORS 97.270:

(a) The spouse.

(b) A son or daughter 18 years of age or older.

(c) Either parent.

(d) A brother or sister 18 years of age or older.

(e) A guardian of the decedent at the time of the death of the decedent.

(f) Any other person authorized or under obligation to dispose of the body.

(3) If the donee has actual notice of contrary indications by the decedent or that a gift by a member of a class is opposed by a member of the same or a prior class, the donee shall not accept the gift. The persons authorized by subsection (2) of this section may make the gift after or immediately before death.

(4) A gift of all or part of a body authorizes any examination necessary to assure medical acceptability of the gift for the purposes intended.

(5) The rights of the donee created by the gift are paramount to the rights of others except as provided by ORS 146.117.

§ 97.268. Death in hospital of person who has not made anatomical gift; request by hospital administrator; exceptions; rules.

(1) When death occurs in a hospital to a person who has not made an anatomical gift, the hospital administrator or designated representative shall request the person described in ORS 97.265(2), in order of priority stated when persons in prior classes are not available at the time of death, and in the absence of actual notice of contrary indication by the decedent or one in a prior class, to consent to the gift of all or any part of the decedent's body as an anatomical gift.

(2) Where such request is made, pursuant to this section, the request and its disposition shall be noted in the patient's medical record and on the death certificate and shall be documented as provided in ORS 97.275(5).

(3) Where, based on medical criteria, such request would not yield a donation which would be suitable for use, the Assistant Director for Health may, by rule, authorize an exception to the request required by this section.

(4) The Assistant Director for Health shall establish rules concerning the training of hospital employees who may be designated to perform the request, and the procedures to be employed in making it. In addition, the assistant director shall establish such rules as are necessary to implement appropriate procedures to facilitate the delivery of donations from receiving hospitals to potential recipients.

(5) The Assistant Director for Health shall establish such additional rules as are necessary for the implementation of this section.

§ 97.270. Who may be donee of anatomical gift.

The following persons may become donees of organs, tissues or parts of bodies for the purposes stated:

(1) Any hospital, surgeon or physician, for medical or dental education, research, advancement of medical or dental science, therapy or transplantation; or

(2) Any accredited medical or dental school, college or university for education, research, advancement of medical or dental science or therapy; or

(3) Any bank or storage facility, for medical or dental education, research, advancement of medical or dental science, therapy or transplantation; or

(4) Any specified individual for therapy or transplantation needed by the individual.

§ 97.275. Manner of executing anatomical gifts.

(1) A gift of all or part of the body under ORS 97.265 (1) may be made by will. The gift becomes effective upon the death of the testator without waiting for probate. If the will is not probated, or if it is declared invalid for testamentary purposes, the gift, to the extent that it has been acted upon in good faith, is nevertheless valid and effective.

(2) A gift of all or part of the body under ORS 97.265 (1) may also be made by document other than a will. The gift becomes effective upon the death of the donor. The document, which may be a card designed to be carried on the person, must be signed by the donor in the presence of two witnesses who must sign the document in the presence of the donor. If the donor cannot sign, the document may be signed for the donor at the direction of the donor and in the presence of the donor in the presence of two witnesses who must sign the document in the presence of the donor. Delivery of the document of gift during the donor's lifetime is not necessary to make the gift valid.

(3) The gift may be made to a specified donee or without specifying a donee. If the latter, the gift may be accepted by the attending physician as donee upon or following death. If the gift is made to a specified donee who is not available at the time and place of death, the attending physician upon or following death, in the absence of any expressed indication that the donor desired otherwise, may accept the gift as donee. The physician who becomes a donee under this subsection shall not participate in the procedures for removing or transplanting a part.

(4) Notwithstanding ORS 97.290 (2), the donor may designate in the will, card, or other document of gift of the donor the surgeon or physician to carry out the appropriate procedures. In the absence of a designation or if the designee is not available, the donee or other person authorized to accept the gift may employ or authorize any surgeon or physician for the purpose. If the part of the body that is the gift is an eye, the donee may authorize or the person authorized to accept the gift may employ or authorize a qualified embalmer licensed under ORS chapter 692 or a qualified eye bank technician to perform the appropriate procedures. The embalmer or technician must have completed a course in eye enucleation and have a certificate of competence from an agency or organization designated by the Board of Medical Examiners for the State of Oregon for the purpose of providing such training.

(5) Any gift by a person designated in ORS 97.265 (2) shall be made by a document signed by the person or made by the telegraphic, recorded telephonic, or other recorded message of the person.

§ 97.280. Delivery, deposit and examination of document of anatomical gift.

If the gift is made by the donor to a specified donee, the will, card, or other document, or an executed copy thereof, may be delivered to the donee to expedite the appropriate procedures immediately after death. Delivery is not necessary to the validity of the gift. The will, card, or other document, or an executed copy thereof, may be deposited in any hospital, bank or storage facility, or county clerk's office that accepts it for safekeeping or for facilitation of procedures after death. On request of any interested party upon or after the donor's death, the person in possession shall produce the document for examination.

§ 97.285. Amendment or revocation of anatomical gift.

(1) If the will, card, or other document or executed copy thereof, has been delivered to a specified donee, the donor may amend or revoke the gift by:

(a) The execution and delivery to the donee of a signed statement; or

(b) An oral statement made in the presence of two persons and communicated to the donee; or

(c) A statement during a terminal illness or injury addressed to an attending physician and communicated to the donee; or

(d) A signed card or document found on the person or in the effects of the person.

(2) Any document of gift which has not been delivered to the donee may be revoked by the donor in the manner set out in subsection (1) of this section or by destruction, cancellation, or mutilation of the document and all executed copies thereof.

(3) Any gift made by a will may also be amended or revoked in the manner provided for amendment or revocation of wills or as provided in subsection (1) of this section.

§ 97.290. Authority of donee who accepts gift; time of death; liability of one acting with probable cause; autopsies.

(1) The donee may accept or reject the gift. If the donee accepts a gift of the entire body, the donee may, subject to the terms of the gift, authorize embalming and the use of the body in funeral services. If the gift is of a part of the body, the donee, upon

the death of the donor and prior to embalming, shall cause the part to be removed without unnecessary mutilation. After removal of the part, custody of the remainder of the body vests in the surviving spouse, next of kin, or other persons under obligation to dispose of the body.

(2) The time of death shall be determined by a physician who attends the donor at the death of the donor, or, if none, the physician who certifies the death. The physician shall not participate in the procedures for removing or transplanting a part.

(3) A person who acts with probable cause in accord with the terms of ORS 97.250 to 97.290 or the anatomical gift laws of another state or a foreign country is not liable for damages in any civil action or subject to prosecution in any criminal proceeding for the act of the person.

(4) The provisions of ORS 97.250 to 97.290 are subject to the laws of this state prescribing powers and duties with respect to autopsies.

§ 97.295. Liability of executor who carries out anatomical gift.

A person named executor who carries out the gift of the testator made under the provisions of ORS 97.250 to 97.290 before issuance of letters testamentary or under a will which is not admitted to probate shall not be liable to the surviving spouse or next of kin for performing acts necessary to carry out the gift of the testator.

§ 97.300. Transplants not covered by implied warranty.

(1) The procuring, processing, furnishing, distributing, administering or using of any part of a human body for the purpose of injecting, transfusing or transplanting that part into a human body is not a sales transaction covered by an implied warranty under the Uniform Commercial Code or otherwise.

(2) As used in this section, "part" means organs, tissues, eyes, bones, arteries, blood, other fluids and any other portions of a human body.

PENNSYLVANIA

UNIFORM ANATOMICAL GIFT ACT

§ 8601. Definitions.

As used in this chapter:

"Bank or storage facility." Means a facility licensed, accredited, or approved under the laws of any state for storage of human bodies or parts thereof.

"Decedent." Means a deceased individual and includes a stillborn infant or fetus.

"Donor." Means an individual who makes a gift of all or part of his body.

"Hospital." Means a hospital licensed, accredited, or approved under the laws of any state; includes a hospital operated by the United States Government, a state, or a subdivision thereof, although not required to be licensed under state laws.

"Part." Means organs, tissues, eyes, bones, arteries, blood, other fluids and any other portions of a human body.

"Person." Means an individual, corporation, government or governmental subdivision or agency, business trust, estate, trust, partnership or association, or any other legal entity.

"Physician" or "surgeon." Means a physician or surgeon licensed or authorized to practice under the laws of any state.

"State." Includes any state, district, commonwealth, territory, insular possession, and any other area subject to the legislative authority of the United States of America.

"Board." Means the Humanity Gifts Registry.

§ 8602. Persons who may execute an anatomical gift.

(a) Any individual of sound mind and 18 years of age or more may give all or any part of his body for any purpose specified in section 8603 of this code (relating to persons who may become donees; purposes for which anatomical gifts may be made), the gift to take effect upon death. A gift of the whole body shall be invalid unless made in writing at least 15 days prior to the date of death.

(b) Any of the following persons, in order of priority stated, when persons in prior classes are not available at the time of death, and in the absence of actual notice of contrary indications by the decedent or actual notice of opposition by a member of the same or a prior class, may give all or any part of the decedent's body for any purpose specified in section 8603 of this code:

(1) the spouse;

(2) an adult son or daughter;

(3) either parent;

(4) an adult brother or sister;

(5) a guardian of the person of the decedent at the time of his death; and

(6) any other person authorized or under obligation to dispose of the body.

(c) If the donee has actual notice of contrary indications by the decedent or that a gift by a member of a class is opposed by a member of the same or a prior class, the donee shall not accept the gift. The persons authorized by subsection (b) of this section may make the gift after or immediately before death.

(d) A gift of all or part of a body authorizes any examination necessary to assure medical acceptability of the gift for the purposes intended.

(e) The rights of the donee created by the gift are paramount to the rights of others except as provided by section 8607(d) of this code (relating to rights and duties at death).

§ 8603. Persons who may become donees; purposes for which anatomical gifts may be made.

The following persons may become donees of gifts of bodies or parts thereof for the purposes stated:

(1) any hospital, surgeon, or physician, for medical or dental education, research, advancement of medical or dental science, therapy, or transplantation; or

(2) any accredited medical or dental school, college or university for education, research, advancement of medical or dental science, or therapy; or

(3) any bank or storage facility, for medical or dental education, research, advancement of medical or dental science, therapy, or transplantation; or

(4) any specified individual for therapy or transplantation needed by him; or

(5) the board.

§ 8604. Manner of executing anatomical gifts.

(a) **Gifts by will.**—A gift of all or part of the body under section 8602(a) (relating to persons who may execute an anatomical gift) may be made by will. The gift becomes effective upon the death of the testator without waiting for probate. If the will is not probated, or if it is declared invalid for testamentary purposes, the gift, to the extent that it has been acted upon in good faith, is nevertheless valid and effective.

(b) **Gifts by other documents.**—A gift of all or part of the body under section 8602(a) may also be made by document other than a will. The gift becomes effective upon the death of the donor. The document, which may be a card designed to be carried on the person, must be signed by the donor in the presence of two witnesses who must sign the document in his presence. If the donor is mentally competent to signify his desire to sign the document but is physically unable to do so, the document may be signed for him by another at his direction and in his presence in the presence of two witnesses who must sign the document in his presence. Delivery of the document of gift during the donor's lifetime is not necessary to make the gift valid.

(c) **Specified and unspecified donees.**—The gift may be made to a specified donee or without specifying a donee. If the latter, the gift may be accepted by the attending physician as donee upon or following death. If the gift is made to a specified donee who is not available at the time and place of death, the attending physician upon or following death, in the absence of any expressed indication that the donor desired otherwise, may accept the gift as donee. The physician who becomes a donee under this subsection shall not participate in the procedures for removing or transplanting a part.

(d) **Designation of person to carry out procedures.**—Notwithstanding section 8607(b) (relating to rights and duties at death), the donor may designate in his will, card, or other document of gift the surgeon or physician to carry out the appropriate procedures. In the absence of a designation or if the designee is not available, the donee or other person authorized to accept the gift may employ or authorize any surgeon or physician for the purpose or, in the case of a gift of eyes, he may employ or authorize a person who is a funeral director licensed by the State Board of Funeral Directors, an eye bank technician or medical student, if said person has successfully completed a course in eye enucleation approved by the State Board of Medical Education and Licensure, or an eye bank technician or medical student trained under a program in the sterile technique for eye enucleation approved by the State Board of Medical Education and Licensure to enucleate eyes for an eye bank for the gift after certification of death by a physician. A qualified funeral director, eye bank technician or medical student acting in accordance with the terms of this subsection shall not have any liability, civil or criminal, for the eye enucleation.

(d.1) **Consent not necessary.**—Where a donor card evidencing a gift of the donor's eyes has been validly executed, consent of any person designated in section 8602(b) at the time of the donor's death or immediately thereafter is not necessary to render the gift valid and effective.

(e) **Documentation of gifts by others.**—Any gift by a person designated in section 8602(b) (relating to persons who may execute an anatomical gift), shall be made by a document signed by him or made by his telegraphic, recorded telephonic, or other recorded message.

§ 8605. Delivery of document of gift.

If the gift is made by the donor to a specified donee, the will, card, or other document, or an executed copy thereof, may be delivered to the donee to expedite the appropriate procedures immediately after death. Delivery is not necessary to the validity of the gift. The will, card, or other document, or an executed copy thereof, may be deposited in any hospital, bank or storage facility or registry office that accepts it for safekeeping or for facilitation of procedures after death. On request of any interested party upon or after the donor's death the person in possession shall produce the document for examination.

§ 8606. Amendment or revocation of the gift.

(a) If the will, card, or other document or executed copy thereof, has been delivered to a specified donee, the donor may amend or revoke the gift by:

 (1) the execution and delivery to the donee of a signed statement; or

 (2) an oral statement made in the presence of two persons and communicated to the donee; or

 (3) a statement during a terminal illness or injury addressed to an attending physician and communicated to the donee; or

 (4) a signed card or document found on his person or in his effects.

(b) Any document of gift which has not been delivered to the donee may be revoked by the donor in the manner set out in subsection (a) of this section, or by destruction, cancellation, or mutilation of the document and all executed copies thereof.

(c) Any gift made by a will may also be amended or revoked in the manner provided for amendment or revocation of wills, or as provided in subsection (a) of this section.

§ 8607. Rights and duties at death.

(a) The donee may accept or reject the gift. If the donee accepts a gift of the entire body, he shall subject to the terms of the gift, authorize embalming and the use of the body in funeral services if the surviving spouse or next of kin as determined in section 8602(b) of this code (relating to persons who may execute an anatomical gift) requests embalming and use of the body for funeral services. If the gift is of a part of the body, the donee, upon the death of the donor and prior to embalming, shall cause the part to be removed without unnecessary mutilation. After removal of the part, custody of the remainder of the body vests in the surviving spouse, next of kin, or other persons under obligation to dispose of the body.

(b) The time of death shall be determined by a physician who tends the donor at his death, or, if none, the physician who certifies the death. The physician who certifies death or any of his professional partners or associates shall not participate in the procedures for removing or transplanting a part.

(c) A person who acts in good faith in accord with the terms of this chapter or with the anatomical gift laws of another state or a foreign country is not liable for damages in any civil action or subject to prosecution in any criminal proceeding for his act.

(d) The provisions of this chapter are subject to the laws of this State prescribing powers and duties with respect to autopsies.

§ 8608. Requests for anatomical gifts.

(a) **Procedure.**—On or before the occurrence of death in an acute care general hospital, the hospital shall request consent to a gift of all or any part of the decedent's body for any purpose specified under this chapter. The request and its disposition shall be noted in the patient's medical record. Whenever medical criteria establishes that a body or body part donation would not be suitable for use, a request need not be made.

(b) **Limitation.**—Where the hospital administrator, or his designee, has received actual notice of opposition from any of the persons named in section 8602(b) (relating to persons who may execute an anatomical gift) and the decedent was not in possession of a validly executed donor card, the gift of all or any part of the decedent's body shall not be requested.

(c) **Donor card.**—Notwithstanding any provision of law to the contrary, the intent of a decedent to participate in an organ donor program as evidenced by the possession of a validly executed donor card shall not be revoked by any member of any of the classes specified in section 8602(b).

(d) **Identification of potential donors.**—Each acute care general hospital shall develop, with the concurrence of the hospital medical staff, a protocol for identifying potential organ and tissue donors. It shall require that, at or near the time of notification of death, persons designated under section 8602(a) and (b) be asked whether the deceased was an organ donor or if the family is a donor family. If not, such persons shall be informed of the option to donate organs and tissues. Pursuant to this chapter, the hospital shall then notify an organ and tissue procurement organization and cooperate in the procurement of the anatomical gift or gifts. The protocol shall encourage discretion and sensitivity to family circumstances in all discussions regarding donations of tissue or organs. The protocol shall take into account the deceased individual's religious beliefs or nonsuitability for organ and tissue donation. In the event an organ and tissue procurement organization does not exist in a region, the hospital shall contact an organ or a tissue procurement organization in an alternative region.

(e) **Exemption.**—The Department of Health is authorized to issue exemptions to any acute care general hospital it deems unable to comply with this section.

(f) **Guidelines.**—The Department of Health shall establish guidelines regarding efficient procedures facilitating the delivery of anatomical gift donations from receiving hospitals to potential recipients and appropriate training concerning the manner and conduct of employees making requests for anatomical gift donations.

RHODE ISLAND

UNIFORM ANATOMICAL GIFT ACT

§ 23-18.6-1. Definitions.

As used in this chapter:

(1) "Anatomical gift" means a donation of all or part of a human body to take effect upon or after death.

(2) "Decedent" means a deceased individual and includes a stillborn infant or fetus.

(3) "Document of gift" means a card, a statement attached to or imprinted on a motor vehicle operator's or chauffeur's license, a will, or other writing used to make an anatomical gift.

(4) "Donor" means an individual who makes an anatomical gift of all or part of the individual's body.

(5) "Enucleator" means an individual who is licensed or certified by the State Board of Medical Examiners and/or department of health and/or federally designated eye procurement organization; to remove or process eyes or parts of eyes.

(6) "Hospital" means a facility licensed, accredited, or approved as a hospital under the law of any state or a facility operated as a hospital by the United States government, a state, or a subdivision of a state.

(7) "Part" means an organ, tissue, eye, bone, artery, blood, fluid, or other portion of a human body.

(8) "Person" means an individual, corporation, business trust, estate, trust, partnership, joint venture, association, government, governmental subdivision or agency, or any other legal or commercial entity.

(9) "Physician" or "surgeon" means an individual licensed or otherwise authorized to practice medicine and surgery or osteopathy and surgery under the laws of any state.

(10) "Procurement organization" means federally designated eye procurement organization accredited, and/or approved under the laws of any state for procurement, distribution, or storage of human bodies or parts.

(11) "State" means a state, territory, or possession of the United States, the district of Columbia, or the commonwealth of Puerto Rico.

(12) "Technician" means an individual who is licensed or certified by the State Board of Medical Examiners and/or department of health and/or federally designated eye procurement organization to remove or process eyes or parts of eyes.

§ 23-18.6-2. Making, amending, revoking, and refusing to make anatomical gifts by individual.

(a) An individual who is at least (18) years of age may (i) make an anatomical gift for any of the purposes stated in § 23-18.6-6(a), (ii) limit an anatomical gift to one or more of those purposes, or (iii) refuse to make an anatomical gift.

(b) An anatomical gift may be made only by a document of gift signed by the donor. If the donor cannot sign, the document of gift must be signed by another individual, the next of kin, or designee and by two witnesses, all of whom have signed at the direction and in the presence of the donor and of each other, and state that it has been so signed.

(c) If a document of gift is attached to or imprinted on a donor's motor vehicle operator's or chauffeur's license, the document of gift must comply with subsection (b). Revocation, suspension, expiration, or cancellation of the license does not invalidate the anatomical gift.

(d) A document of gift may designate a particular physician or surgeon in cases of living relation donation and transplantation to carry out the appropriate procedures. In the absence of a designation or if the designee is not available, the donee or other person authorized to accept the anatomical gift may employ or authorize any physician, surgeon, technician, or enucleator to carry out the appropriate procedures.

(e) An anatomical gift by will takes effect upon death of the testator, whether or not the will is probated. If, after death, the will is declared invalid for testamentary purposes, the validity of the anatomical fight is unaffected.

(f) A donor may amend or revoke an anatomical gift, not made by will, only by:

(1) A signed statement;

(2) An oral statement made in the presence of two (2) individuals;

(3) Any form of communication during a terminal illness or injury addressed to a physician or surgeon; or

(4) The delivery of a signed statement to a specified donee to whom a document of gift had been delivered.

(g) The donor of an anatomical gift made by will may amend or revoke the gift in the manner provided for amendment or revocation of will, or as provided for amendment or revocation of will, or as provided in subsection (f).

(h) An anatomical gift that is not revoked by the donor before death is irrevocable and does not required the consent or concurrence of any person after the donor's death.

(i) An individual may refuse to make an anatomical gift of the individual's body or party by (i) a writing signed in the same manner as a document of gift, (ii) a statement attached to or imprinted on a donor's motor vehicle operator's or chauffeur's license, or (iii) any other writing used to identify the individual as refusing to make an anatomical gift. During a terminal illness or injury, the refusal may be an oral statement or other form of communication.

(j) In the absence of contrary indications by the donor, an anatomical gift of a part is neither a refusal to give other parts nor a limitation on an anatomical gift under § 23-18.6-3 or on a removal or release of other parts under § 23-18.6-4.

(k) In the absence of contrary indications by the donor, a revocation or amendment of an anatomical gift is not a refusal to make another anatomical gift. If the donor intends a revocation to be a refusal to make an anatomical gift, the donor shall make the refusal pursuant to subsection (i).

§ 23-18.6-3. Making, revoking, and objecting to anatomical gifts by others.

(a) Any member of the following classes of persons, in the order of priority listed, may make an anatomical gift of all or a part of the decedent's body for an authorized purpose, unless the decedent, at the time of death, has made an unrevoked refusal to make that anatomical gift:

(1) The spouse of the decedent;

(2) An adult son or daughter of the decedent;

(3) Either parent of the decedent;

(4) An adult brother or sister of the decedent;

(5) A grandparent of the decedent; and

(6) A guardian of the person of the decedent at the time of death.

(b) An anatomical gift may not be made by a person listed in subsection (a) if:

(1) A person in a prior class is available at the time of death to make an anatomical gift;

(2) The person proposing to make an anatomical gift knows of a refusal or contrary indications by the decedent; or

(3) The person proposing to make an anatomical gift knows of an objection to making an anatomical gift by a member of the person's same class or a prior class.

(c) An anatomical gift by a person authorized under subsection (a) must be made by (i) a document of gifts signed by the person or (ii) the person's telegraphic, recorded telephonic, or other recorded message, or other form of communication from the person that is contemporaneously reduced to writing and signed by the recipient.

(d) An anatomical gift by a person authorized under subsection (a) may be revoked by any member of the same or a prior class before procedures have begun for the removal from the body of the decedent, the physician, surgeon, technician, or enucleator removing the part.

(e) A failure to make an anatomical gift under subsection (a) is not an objection to the making of an anatomical gift.

§ 23-18.6-4. Authorization by medical examiner.

(a) The medical examiner may release and permit the removal of a part from a body within that official's custody, for transplantation or therapy, if:

(1) The official has received a request for the part from a hospital, physician, surgeon, or procurement organization;

(2) The hospital staff "transplant team" has made a reasonable effort, taking into account the useful life to the part, to locate and examine the decedent's medical records and inform persons listed in § 23-18.6-3(a) of their option to make, or object to making, an anatomical gift;

(3) The official does not know of a refusal or contrary indication by the decedent or objection by a person having priority to act as listed in § 23-18.6-3(a);

(4) The removal will be by a physician, surgeon, or technician; but in the case of eyes, by one of them or by an enucleator;

(5) The removal will not interfere with any autopsy, investigation, procedure, or other additional activity as deemed necessary by the Medical Examiner to arrive at a reasonable cause and manner of death.

(6) The removal will be in accordance with accepted medical standards; and

(7) Cosmetic restoration will be done, if appropriate.

(b) A permanent record of the names of the decedent, the person making the request, the date and purpose of the request, the part requested, and the person to whom it was released should be made by the hospital/physician/technician (enucleator) and forwarded to the Medical Examiner for his or her records.

§ 23-18.6-5. Routine inquiry and required request — Search and notification.

(a) When, in the opinion of the attending physician or other competent medical personnel that the death of any patient is imminent or has occurred, a representative designated by the hospital administration, shall notify the federally designated organ/tissue procurement organization of pending death. Except in cases in which the patient is obviously unsuited for donorship, a discussion of possible donation of organs/tissues shall take place according to medical criteria established by the federally designated organ/tissue procurement organization and documentation of notification and resultant options shall take place in the patient's medical record. The hospital administration shall actively support the education of all appropriate hospital personnel concerning organ and tissue donation on a regular basis, and shall take all steps necessary to assure full compliance with this chapter. The federally approved Organ Procurement Organization shall from time to time be asked to render opinion to the state hospital authority as to the adequacy of hospital efforts in this area.

(b) If, at or near the time of death of a patient, there is no medical record that the patient has made or refused to make an anatomical gift, the hospital administrator or a representative designated by the administrator shall discuss the option to make or refuse to make an anatomical gift and request the making of an anatomical gift pursuant to § 23-18.6-3(a). The request must be made with reasonable discretion and sensitivity to the circumstances of the family. A request is not required if the gift is not suitable, based upon accepted medical standards, established by the federally designated organ/tissue procurement agency, for a purpose specified in § 23-18.6-6. An entry must be made in the medical record of the patient, stating the name and affiliation of the individual making the request, and of the name, response, reason for not asking the next of kin or designee, and relationship to the patient of the person to whom the request was made. The director of the department of health in conjunction with the federally designated organ/tissue procurement organization shall adopt regulations to implement this subsection.

(c) The following persons shall make a reasonable search for a document of gift or other information identifying the bearer as a donor or as an individual who has refused to make an anatomical gift:

(1) A law enforcement officer, fireman, paramedic, or other emergency rescuer finding an individual who the searcher believes is dead or near death; and

(2) A hospital, upon the admission of an individual at or near the time of death, if there is not immediately available any other source of that information.

(d) If a document of gift or evidence of refusal to make an anatomical gift is located by the search required by subsection (c)(1), and the individual or body to whom it relates is taken to a hospital, the hospital must be notified of the contents and the document or other evidence must be sent to the hospital.

(e) If, at or near the time of death of a patient, a hospital knows that an anatomical gift has been made pursuant to § 23-18.6-3(a) of a release and removal of a part has been permitted pursuant to § 23-18.6-4, or that a patient or an individual identified as in transit to the hospital is a donor, the hospital shall notify the donee. The hospital shall cooperate in the implementation of the anatomical gift or release and removal of a part.

(f) A person who fails to discharge the duties imposed by this section is not subject to criminal or civil liability but is subject to appropriate administrative sanctions.

(g) Each hospital shall develop a protocol for addressing the issue of organ and tissue donation whenever a death occurs in a hospital and the intention of the deceased is unknown. The protocol shall require that any deceased individual's next of kin or other individual, as specified in § 23-18.6-2, shall be informed of the option to donate organs and tissue pursuant to chapter 18 of this title for any purpose specified in § 23-18.6-3. The protocol shall encourage reasonable discretion and sensitivity to the family circumstances in all discussions regarding donations of tissue or organs and may take into account the deceased individual's religious beliefs or obvious nonsuitability for organ and tissue donation in determining whether or not to make the request.

(h) The protocol shall require documentation of the request in the decedent's medical record and, if no request has been made, of the reasons therefor. Whether or not consent is granted, the statement shall indicate the name of the person granting or refusing the consent, and his or her relationship to the decedent.

(i) Each hospital shall submit a copy of the protocol to the department of health.

§ 23-18.6-6. Persons who may become donees — Purposes for which anatomical gifts may be made.

(a) The following persons may become donees of anatomical gifts for the purposes stated:

(1) A hospital, physician, surgeon, or federally designated organ/tissue procurement organization, for transplantation, therapy, medical or dental education, research, or advancement of medical or dental science;

(2) An accredited medical or dental school, college, or university for education, research, advancement of medical or dental science; or

(3) A designated individual for transplantation or therapy needed by that individual.

(b) An anatomical gift may be made to designated donee in the case of living related donor/donee or donation of entire body to a medical school for research prior to and well in advance of death. If a donee is not designated or if the donee is not available or rejects the anatomical gift, the anatomical gift may be accepted by any hospital.

(c) If the donee knows of the decedent's refusal or contrary indications to make an anatomical gift or that an anatomical gift by a member of a class having priority to act is opposed by a member of the same class or a prior class under § 23-18.6-3(a), the donee may not accept the anatomical gift.

§ 23-18.6-7. Delivery of document of gift.

(a) Delivery of a document of gift during the donor's lifetime is not required for the validity of an anatomical gift.

(b) If an anatomical gift is made to a designated donee, the document of gift, or a copy, may be delivered to the donee to expedite the appropriate procedures at the time of death.

§ 23-18.6-8. Rights and duties at death.

(a) Rights of a donee created by an anatomical gift are superior to rights of others except with respect to autopsies under § 23-18.6-11(b). A donee may accept or reject an anatomical gift. If a donee accepts an anatomical gift of an entire body, the donee, subject to the terms of the gift, may allow embalming and use of the body in funeral services. If the gift is of a part of a body, the donee, upon the death of the donor and before embalming, shall cause the part to be removed without unnecessary mutilation. After removal of the part, custody of the remainder of the body vests in the person under obligation to dispose of the body.

(b) The time of death must be determined by a physician or surgeon who attends the donor at death or, if none, the physician or surgeon who certifies the death. Neither the physician or surgeon who attends the donor at death nor the physician or surgeon who determines the time of death may participate in the procedures for removing or transplanting a part unless the document of gift designates a particular physician or surgeon pursuant to § 23-18.6-2(d).

(c) If there has been an anatomical gift, a technician may remove any donated parts and an enucleator may remove any donated eyes or parts of eyes, after determination of death by a physician or surgeon.

§ 23-18.6-9. Coordination of procurement and use.

Each hospital in this state shall establish agreements or affiliations with the federally designated organ/tissue procurement organization for coordination of procurement and use of human bodies and parts.

§ 28-18.6-10. Sale or purchase of parts prohibited.

(a) A person may not knowingly, for valuable consideration, purchase or sell a part for transplantation or therapy, if removal of the part is intended to occur after the death of the decedent.

(b) Valuable consideration does not include reasonable payment for the removal, processing, disposal, preservation, quality control, storage, transportation, or implantation of a part.

(c) A person who violates this section is guilty of a felony and upon conviction is subject to a fine not exceeding fifty thousand dollars ($50,000) or imprisonment not exceeding five (5) years, or both.

§ 23-18.6-11. Examination, autopsy, liability.

(a) An anatomical gift authorizes any reasonable examination necessary to assure medical acceptability of the gift for the purposes intended.

(b) The provisions of this chapter are subject to the laws of this state governing autopsies.

(c) A hospital, physician, surgeon, medical examiner, local public health officer, enucleator, technician, or other person, who acts in accordance with this chapter or with the applicable anatomical gift law of another state or a foreign country or attempt in good faith to do so is not liable for that act in a civil action or criminal proceeding.

(d) An individual who makes an anatomical gift pursuant to § 23-18.6-2 or 23-18.6-3 and the individual's estate are not liable for any injury or damage that may result from the making or the use of the anatomical gift.

§ 23-18.6-12. Acquired immune deficiency syndrome testing.

Prior to any organ, tissue, or part of a human body being transplanted in any human being, the donor shall be tested for the presence of antibodies to the probable causative agent for acquired immune deficiency syndrome (AIDS), provided that this condition shall not apply if there is a bona fide documentable medical emergency which endangers the life of any person. If the test for the presence of the antibodies is positive, the organ, tissue, or body part shall not be used.

§ 23-18.6-13. Transitional provisions.

This chapter applies to a document of gift, revocation, or refusal to make an anatomical gift signed by the donor or a person authorized to make or object to making an anatomical gift before, on, or after [July 1, 1989].

§ 23-18.6-14. Uniformity of application and construction.

This chapter shall be applied and construed to effectuate its general purpose to make uniform the law with respect to the subject of this chapter among states enacting it.

§ 23-18.6-15. Severability.

If any provision of this chapter or its application thereof to any person or circumstance is held invalid, the invalidity does not affect other provisions or application of this chapter which can be given effect without the invalid provision or application, and to this end the provisions of this chapter are severable.

SOUTH CAROLINA

UNIFORM ANATOMICAL GIFT ACT

§ 44-43-310. Short title.
This article may be cited as the Uniform Anatomical Gift Act.

§ 44-43-320. Definitions.
(a) "Bank or storage facility" means a facility licensed, accredited or approved under the laws of any state for storage of human bodies or parts thereof.

(b) "Decedent" means a deceased individual and includes a stillborn infant or fetus.

(c) "Donor" means an individual who makes a gift of all or part of his body.

(d) "Hospital" means a hospital licensed, accredited or approved under the laws of any state and includes a hospital operated by the United States Government, a state, or a subdivision thereof, although not required to be licensed under State laws.

(e) "Part" includes organs, tissues, eyes, bones, arteries, blood, other fluids and other portions of a human body, and "part" includes "parts."

(f) "Person" means an individual, corporation, government or governmental subdivision or agency, business trust, estate, trust, partnership or association or any other legal entity.

(g) "Physician" or "surgeon" means a physician or surgeon licensed or authorized to practice under the laws of any state.

(h) "State" includes any state, district, commonwealth, territory, insular possession, and any other area subject to the legislative authority of the United States of America.

§ 44-43-330. Persons who may make gift; situation in which donee may not accept; examination to determine medical acceptability; rights of donee shall be paramount.
(a) Any individual of sound mind and eighteen years of age or more may give all or any part of his body for any purposes specified in § 44-43-340, the gift to take effect upon death.

(b) Any of the following persons, in order of priority stated, when persons in prior classes are not available at the time of death, and in the absence of actual notice of contrary indications by the decedent, or actual notice of opposition by a member of the same or a prior class, may give all or any part of the decedent's body for any purposes specified in § 44-43-340:
(1) The spouse,
(2) An adult son or daughter,
(3) Either parent,
(4) An adult brother or sister,
(5) A guardian of the person of the decedent at the time of his death,
(6) Any other person authorized or under obligation to dispose of the body.

(c) If the donee has actual notice of contrary indications by the decedent, or that a gift by a member of a class is opposed by a member of the same or a prior class, the donee shall not accept the gift. The persons authorized by this subsection may make the gift after death or immediately before death.

(d) A gift of all or part of a body authorizes any examination necessary to assure medical acceptability of the gift for the purposes intended.

(e) The rights of the donee created by the gift are paramount to the rights of others except as provided by § 44-43-380(d).

§ 44-43-340. Persons who may become donee.
The following persons may become donees of gifts of bodies or parts thereof for the purposes stated:
(1) Any hospital, surgeon, or physician, for medical or dental education, research, advancement of medical or dental science, therapy or transplantation; or
(2) Any accredited medical or dental school, college or university for education, research, advancement of medical or dental science or therapy; or
(3) Any bank or storage facility for medical or dental education, research, advancement of medical or dental science, therapy or transplantation; or
(4) Any specified individual for therapy or transplantation needed by him.

§ 44-43-350. Manner in which gift may be made.
(a) A gift of all or part of the body under § 44-43-330(a) may be made by will. The gift becomes effective upon the death of the testator without waiting for probate. If the will is not probated, or if it is declared invalid for testamentary purposes, the gift, to the extent that it has been acted upon in good faith, is nevertheless valid and effective.

(b) A gift of all or part of the body under § 44-43-330(a) may also be made by document other than a will. The gift becomes effective upon the death of the donor. The document, which may be a card designed to be carried on the person, must be signed by the donor, in the presence of two witnesses who must sign the document in his presence. If the donor cannot sign, the document may be signed for him at his direction and in his presence, and in the presence of two witnesses who must sign the document in his presence. Delivery of the document of gift during the donor's lifetime is not necessary to make the gift valid.

(c) The gift may be made to a specified donee or without specifying a donee. If the latter, the gift may be accepted by the attending physician as donee upon or following death. If the gift is made to a specified donee who is not available at the time and place of death, the attending physician upon or following death, in the absence of any expressed indication that the donor desired otherwise, may accept the gift as donee. The physician who becomes a donee under this subsection shall not participate in the procedures for removing or transplanting a part.

(d) Notwithstanding § 44-43-380(b), the donor may designate in his will, card or other document of gift the surgeon or physician to carry out the appropriate procedures. In the absence of a designation, or if the designee is not available, the donee or other person authorized to accept the gift may employ or authorize any surgeon or physician for the purpose.

(e) Any gift by a person designated in § 44-43-330(b) shall be made by a document signed by him, or made by his telegraphic, recorded telephonic or other recorded message.

§ 44-43-360. Delivery or deposit of document of gift or copy thereof.

If the gift is made by the donor to a specified donee, the will, card or other document, or an executed copy thereof, may be delivered to the donee to expedite the appropriate procedures immediately after death, but delivery is not necessary to the validity of the gift. The will, card or other document, or an executed copy thereof, may be deposited in any hospital, bank or storage facility or registry office that accepts them for safekeeping or for facilitation of procedures after death. On request of any interested party upon or after the donor's death, the person in possession shall produce the document for examination.

§ 44-43-370. Amendment or revocation of gift.

(a) If the will, card or other document or executed copy thereof, has been delivered to a specified donee, the donor may amend or revoke the gift by:

(1) The execution and delivery to the donee of a signed statement, or

(2) An oral statement made in the presence of two persons and communicated to the donee, or

(3) A statement during a terminal illness or injury addressed to an attending physician and communicated to the donee, or

(4) A signed card or document found on his person or in his effects.

(b) Any document of gift which has not been delivered to the donee may be revoked by the donor in the manner set out in subsection (a) or by destruction, cancellation, or mutilation of the document and all executed copies thereof.

(c) Any gift made by a will may also be amended or revoked in the manner provided for amendment or revocation of wills, or as provided in subsection (a).

§ 44-43-380. Acceptance or rejection of gift; disposition of remainder of body; determination of time of death; immunity from liability; article subject to laws with respect to autopsies.

(a) The donee may accept or reject the gift. If the donee accepts a gift of the entire body, he may, subject to the terms of the gift, authorize embalming and the use of the body in funeral services. If the gift is of a part of the body, the donee, upon the death of the donor and prior to embalming, shall cause the part to be removed without unnecessary mutilation. After removal of the part, custody of the remainder of the body vests in the surviving spouse, next of kin or other persons under obligation to dispose of the body.

(b) The time of death shall be determined by a physician who attends the donor at his death, or, if none, the physician who certifies the death. This physician shall not participate in the procedures for removing or transplanting a part.

(c) A person who acts in good faith in accord with the terms of this article, or under the anatomical gift laws of another state is not liable for damages in any civil action or subject to prosecution in any criminal proceeding for his act. Provided, however, that such immunity from civil liability shall not extend to cases of provable malpractice on the part of any physician, surgeon or other medical attendant.

(d) The provisions of this article are subject to the laws of this State prescribing powers and duties with respect to autopsies.

§ 44-43-390. This article supplemental to Article 3 of this chapter.

The provisions of this article are supplementary to Article 3 of this chapter, relating to the donation of eyes for the restoration of sight, and shall not be construed to in any manner repeal or replace that article. The restriction against a physician donee participating in removal or transplant of a body part in subsection (c) of § 44-43-350 shall not apply in the case of eyes or parts thereof.

§ 44-43-400. Construction.

This article shall be so construed as to effectuate its general purpose to make uniform the law of those states which enact it.

SOUTH DAKOTA

ANATOMICAL GIFTS

§ 34-26-20. Anatomical gifts — Definition of terms.

Terms used in §§ 34-26-20 to 34-26-41, inclusive, mean:

(1) "Bank" or "storage facility," a facility licensed, accredited, or approved under the laws of any state for storage of human bodies or parts thereof.

(2) "Decedent," a deceased individual and includes a stillborn infant or fetus.

(3) "Donor," an individual who makes a gift of all or part of his body.

(4) "Hospital," a hospital licensed, accredited, or approved under the laws of any state, and includes a hospital operated by the United States government, a state, or a subdivision thereof, although not required to be licensed under state laws.

(5) "Part," organs, tissues, eyes, bones, arteries, blood, other fluids and any other portions of a human body.

(6) "Person," an individual, corporation, government or governmental subdivision or agency, business trust, estate, trust, partnership or association, or any other legal entity.

(7) "Physician" or "surgeon," a physician or surgeon licensed or authorized to practice under the laws of any state.

(8) "State" includes any state, district, commonwealth, territory, insular possession, and any other area subject to the legislative authority of the United States of America.

§ 34-26-21. Eligibility to make gifts of own body.

Any individual of sound mind and eighteen years of age or more may give all or any part of his body for any purpose specified in § 34-26-27, the gift to take effect upon death.

§ 34-26-22. Anatomical gift by will.

A gift of all or part of the body under § 34-26-21 may be made by will. The gift becomes effective upon the death of the testator without waiting for probate. If the will is not probated, or if it is declared invalid for testamentary purposes, the gift, to the extent that it has been acted upon in good faith, is nevertheless valid and effective.

§ 34-26-23. Anatomical gift by document other than will — Execution and effectiveness of document.

A gift of all or part of the body under § 34-26-21 may also be made by document other than a will. The gift becomes effective upon the death of the donor. The document, which may be a card designed to be carried on the person, must be signed by the donor in the presence of two witnesses who must sign the document in his presence. If the donor cannot sign, the document may be signed for him at his direction and in his presence of two witnesses who must sign the document in his presence. Delivery of the document of gift during the donor's lifetime is not necessary to make the gift valid.

§ 34-26-24. Anatomical gifts by spouse, kin, guardian, or authorized person — Priority of authority to make gift — Time of gift.

Any of the following persons, in order of priority stated, when persons in prior classes are not available at the time of death, and in the absence of actual notice of contrary indications by the decedent or actual notice of opposition by a member of the same or a prior class, may give all or any part of the decedent's body for any purpose specified in § 34-26-27:

(1) The spouse,

(2) An adult son or daughter,

(3) Either parent,

(4) An adult brother or sister,

(5) A guardian of the person of the decedent at the time of his death,

(6) Any other person authorized or under obligation to dispose of the body.

The persons authorized may make the gift after or immediately before death.

§ 34-26-25. Execution of anatomical gift by spouse, kin, guardian or authorized person.

Any gift by a person designated in § 34-26-24 shall be made by a document signed by him or made by his telegraphic, recorded telephonic, or other recorded message.

§ 34-26-26. Donee not to accept unauthorized anatomical gift.

If the donee has actual notice of contrary indications by the decedent or that a gift by a member of a class is opposed by a member of the same or a prior class, the donee shall not accept the gift.

§ 34-26-27. Authorized donees of anatomical gifts — Authorized purposes.

The following persons may become donees of gifts of bodies or parts thereof for the purposes stated:

(1) Any hospital, surgeon, or physician, for medical or dental education, research, advancement of medical or dental science, therapy or transplantation; or

(2) Any accredited medical or dental school, college or university for education, research, advancement of medical or dental science, or therapy; or

(3) Any bank or storage facility, for medical or dental education, research, advancement of medical or dental science, therapy, or transplantation; or

(4) Any specified individual for therapy or transplantation needed by him.

§ 34-26-28. Anatomical gift to specified donee or without specifying donee — Acceptance of gift by attending physician.

The gift may be made to a specified donee or without specifying a donee. If the latter, the gift may be accepted by the attending physician as donee upon or following death. If the gift is made to a specified donee who is not available at the time and place of death, the attending physician upon or following death, in the absence of any expressed indication that the donor desired otherwise, may accept the gift as donee. The physician who becomes a donee under this section shall not participate in the procedures for removing or transplanting a part.

§ 34-26-29. Designation of surgeon or physician to carry out purposes of anatomical gift.

Notwithstanding § 34-26-34, the donor may designate in his will, card, or other document of gift the surgeon or physician to carry out the appropriate procedures. In the absence of a designation or if the designee is not available, the donee or other person authorized to accept the gift may employ or authorize any surgeon or physician for the purpose.

§ 34-26-29.1. Enucleation of eye by properly certified person — Immunity from liability.

In respect to a gift of an eye as provided for in § 34-26-21, a licensed funeral director, as defined in § 36-19-14, or any other person who has completed a course in eye enucleation and has received a certificate of competence from a university medical school, a university medical school of ophthalmology, or a training unit approved by a university medical school or university medical school of ophthalmology, may, at the direction of a physician, enucleate eyes for such gift after proper certification of death by a physician and compliance with the intent of such gift as defined in this chapter. No such properly certified funeral director or other person acting in accordance with the terms of this chapter may be liable, civilly or criminally, for such eye enucleation.

§ 34-26-30. Delivery of document of anatomical gift.

If the gift is made by the donor to a specified donee, the will, card, or other document, or an executed copy thereof, may be delivered to the donee to expedite the appropriate procedures immediately after death. Delivery is not necessary to the validity of the gift. The will, card, or other document, or an executed copy thereof, may be deposited in any hospital, bank or storage facility, or registry office that accepts it for safekeeping or for facilitation of procedures after death. On request of any interested party upon or after the donor's death, the person in possession shall produce the document for examination.

§ 34-26-31. Amendment or revocation of anatomical gift delivered to specified donee.

If the will, card, or other document or executed copy thereof, has been delivered to a specified donee, the donor may amend or revoke the gift by:

(1) The execution and delivery to the donee or a signed statement, or

(2) An oral statement made in the presence of two persons and communicated to the donee, or

(3) A statement during a terminal illness or injury addressed to an attending physician and communicated to the donee, or

(4) A signed card or document found on his person or in his effects.

§ 34-26-32. Revocation of undelivered document of anatomical gift.

Any document of gift which has not been delivered to the donee may be revoked by the donor in the manner set out in § 34-26-31 or by destruction, cancellation, or mutilation of the document and all executed copies thereof.

§ 34-26-33. Amendment or revocation of anatomical gift by will.

Any gift made by a will may also be amended or revoked in the manner provided for amendment or revocation of wills or as provided in § 34-26-31.

§ 34-26-34. Determination of time of death of donor of anatomical gift — Attending physician not to participate in removal or transplant of part.

The time of death shall be determined by a physician who attends the donor at his death or, if none, the physician who certifies the death. The physician shall not participate in the procedures for removing or transplanting a part.

§ 34-26-35. Rights of donee paramount — Exception.

The rights of the donee created by the gift are paramount to the rights of others except as provided by § 34-26-38.

§ 34-26-36. Examination for medical acceptability authorized by anatomical gift.

A gift of all or part of a body authorizes any examination necessary to assure medical acceptability of the gift for the purposes intended.

§ 34-26-37. Acceptance or rejection of anatomical gift by donee — Removal of part of body.

The donee may accept or reject the gift. If the donee accepts a gift of the entire body, he may, subject to the terms of the gift, authorize embalming and the use of the body in funeral services. If the gift is of a part of the body, the donee, upon the death of the donor and prior to embalming, shall cause the part to be removed without unnecessary mutilation. After removal of the part, custody of the remainder of the body vests in the surviving spouse, next of kin, or other persons under obligation to dispose of the body.

§ 34-26-38. Anatomical gift provisions subject to autopsy laws.

The provisions of §§ 34-26-20 to 34-26-41, inclusive, are subject to the laws of this state prescribing powers and duties with respect to autopsies.

§ 34-26-39. Exemption from civil or criminal liability for good faith actions under anatomical gift laws.

A person who acts in good faith in accord with the terms of §§ 34-26-20 to 34-26-41, inclusive, or the anatomical gift laws of another state or a foreign country is not liable for damages in any civil action or subject to prosecution in any criminal proceeding for his act.

§ 34-26-40. Uniformity of interpretation of anatomical gift provisions.

Sections 34-26-20 to 34-26-41, inclusive, shall be so construed as to effectuate their general purpose to make uniform the law of those states which enact them.

§ 34-26-41. Citation of anatomical gift provisions.

Sections 34-26-20 to 34-26-41, inclusive, may be cited as the Uniform Anatomical Gift Act.

TENNESSEE

UNIFORM ANATOMICAL GIFT ACT

§ 68-30-101. Title.
This part may be cited as the "Uniform Anatomical Gift Act."

§ 68-30-102. Definitions.
As used in this part:

(1) "Bank or storage facility" means a facility licensed, accredited, or approved under the laws of any state for storage of human bodies or parts thereof;

(2) "Decedent" means a deceased individual and includes a stillborn infant or fetus;

(3) "Donor" means an individual who makes a gift of all or part of his body;

(4) "Eye bank" means any not-for-profit agency certified by the Eye Bank Association of America to procure eye tissue for the purpose of transplantation or research;

(5) "Hospital" means a hospital licensed, accredited, or approved under the laws of any state; the term includes a hospital operated by the United States government, a state, or a subdivision thereof, although not required to be licensed under state laws;

(6) "Organ procurement agency" means any not-for-profit agency approved by the health care financing administration to procure and place human organs for transplantation, therapy, or research;

(7) "Part" means organs, tissues, eyes, bones, arteries, blood, other fluids and any other portions of a human body;

(8) "Person" means an individual, corporation, government or governmental subdivision or agency, business trust, estate, trust, partnership or association, or any other legal entity;

(9) "Physician" or "surgeon" means a physician or surgeon licensed or authorized to practice under the laws of any state;

(10) "State" includes any state, district, commonwealth, territory, insular possession, and any other area subject to the legislative authority of the United States of America; and

(11) "Terminal patient" means any human being afflicted with any disease, illness, injury, or condition from which there is no reasonable medical expectation of recovery and which disease, injury, illness or condition will as a medical probability, result in the death of such human being within a short period of time regardless of the use or discontinuance of medical treatment implemented for the purpose of sustaining life, or the life processes.

§ 68-30-103. Persons who may execute an anatomical gift.
(a) Any individual of sound mind and eighteen (18) years of age or more may give all or any part of his body for any purpose specified in § 68-30-104, the gift to take effect upon death.

(b) Any of the following persons, in order of priority stated, when persons in prior classes are not available at the time of death, and in the absence of actual notice of contrary indications by the decedent or actual notice of opposition by a member of the same or a prior class, may give all or any part of the decedent's body for any purpose specified in § 68-30-104:

(1) The spouse;

(2) An adult son or daughter;

(3) Either parent;

(4) An adult brother or sister;

(5) A guardian of the person of the decedent at the time of his death; or

(6) Any other person authorized or under obligation to dispose of the body.

(c) If the donee has actual notice of contrary indications by the decedent or actual notice that a gift by a member of a class is opposed by a member of the same or a prior class, the donee shall not accept the gift. The persons authorized by subsection (b) may make the gift after or immediately before death.

(d) A gift of all or part of a body authorizes any examination necessary to assure medical acceptability of the gift for the purposes intended.

(e) The rights of the donee created by the gift are paramount to the rights of others except as provided by § 68-30-108(d).

§ 68-30-104. Persons who may become donees — Purposes for which anatomical gifts may be made.
The following persons may become donees of gifts of bodies or parts thereof for the purposes stated:

(1) Any hospital, surgeon, or physician, for medical or dental education, research, advancement of medical or dental science, therapy, or transplantation;

(2) Any accredited medical or dental school, college or university for education, research, advancement of medical or dental science, or therapy;

(3) Any bank or storage facility, for medical or dental education, research, advancement of medical or dental science, therapy, or transplantation; or

(4) Any specified individual for therapy or transplantation needed by him.

§ 68-30-105. Method of executing anatomical gifts.

(a) A gift of all or part of the body under § 68-30-103(a) may be made by will. The gift becomes effective upon the death of the testator without waiting for probate. If the will is not probated, or if it is declared invalid for testamentary purposes, the gift, to the extent that it has been acted upon in good faith, is nevertheless valid and effective.

(b) A gift of all or part of the body under § 68-30-103(a) may also be made by document other than a will. The gift becomes effective upon the death of the donor. The document, which may be a card designed to be carried on the person, must be signed by the donor in the presence of two (2) witnesses who must sign the document in his presence. If the donor cannot sign, the document may be signed for him at his direction and in his presence in the presence of two (2) witnesses who must sign the document in his presence. Delivery of the document of gift during the donor's lifetime is not necessary to make the gift valid.

(c) The gift may be made to a specified donee or without specifying a donee. If the latter, the gift may be accepted by the attending physician as donee upon or following death. If the gift is made to a specified donee who is not available at the time and place of death, the attending physician upon or following death, in the absence of any expressed indication that the donor desired otherwise, may accept the gift as donee. The physician who becomes a donee under this subsection shall not participate in the procedures for removing or transplanting a part.

(d) Notwithstanding § 68-30-108(b), the donor may designate in his will, card, or other document of gift the surgeon or physician to carry out the appropriate procedures. In the absence of a designation or if the designee is not available, the donee or other person authorized to accept the gift may employ or authorize any surgeon or physician for the purpose. In the case of a gift of eyes, in the absence of a designation by the donor or if such designee is not available, the donee or other person authorized to accept the gift may employ or authorize an ophthalmic technician trained in eye enucleation.

(e) Any gift by a person designated in § 68-30-103(a) may also be made by a statement provided for on the reverse side of all Tennessee operators' and chauffeurs' licenses. The gift becomes effective upon the death of the donor. The statement must be signed by the owner of the operator's or chauffeur's license in the presence of two (2) witnesses, who must sign the statement in the presence of the donor. Delivery of the license during the donor's lifetime is not necessary to make the gift valid. The gift shall become invalidated upon expiration, cancellation, revocation, or suspension of the license, and the gift must be renewed upon renewal of each license. Any hospital, hospital personnel, physician, surgeon, undertaker, law enforcement officer, or other person may rely upon such statement when signed by the owner of such license and two (2) witnesses as a properly executed legal document, and shall be immune from civil or criminal liability when acting in good faith upon the anatomical gift made pursuant thereto.

§ 68-30-106. Delivery of document of gift.

If the gift is made by the donor to a specified donee, the will, card, or other document, or an executed copy thereof, may be delivered to the donee to expedite the appropriate procedures immediately after death. Delivery is not necessary to the validity of the gift. The will, card, or other document, or an executed copy thereof, may be deposited in any hospital, bank or storage facility or registry office that accepts it for safekeeping or for facilitation of procedures after death. On request of any interested party upon or after the donor's death, the person in possession shall produce the document for examination.

§ 68-30-107. Amendment or revocation of the gift.

(a) If the will, card, or other document or executed copy thereof, has been delivered to a specified donee, the donor may amend or revoke the gift by:

(1) The execution and delivery to the donee of a signed statement;

(2) An oral statement made in the presence of two (2) persons and communicated to the donee;

(3) A statement during a terminal illness or injury addressed to an attending physician and communicated to the donee; or

(4) A signed card or document found on his person or in his effects.

(b) Any document of gift which has not been delivered to the donee may be revoked by the donor in the manner set out in subsection (a), or by destruction, cancellation, or mutilation of the document and all executed copies thereof.

(c) Any gift made by a will may also be amended or revoked in the manner provided for amendment or revocation of wills, or as provided in subsection (a).

§ 68-30-108. Rights and duties at death — Embalming — Disposition of body.

(a) The donee may accept or reject the gift. If the donee accepts a gift of the entire body , he may, subject to the terms of the gift, authorize embalming and the use of the body in funeral services. If the gift is of a part of the body, the donee, upon the death of the donor and prior to embalming, shall cause the part to be removed without unnecessary mutilation. After removal of the part, custody of the remainder of the body vests in the surviving spouse, next of kin, or other persons under obligation to dispose of the body.

(b) The time of death shall be determined by a physician who tends the donor at his death, or, if none, the physician who certifies the death. The physician shall not participate in the procedures for removing or transplanting a part.

(c) A person who acts in good faith in accordance with the terms of this part or with the anatomical gift laws of another state (or a foreign country) is not liable for damages in any civil action or subject to prosecution in any criminal proceeding for his act.

(d) The provisions of this part are subject to the laws of this state prescribing powers and duties with respect to autopsies.

§ 68-30-109. Uniformity of interpretation.

This part shall be so construed as to effectuate its general purpose to make uniform the laws of those states which enact it.

§ 68-30-110. Conveyance of patient's wishes — Acute care hospitals — Organ and tissue donation policies and procedures.

(a) All physicians, surgeons, or hospital personnel shall make every reasonable effort to convey to the appropriate hospital department the wishes of a hospitalized patient to make an anatomical donation of his body or part thereof, in order that the necessary documents are properly executed in accordance with this part.

(b) Failure to comply with the provisions of this section shall not subject any hospital, hospital personnel, physician, surgeon, or other person to civil or criminal liability for any such failure.

(c) Every acute care hospital in the state of Tennessee will establish a committee to develop and implement an organ and tissue donation policy and procedure to assist the physicians in identifying and evaluating terminal patients who may be suitable organ or tissue donors. The committee will include members of the administrative, medical, and nursing staffs and will appoint a member to act as a liaison between the hospital and the local organ procurement agency and eye bank.

(d) The organ and tissue donation policy and procedure will contain information on acceptable donor criteria, the name and number of the local organ procurement agency and eye bank, a standard organ and tissue donation consent form, mechanisms for informing the next of kin of the potential donor about organ and tissue donation options, provisions for the maintenance and procurement of donated organs and tissues, and methods for routine education of the hospital staff about the policy and procedure.

(e) Each hospital organ and tissue donation policy and procedure will include provisions for the identification of every terminal patient who, in the opinion of the attending physician, meets the criteria established in the policy and the subsequent notification to the local organ procurement agency and/or eye bank for evaluation of the suitability of the organs or tissues. Notification concerning patients who are eligible for a declaration of death abased on irreversible cessation of brain function according to § 68-3-501(b)(2), upon recommendation of the attending physician, shall be made to the local organ procurement agency for evaluation prior to a declaration of death or termination of medical treatment. Notification concerning patients who are eligible for a declaration of death based on irreversible cessation of cardiorespiratory function according to § 68-3-501(b)(1), upon recommendation of the attending physician, shall be made to the local organ procurement agency for evaluation, if possible, prior to the declaration of death. In the event that death is sudden and unpredictable, such notification to the eye bank will be accomplished immediately following declaration of death.

(f) Every acute care hospital will develop and implement a protocol for the determination of death pursuant to § 68-3-501.

(g) All physicians, surgeons, and hospital personnel will make every reasonable effort to identify terminal patients who satisfy the donor criteria and to notify the appropriate agency regarding the potential donor.

(h) The commissioner of health and environment shall prepare and issue an annual report summarizing existing data pertaining to organ donation and transplantation activity in Tennessee hospitals.

§ 68-30-111. Source of body parts for transplantation — Confidentiality.

It is the intent and purpose of the legislature that for the public welfare, the general public be encouraged to donate body parts for the purpose of transplantation. To this end all records containing the source of body parts for transplantation or any information concerning persons donating body parts for transplantation shall be made confidential under § 10-7-504(a).

TEXAS

UNIFORM ANATOMICAL GIFT ACT (1968)

§ 692.002. Definitions.

In this chapter:

(1) "Bank or storage facility" means a facility licensed, accredited, or approved under the laws of any state to store human bodies or body parts.

(2) "Decedent" means a deceased person and includes a stillborn infant or fetus.

(3) "Donor" means a person who makes a gift of all or part of the person's body.

(4) "Eye bank" means a nonprofit corporation chartered under the laws of this state to obtain, store, and distribute donor eyes to be used by ophthalmologists for corneal transplants, research, or other medical purposes.

(5) "Hospital" means a hospital:

    (A) licensed, accredited, or approved under the laws of any state; or

    (B) operated by the federal government, a state government, or a political subdivision of a state government.

(6) "Part" includes an organ, tissue, eye, bone, artery, blood, other fluid, and other parts of a human body.

(7) "Physician" means a physician licensed or authorized to practice under the laws of any state.

(8) "Qualified organ or tissue procurement organization" means an organization that procures and distributes organs or tissues for transplantation, research, or other medical purposes and is:

    (A) affiliated with a university or hospital; or

    (B) registered to operate as a nonprofit organization in this state for the primary purpose of organ or tissue procurement.

§ 692.003. Manner of Executing Gift of Own Body.

(a) A person who has testamentary capacity under the Texas Probate Code may give all or part of the person's body for a purpose specified by Section 692.005.

(b) A person may make a gift under this section by will or by use of a document other than a will.

(c) A gift made by will is effective on the death of the testator without the necessity of probate. If the will is not probated or if the will is declared invalid for testamentary purposes, the gift is valid to the extent to which it has been acted on in good faith.

(d) A gift made by a document other than a will is effective on the death of the donor. The document may be a card designed to be carried by the donor. To be effective, the document must be signed by the donor in the presence of two witnesses. If the donor cannot sign the document, a person may sign the document for the donor at the donor's direction and in the presence of the donor and two witnesses. The witnesses to the signing of a document under this subsection must sign the document in the presence of the donor. Delivery of the document during the donor's lifetime is not necessary to make the gift valid.

§ 692.004. Persons Who May Execute Gift.

(a) The following persons, in the following priority, may give all or any part of a decedent's body for a purpose specified by Section 692.005:

    (1) the decedent's spouse;

    (2) the decedent's adult child;

    (3) either of the decedent's parents;

    (4) the decedent's adult brother or sister;

    (5) the guardian of the person of the decedent at the time of death; or

    (6) any other person authorized or under an obligation to dispose of the body.

(b) A person listed in Subsection (a) may make the gift only if:

    (1) a person in a higher priority class is not available at the time of death;

    (2) there is no actual notice of contrary indications by the decedent; and

    (3) there is no actual notice of opposition by a member of the same or a higher priority class.

(c) A person listed in Subsection (a) may make the gift after death or immediately before death. The person must make the gift by a document signed by the person or by a telegraphic, recorded telephonic, or other recorded message.

§ 692.005. Persons Who May Become Donees.

The following persons may be donees of gifts of bodies or parts:

(1) a hospital or physician, to be used only for medical or dental education, research, therapy, transplantation, or the advancement of medical or dental science;

(2) an accredited medical, chiropractic, or dental school, college, or university, to be used only for education, research, therapy, or the advancement of medical or dental science;

(3) a bank or storage facility, to be used only for medical or dental education, research, therapy, transplantation, or the advancement of medical or dental science;

(4) a person specified by a physician, to be used only for therapy or transplantation needed by the person;

(5) an eye bank the medical activities of which are directed by a physician; or

(6) the Anatomical Board of the State of Texas.

§ 692.006. Designation of Donee or Physician.

(a) A person may make a gift to a specified donee. If the gift is not made to a specified donee, the attending physician may accept the gift as donee at the time of death or after death.

(b) If the gift is made to a specified donee who is not available at the time and place of death, the attending physician may accept the gift as donee at the time of death or after death unless the donor expressed an indication that the donor desired a different procedure.

(c) A physician who becomes a donee under Subsection (a) or (b) may not participate in the procedures for removing or transplanting a part.

(d) Notwithstanding Section 692.009, a donor may designate in the donor's will or document of gift the physician to perform the appropriate procedures. If the donor does not designate the physician, or if the physician is not available, the donee or other person authorized to accept the gift may employ or authorize any physician to perform the appropriate procedures.

§ 692.007. Delivery of Document.

(a) If a donor makes a gift to a specified donee, the donor may deliver the will or document, or an executed copy, to the donee to expedite the appropriate procedures immediately after death. Delivery is not necessary to make the gift valid.

(b) The donor may deposit the will or other document, or an executed copy, in a hospital, registry office, or bank or storage facility that accepts the document for safekeeping or to facilitate the procedures after death.

(c) On or after the donor's death and on the request of an interested party, the person in possession of the document shall produce the document for examination.

§ 692.008. Amendment or Revocation of Gift.

(a) If the donor has delivered the will or other document, or executed copy, to a specified donee, the donor may amend or revoke the gift by:

(1) executing and delivering to the donee a signed statement;

(2) making an oral statement in the presence of two persons that is communicated to the donee;

(3) making a statement to an attending physician that is communicated to the donee; or

(4) executing a signed document that is found on the donor or found in the donor's effects.

(b) If the donor has not delivered the document of gift to the donee, the donor may revoke the gift in a manner prescribed by Subsection (a) or by destroying, canceling, or mutilating the document and each executed copy of the document.

(c) If the donor made the gift by will, the donor may revoke or amend the gift in a manner prescribed by Subsection (a) or in a manner prescribed for the amendment or revocation of a will.

§ 692.009. Determination of Time of Death.

The attending physician or, if none, the physician who certifies the death shall determine the time of death. That physician may not participate in the procedures for removing or transplanting a part.

§ 692.010. Acceptance or Rejection of Gift.

(a) A donee may accept or reject a gift.

(b) If the donee or the donee's physician has actual notice of contrary indications by the decedent or has actual notice that a gift made under Section 692.004 is opposed by a member of the same or a higher priority class, the donee may not accept the gift.

(c) If a donee accepts a gift of an entire body, the decedent's surviving spouse or any other person authorized to give all or part of the body may authorize the body's embalming and have the use of the body for funeral services, subject to the terms of the gift.

(d) If a donee accepts a gift of a part, the donee shall cause the part to be removed from the body without unnecessary mutilation after death occurs and before the body is embalmed. After the part is removed, the surviving spouse, next of kin, or other person under obligation to dispose of the body has custody of the body.

§ 692.011. Examination for Medical Acceptability Authorized.

A gift of all or part of a body authorizes any examination necessary to assure medical acceptability of the gift for the intended purposes.

§ 692.012. Donee's Rights Superior.

Except as prescribed by Section 692.015(a), a donee's rights that are created by a gift are superior to the rights of other persons.

§ 692.013. Hospital Protocol.

(a) Each hospital shall develop a protocol for identifying potential organ and tissue donors from among those persons who die in the hospital. The hospital shall make its protocol available to the public during the hospital's normal business hours.

(b) The protocol must:

(1) provide that the hospital use appropriately trained persons to make inquiries relating to donations;

(2) encourage sensitivity to families' beliefs and circumstances in all discussions relating to the donations;

(3) establish guidelines based on accepted medical standards for determining if a person is medically suitable to donate organs or tissues; and

(4) provide for documentation of the inquiry and of its disposition in the decedent's medical records.

(c) The protocol must provide that a hospital is not required to make an inquiry under Section 692.014 if:

(1) the decedent is not medically suitable for donation based on the suitability guidelines established by protocol;

(2) the hospital has actual notice of an objection to the donation made by:

(A) the decedent;

(B) the person authorized to make the donation under Section 692.004, according to the priority established by that section; or

(C) an unavailable member of a higher priority class; or

(3) the hospital administrator has not been notified by a qualified organ or tissue procurement organization that:

(A) there is a current medical need for organs or tissues; and

(B) the organization is available to retrieve the organs or tissues in a manner consistent with accepted medical standards.

§ 692.014. Hospital Procedures.

(a) In accordance with the protocol established under Section 692.013, at or near the time of notification of death, the hospital shall ask the person authorized to make an anatomical gift on behalf of the decedent under Section 692.004, according to the priority established by that section, if the decedent is a donor.

(b) If there are two or more persons in the same priority class authorized to make a gift under Section 692.004, the hospital shall ask those class members reasonably available at or near the time of notification of death.

(c) If the decedent is not a donor, the hospital shall inform the person of the option to donate the decedent's organs and tissues. If the person approves the donation, the hospital shall notify a qualified organ or tissues procurement organization of the potential donation.

§ 692.015. Effect of Other Laws.

(a) This chapter is subject to the laws of this state prescribing the powers and duties relating to autopsies.

(b) Sections 692.013 and 692.014 do not affect the laws relating to notification of the medical examiner or justice of the peace of each case of reportable death.

§ 692.016. Limitation of Liability.

(a) A person who acts in good faith in accordance with this chapter is not liable for civil damages or subject to criminal prosecution for the person's action if the prerequisites for an anatomical gift are met under the laws applicable at the time and place the gift is made.

(b) A person who acts in good faith in accordance with Sections 692.013 and 692.014 is not liable as a result of the action except in the case of the person's own negligence. For purposes of this subsection, "good faith" in determining the appropriate person authorized to make a donation under Section 692.004 means making a reasonable effort to locate and contact the member or members of the highest priority class who are available at or near the time of death.

UTAH

ANATOMICAL GIFT ACT

§ 26-28-1. Gifts or parts of the body — Eligibility to make — Procedure.

Any person 18 years of age or older, or less than 18 years if legally married with the consent in writing of the parent or parents or guardian of such person, may make a gift of any part of his body, or of any organ or tissue thereof, effective upon his death, by a written or printed statement of gift signed by him or his legally appointed representative in the presence of at least one attesting witness. The gift shall be deemed effective without delivery or notification to, or acceptance by, the donee and may be revoked by the donor at any time by a written revocation statement executed in like manner, subject to the provisions of Sections 26-28-5 and 26-28-6.

§ 26-28-2. Eligible donees — Failure to designate or incapacity of donee — Eye enucleation by qualified funeral service practitioner.

(1) A gift made under this chapter may designate as donee:

(a) a licensed physician or surgeon;

(b) a hospital;

(c) a medical school, college, or university engaged in medical education and research;

(d) a blood bank, artery bank, eye bank, or other storage facility for human parts or tissues to be used for transplantation or therapy; or

(e) any licensed physician or surgeon claiming the body, not naming him.

(2) If a statement of gift fails to designate a donee, or the donee designated is incapable of accepting the gift upon the donor's death, the statement of gift shall be deemed to designate any licensed physician or surgeon claiming the body as an alternate solely for the purpose of carrying out the purposes of the gift.

(3) If the part of the body that is the gift is eye tissue, the donee or the person authorized to accept the gift may employ or authorize a certified individual, licensed in the practice of funeral service under Chapter 9, Title 58, to enucleate the eye.

§ 26-28-3. Purpose of gift — Donor may designate.

(1) A gift made under this chapter may designate and limit the purpose for which the gift is made to any one or more of the following:

(a) for transplantation to replace diseased, deteriorated, or malfunctioning parts of living persons;

(b) for use or aid in therapy or in the production of therapeutic substances; or

(c) for medical education or scientific research in medicine.

(2) A statement of gift which fails to designate a purpose, or which states that the gift is for any lawful purpose, shall be construed as a gift for all of the purposes stated in this section.

§ 26-28-4. Necessary surgery and temporary custody of body authorized — Liability for costs of procedures.

(1) A gift made under this chapter, in addition to the authorizations contained in the statement of gift, authorizes the donee or his agent to perform any surgical procedure necessary to make the gift effective, and authorizes the donee or his agent to take and maintain custody of the donor's body immediately after death for a reasonable period of time, not exceeding 24 hours, for the purpose of performing necessary surgical procedures. Immediately following the removal of the parts of the body, or organs or tissues, designated in the statement of gift, custody of the donor's remains shall be transferred to the next of kin or his agent.

(2) In no instance may the donor, his insurance, or his estate be held liable for the costs of surgical or other procedures necessary to effectuate the gift.

§ 26-28-5. Rights of donee — Immunity from liability.

(1) The rights of a donee or his agent with respect to a gift made under this chapter are superior to those of any person claiming as spouse, relative, guardian, or in any other relationship.

(2) A person who, in good-faith reliance upon a statement of gift or upon prima facie evidence of a gift as defined in Section 26-28-7, and without actual notice of revocation thereof, takes possession of, performs or causes to be performed surgical operations upon, or removes or causes to be removed organs, tissues, or parts from a human body shall not be liable in damages in any suit brought against him for such act.

(3) Any donee who refuses such gift or in good faith fails to carry out the wishes of the donor as designated in the statement of gift, shall not be liable in damages on account thereof.

§ 26-28-6. Registration of gift — Information available without charge — Regulation by department.

Registration of a statement of gift shall remain effective for all purposes until a duly executed statement of revocation of the same gift is filed with the registration service. All information in the registry shall be of public record and available for inspection on request by any member of the public. No fees shall be charged or collected for registering or revoking a statement of gift, nor shall any fees be assessed for providing information or data in the registry to any licensed physician or surgeon, or representative of any hospital, medical school organ or tissue bank, or other person or institution authorized to be designated as a donee under this chapter. The department may establish a registration and indexing service to provide for the preservation and identification of statement of gift and may adopt, amend or rescind rules necessary to effectuate the registration provisions of this chapter.

§ 26-28-7. Prima facie evidence of gift.

Prima facie evidence that a valid and effective gift has been made consists of:

(1) an instrument or statement of gift in substantial conformity with Section 26-28-1, found on the person or among the personal effects of the donor at the time of his death;

(2) an instrument or statement of gift in substantial conformity with Section 26-28-1 found in the possession of the donee or his agent at the time of the donor's death; or

(3) an unrevoked registration of a statement of gift in the records of an authorized state or local registration service.

§ 26-28-8. Act to be liberally construed — Gifts made in other states.

This chapter shall be liberally construed and applied in order to carry out the purpose of providing legal procedures and safeguards by which effective gifts of parts of the human body may be made effective at death for medical, humanitarian, and scientific purposes. A gift within the purview of this chapter, made by any donor who dies within the state, shall be deemed valid and effective if valid under the law of this state or under the laws of the place where the instrument of gift was executed, and this chapter shall be fully applicable thereto.

VERMONT

UNIFORM ANATOMICAL GIFT ACT

§ 5231. Definitions.

(a) "Bank or storage facility" means a facility licensed, accredited, or approved under the laws of any state for storage of human bodies or parts thereof.

(b) "Decedent" means a deceased individual and includes a stillborn infant or fetus.

(c) "Donor" means an individual who makes a gift of all or part of his body.

(d) "Hospital" means a hospital licensed, accredited, or approved under the laws of any state, or a hospital operated by the United States government, a state, or a subdivision thereof, although not required to be licensed under state laws.

(e) "Part" means organs, tissues, eyes, bones, arteries, blood, other fluids and any other portions of a human body.

(f) "Person" means an individual, corporation, government or governmental subdivision or agency, business trust, estate, trust, partnership or association, or any other legal entity.

(g) "Physician" or "surgeon" means a physician or surgeon licensed or authorized to practice under the laws of any state.

(h) "State" means any state, district, commonwealth, territory, insular possession, and any other area subject to the legislative authority of the United States of America.

§ 5232. Persons who may execute an anatomical gift.

(a) Any individual of sound mind and who has attained the age of majority may give all or any part of his body for any purpose specified in section 5233 of this title, the gift to take effect upon death.

(b) Any of the following persons, in order of priority stated, when persons in prior classes are not available at the time of death, and in the absence of actual notice of contrary indications by the decedent or actual notice of opposition by a member of the same or a prior class, may give all or any part of the decedent's body for any purpose specified in section 5233 of this title:

(1) The spouse;

(2) An adult son or daughter;

(3) Either parent;

(4) An adult brother or sister;

(5) A guardian of the person of the decedent at the time of his death;

(6) Any other person authorized or under obligation to dispose of the body.

(c) If the donee has actual notice of a contrary indication by the decedent or that a gift by a member of a class is opposed by a member of the same or a prior class, the donee shall not accept the gift. The persons authorized by subsection (b) of this section may make the gift after or immediately before death.

(d) A gift of all or part of a body authorizes any examination necessary to assure medical acceptability of the gift for the purposes intended.

(e) The rights of the donee created by the gift are paramount to the rights of others except as provided by section 5237(d) of this title.

§ 5233. Persons who may become donees; purposes for which anatomical gifts may be made.

The following persons may become donees of gifts of bodies or parts thereof for the purposes stated:

(1) Any hospital, surgeon, or physician, for medical or dental education, research, advancement of medical or dental science, therapy, or transplantation; or

(2) Any accredited medical or dental school, college or university for education, research, advancement of medical or dental science, or therapy; or

(3) Any bank or storage facility, for medical or dental education, research, advancement of medical or dental science, therapy or transplantation; or

(4) Any specified individual for therapy or transplantation needed by him.

§ 5234. Manner of executing anatomical gifts.

(a) A gift of all or part of the body under section 5232(a) of this title may be made by will. The gift becomes effective upon the death of the testator without waiting for probate. If the will is not probated, or if it is declared invalid for testamentary purposes, the gift, to the extent that it has been acted upon in good faith, is nevertheless valid and effective.

(b) A gift of all or part of the body under section 5232(a) of this title may also be made by document other than a will. The gift becomes effective upon the death of the donor. The document, which may be a card designed to be carried on the person, must be signed by the donor in the presence of two witnesses who must sign the document in his presence. If the donor cannot sign, the document may be signed for him at his direction and in his presence in the presence of two witnesses who must sign the document in his presence. Delivery of the document of gift during the donor's lifetime is not necessary to make the gift valid.

(c) The gift may be made to a specified donee or without specifying a donee. If the latter, the gift may be accepted by the attending physician as donee upon or following death. If the gift is made to a specified donee who is not available at the time and place of death, the attending physician upon or following death, in the absence of any expressed indication that the donor desired otherwise, may accept the gift as donee. The physician who becomes a donee under this subsection shall not participate in the procedures for removing or transplanting a part.

(d) Notwithstanding section 5237(b) of this title, the donor may designate in his will, card, or other document of gift the surgeon or physician to carry out the appropriate procedures; provided, however, that eye enucleations may also be performed by a person who has successfully completed a course of training acceptable to the New England Eye Bank at the Massachusetts Eye and Ear Infirmary. In the absence of a designation or if the designee is not available, the donee or other person authorized to accept the gift may employ or authorize any surgeon or physician for the purpose.

(e) Any gift by a person designated in section 5232(b) of this title, shall be made by a document signed by him or made by his telegraphic, recorded telephonic, or other recorded message.

(f) A statement may be made by the holder of an operator's license that he is, by separate instrument, an anatomical gift donor.

§ 5235. Delivery of document of gift.

If the gift is made by the donor to a specified donee, the will, card, or other document, or an executed copy thereof, may be delivered to the donee to expedite the appropriate procedures immediately after death. Delivery is not necessary to the validity of the gift. The will, card, or other document, or an executed copy thereof, may be deposited in any hospital bank or storage facility or registry office that accepts it for safekeeping or for facilitation of procedures after death. On request of any interested party upon or after the donor's death, the person in possession shall produce the document for examination.

§ 5236. Amendment or revocation of the gift.

(a) If the will, card, or other document or executed copy thereof, has been delivered to a specified donee, the donor may amend or revoke the gift by:

(1) The execution and delivery to the donee of a signed statement, or

(2) An oral statement made in the presence of two persons and communicated to the donee, or

(3) A statement during a terminal illness or injury addressed to an attending physician and communicated to the donee, or

(4) A signed card or document found on his person or in his effects.

(b) Any document of gift which has not been delivered to the donee may be revoked by the donor in the manner set out in subsection (a) of this section, or by destruction or cancellation of the document and all executed copies thereof.

(c) Any gift made by a will may also be amended or revoked in the manner provided for amendment or revocation of wills, or as provided in subsection (a) of this section — 1969, No. 53, § 6.

§ 5237. Rights and duties at death.

(a) The donee may accept or reject the gift. If the donee accepts a gift of the entire body, he may, subject to the terms of the gift, authorize embalming and the use of the body in funeral services. If the gift is of a part of the body, the donee, upon the death of the donor and prior to embalming, shall cause the part to be removed without unnecessary mutilation. After removal of the part, custody of the remainder of the body vests in the surviving spouse, next of kin, or other persons under obligation to dispose of the body.

(b) The time of death shall be determined by a physician who tends the donor at his death, or, if none, the physician who certifies the death. The physician shall not participate in the procedures for removing or transplanting a part.

(c) A person who acts in good faith in accord with the terms of this chapter or with the anatomical gift laws of another state or foreign country is not liable for damages in any civil action or subject to prosecution in any criminal proceeding for his act.

(d) The provisions of this chapter are subject to the laws of this state prescribing powers and duties with respect to autopsies.

VIRGINIA

ANATOMICAL GIFTS

§ 32.1-289. Definitions.

As used in this article:

1. "Bank or storage facility" means a facility licensed, accredited or approved under the laws of any state for storage of human bodies or parts thereof.

2. "Decedent" means a deceased individual and includes a stillborn infant or fetus.

3. "Donor" means an individual who makes a gift of all or part of his body.

4. "Hospital" means a hospital licensed, accredited or approved under the laws of any state and a hospital operated by the United States government, a state, or a subdivision thereof which is not required to be licensed under state laws.

5. "Part" includes organs, tissue, eyes, bones, glands, arteries, blood, other fluids and other portions of a human body, and "part" includes "parts."

6. "Person" includes, in addition to the entities enumerated in paragraph 4 of § 32.1-3, a government and a governmental subdivision or agency.

7. "Physician" or "surgeon" means a physician or surgeon licensed or authorized to practice under the laws of any state.

8. "State" includes any state, district, commonwealth, territory, insular possession, and any other area subject to the legislative authority of the United States of America.

§ 32.1-289.1. Sale of body parts prohibited; exceptions; penalty.

With the exception of hair, blood and other self-replicating body fluids, it shall be unlawful for any person to sell, to offer to sell, to buy, to offer to buy or to procure through purchase any natural body part for any reason including, but not limited to, medical and scientific uses such as transplantation, implantation, infusion or injection. Nothing in this section shall prohibit the reimbursement of expenses associated with the removal and preservation of any natural body parts for medical and scientific purposes. This section shall not apply to any transaction pursuant to Article 3 (§ 32.1-298 et seq.), Chapter 8 of this title.

Any person engaging in any of these prohibited activities shall be guilty of a Class 6 felony.

§ 32.10289.2. Donation or sale of blood, body fluids, organs and tissues by persons infected with human immunodeficiency virus.

Any person who donates or sells, who attempts to donate or sell, or who consents to the donation or sale of blood, other body fluids, organs and tissues, knowing that the donor is, or was, infected with human immunodeficiency virus, and who has been instructed that such blood, body fluids, organs or tissues may transmit the infection, shall be guilty, upon conviction, of a Class 6 felony.

This section shall not be construed to prohibit the donation of infected blood, other body fluids, organs and tissues for use in medical or scientific research.

§ 32.1-290. Persons who may execute anatomical gift; when gift may be executed; examination of body authorized; rights of donee paramount.

A. Any individual of sound mind and eighteen years of age or more may give all or any part of his body for any purposes specified in § 32.1-291, the gift to take effect upon death.

B. Any of the following persons, in order of priority stated, when persons in prior classes are not available at the time of death and there is no actual notice of contrary indications by the decedent and no actual notice of opposition by a member of the same or a prior class, may give all or any part of the decedent's body for any purposes specified in § 32.1-291:

1. The spouse,

2. An adult son or daughter,

3. Either parent,

4. An adult brother or sister,

5. A guardian of the person of the decedent at the time of his death, or

6. Any other person authorized or under obligation to dispose of the body.

C. If the donee has actual notice of contrary indications by the decedent or that a gift by a member of a class is opposed by a member of the same or a prior class, the donee shall not accept the gift. The persons authorized by subsection B may make the gift after death or immediately before death.

D. A gift of all or part of a body authorizes any examination necessary to assure medical acceptability of the gift for the purposes intended.

E. The rights of the donee created by the gift are paramount to the rights of others except as provided by subsection E of § 32.1-295.

§ 32.1-291. Persons who may become donees; purposes for which anatomical gifts may be made.

The following persons may becomes donees of gifts of bodies or parts thereof for the purposes stated:

1. Any hospital, surgeon or physician, for medical or dental education, research, advancement of medical or dental science, therapy or transplantation; or

2. Any accredited medical or dental school, college or university, for education, research, advancement of medical or dental science or therapy; or

3. Any bank or storage facility, for medical or dental education, research, advancement of medical or dental science, therapy or transplantation; or

4. Any specified individual for therapy or transplantation needed by him.

§ 32.1-292. Manner of executing anatomical gifts.

A. A gift of all or part of the body under subsection A of § 32.1-290 may be made by will. The gift becomes effective upon the death of the testator without waiting for probate. If the will is not probated or if it is declared invalid for testamentary purposes, the gift, to the extent that it has been acted upon in good faith, is nevertheless valid and effective.

B. A gift of all or part of the body under subsection A of § 32.1-290 may also be made by document other than a will. The gift becomes effective upon the death of the donor. The document, which may be a card designed to be carried on the person, must be signed by the donor in the presence of two witnesses who must sign the document in his presence. If the donor cannot sign, the document may be signed for him at his direction and in his presence and in the presence of two witnesses who must sign the document in his presence. Delivery of the document of gift during the donor's lifetime is not necessary to make the gift valid.

C. The gift may be made to a specified donee or without specifying a donee. If the latter, the gift may be accepted by the attending physician as donee upon or following death. If the gift is made to a specified donee who is not available at the time and place of death, the attending physician upon or following death, in the absence of any expressed indication that the donor desired otherwise, may accept the gift as donee. Any physician who becomes a donee under this subsection shall not participate in the determination of death.

D. Except as provided in subsection C of this section and subsection C of § 32.1-295, the donor may designate in his will, card or other document of gift the surgeon or physician to carry out the appropriate procedures. In the absence of a designation, or if the designee is not available, the donee or other person authorized to accept the gift may employ or authorize any surgeon or physician for the purpose. In the case of a gift of eyes, in the absence of a designation by the donor or if such designee is not available, the donee or other person authorized to accept the gift may employ or authorize:

1. Any surgeon or physician; or

2. Any funeral service licensee or embalmer licensed in this Commonwealth who has successfully completed a course in eye enucleation in any accredited medical school in the United States; or

3. Any technicians who can document the successful completion of a course for ophthalmic medical assistance, provided by the American Association of Ophthalmology, and in addition has proof of successful completion of a course in eye enucleation as outlined in subdivision D 2 above, to enucleate eyes for such purpose.

In the case of a gift of skin, temporal bone or other bone, in the absence of a designation by the donor or if such designee is not available, the donee or other person authorized to accept the gift may employ or authorize to perform the appropriate procedures: (i) any physician or surgeon or in the case of temporal bone, any otolaryngologist or otorhinolaryngologist; (ii) any technician approved by the University of Virginia Skin Bank as qualified to perform the act of skin harvesting; (iii) any technician approved by the Virginia Tissue Bank as qualified to perform the act of skin or bone harvesting; or (iv) any funeral director or embalmer licensed in this Commonwealth who has completed a course for harvesting temporal bones as provided by the University of Virginia Hospital.

In the case of a gift of the brain to be used for confirmation of diagnosis and research into the etiology of any organic brain disease, the donee or other person authorized to receive the organ may employ or authorize a laboratory technician trained by a licensed neuropathologist to recover the brain.

Any person authorized by this section to perform eye enucleation, or recovery of skin, temporal bone and other bone or tissue or vascular organs may draw blood from the donor and order such tests as may be appropriate to protect his health and the health of the potential recipients of the tissues or organs.

E. A surgeon, physician, otolaryngologist, otorhinolaryngologist, funeral service licensee, embalmer, technician or ophthalmic assistant acting in accordance with the terms of this section shall not have any liability, civil or criminal, for the eye enucleation, recovery of the brain or other organ or harvesting of skin or bones.

§ 32.1-293. Delivery of document of gift.

If the gift is made by the donor to a specified donee, the will, card or other document, or an executed copy thereof, may be delivered to the donee to expedite the appropriate procedures immediately after death, but delivery is not necessary to the validity of the gift. The will, card or other document, or an executed copy thereof, may be deposited in any hospital, bank or storage facility or registry office that accepts them for safekeeping or for facilitation of procedures after death. On request of any interested party upon or after the donor's death, the person in possession shall produce the document for examination.

§ 32.1-294. Amendment or revocation of gift.

A. If the will, card or other document or executed copy thereof, has been delivered to a specified donee, the donor may amend or revoke the gift by:

1. The execution and delivery to the donee of a signed statement, or
2. An oral statement made in the presence of two persons and communicated to the donee, or
3. A statement during a terminal illness or injury addressed to an attending physician and communicated to the donee, or
4. A signed card or document found on his person or in his effects.

B. Any document of gift which has not been delivered to the donee may be revoked by the donor in the manner set out in subsection A or by destruction, cancellation, or mutilation of the document and all executed copies thereof.

C. Any gift made by a will may also be amended or revoked in the manner provided for amendment or revocation of wills or as provided in subsection A.

§ 32.1-295. Rights and duties at death.

A. The donee may accept or reject the gift. If the donee accepts a gift of the entire body, he may, subject to the terms of the gift, authorize embalming and the use of the body in funeral services. If the gift is of a part of the body, the donee, upon the death of the donor and prior to embalming, shall cause the part to be removed without unnecessary mutilation. After removal of the part, custody of the remainder of the body shall vest in the surviving spouse, next of kin or other persons under obligation to dispose of the body.

B. The provisions of Article 3 (§ 32.1-298 et seq.) of this chapter shall be applicable whenever a gift is made of a body for the purpose of medical or dental education, scientific study, research or advancement of medical or dental science and (i) no donee is specified or (ii) the donee requests the Commissioner to accept the body for distribution as provided in such article and the Commissioner accepts the body.

C. The time of death shall be determined by a physician who attends the donor at his death or, if none, the physician who certifies the death. This physician shall not participate in the procedures for removing or transplanting a part.

D. A person who acts in good faith in accord with the terms of this article, or under the anatomical gift laws of another state or a foreign country is not liable for damages in any civil action or subject to prosecution in any criminal proceeding for his act.

E. The provisions of this article are subject to the provisions of § 32.1-285.

§ 32.1-296. Determination of death.

The provisions of § 54-325.7 shall be applicable for the purposes of this article.

§ 32.1-297. Action for implied warranty in connection with transfer of blood or human tissue.

No action for implied warranty shall lie for the procurement, processing, distribution or use of whole blood, plasma, blood products, blood derivatives and other human tissue such as corneas, bones, or organs for the purpose of injecting, transfusing or transplanting any of them into the human body except where any defects or impurities in the said whole blood, plasma, blood products, blood derivatives and other human tissue such as corneas, bones, or organs are detectable by the use of established medical and technological procedures employed pursuant to the standards of local medical practice.

§ 32.1-297.1. (Effective July 1, 1986) The Virginia Transplant Council.

For the purpose of conducting educational and informational activities and coordinating such activities as they relate to organ and tissue procurement and transplantation efforts in the Commonwealth, there is hereby established the Virginia Transplant Council. The membership of the Council shall initially consist of the following organizations, each of whom shall have one vote: the University of Virginia Medical Center, the Medical College of Virginia, the Virginia Organ Procurement Agency, the Eastern Virginia Renal Transplant Program, the Eastern Virginia Tissue Bank, the Old Dominion Eye Bank, the Lion's Eye and Research Center of Eastern Virginia, the Eye Bank and Research Foundation of Virginia and the South-Eastern Organ Procurement Foundation. In order to provide flexibility, viable coordination and prevent duplication of efforts, the member organizations may agree to include as members of the Council other organizations directly involved in organ or tissue procurement or transplantation as they deem appropriate.

The Board of Health shall be designated as budgetary administrator of the Council and shall receive such funds as may be provided by the General Assembly in the appropriations act. The Board shall provide technical oversight for the Commonwealth of the activities of the Council and shall require such fiscal and substantive reports of the Council as it deems necessary. The Board shall report to the 1988 and 1991 Sessions of the General Assembly on the activities of the Council.

The Council shall conduct its activities in consultation and coordination with other organizations whose goals are related to organ or tissue procurement or transplantation including, but not limited to the End Stage Renal Disease Network of the Virginias, the North American Transplant Coordinators' Organization, the National Kidney Foundation of Virginia, the American Liver Foundation, the United Network for Organ Sharing and the Virginia Heart Association. To achieve its purpose efficiently and effectively, the Council may conduct its activities through its member organizations or may contract for services with appropriate parties.

WASHINGTON

ANATOMICAL GIFT LAW

§ 68.50.340. Definitions.

(1) "Bank or storage facility" means a facility licensed, accredited, or approved under the laws of any state for storage of human bodies or parts thereof including pacemakers.

(2) "Decedent" means a deceased individual and includes a stillborn infant or fetus.

(3) "Donor" means an individual who makes a gift of all or part of his body.

(4) "Hospital" means a hospital licensed, accredited, or approved under the laws of any state; includes a hospital operated by the United States government, a state, or a subdivision thereof, although not required to be licensed under state laws.

(5) "Part" means pacemakers, organs, tissues, eyes, bones, arteries, blood, other fluids and any other portions of a human body including artificial parts.

(6) "Person" means an individual, corporation, government or governmental subdivision or agency, business trust, estate, trust, partnership or association, or any other legal entity.

(7) "Physician" or "surgeon" means a physician or surgeon licensed or authorized to practice under the laws of any state.

(8) "State" includes any state, district, commonwealth, territory, insular possession, and any other area subject to the legislative authority of the United States of America.

§ 68.50.350. Gift of any part of body to take effect upon death authorized — Who may make — Priorities — Examination — Rights of donee paramount.

(1) Any individual of sound mind and eighteen years of age or more may give all or any part of his body for any purpose specified in RCW 68.50.360, the gift to take effect upon death.

(2) Any of the following persons, in order of priority stated, when persons in prior classes are not available at the time of death, and in the absence of actual notice of contrary indications by the decedent or actual notice of opposition by a member of the same or a prior class, may give all or any part of the decedent's body for any purpose specified in RCW 68.50.360:

(a) the spouse,

(b) an adult son or daughter,

(c) either parent,

(d) an adult brother or sister,

(e) a guardian of the person of the decedent at the time of his death,

(f) any other person authorized or under obligation to dispose of the body.

(3) If the donee has actual notice of contrary indications by the decedent or that a gift by a member of a class is opposed by a member of the same or a prior class, the donee shall not accept the gift. The persons authorized by subsection (2) may make the gift after death or during the terminal illness.

(4) A gift of all or part of a body authorizes any examination necessary to assure medical acceptability of the gift for the purposes intended.

(5) The rights of the donee created by the gift are paramount to the rights of others except as provided by RCW 68.50.400(4).

§ 68.50.360. Eligible donees — Eye removal by embalmers.

(1) The following persons may become donees of gifts of bodies or parts thereof for the purposes stated:

(a) Any hospital, surgeon, physician, or other entity which has a physician or surgeon as a regular full-time employee, for medical or dental education, research, advancement of medical or dental science, therapy, or transplantation;

(b) Any accredited medical or dental school, college or university for education, research, advancement of medical or dental science, or therapy;

(c) Any bank or storage facility, for medical or dental education, research, advancement of medical or dental science, therapy, or transplantation; or

(d) Any specified individual for therapy or transplantation needed by him.

(2) If the part of the body that is the gift is an eye, the donee or the person authorized to accept the gift may employ or authorize a qualified embalmer, licensed under chapter 18.39 RCW, to remove the eye.

§ 68.50.370. Gift by will, card, document, or driver's license — Procedures.

(1) A gift of all or part of the body under RCW 68.50.350(1), may be made by will. The gift becomes effective upon the death of the testator without waiting for probate. If the will is not probated, or if it is declared invalid for testamentary purposes, the gift, to the extent that it has been acted upon in good faith, is nevertheless valid and effective.

(2) A gift of all or part of the body under RCW 68.50.350(1), may also be made by document other than a will. The gift becomes effective upon the death of the donor. The document, which may be a card designed to be carried on the person, must be signed

by the donor in the presence of two witnesses who must sign the document in his presence. If the donor cannot sign, the document may be signed for him at his direction and in his presence in the presence of two witnesses who must sign the document in his presence. Delivery of the document of gift during the donor's lifetime is not necessary to make the gift valid.

(3) A gift of all or part of the body under RCW 68.50.350(1) may also be made by a statement provided for on Washington state driver's licenses. The gift becomes effective upon the death of the licensee. The statement must be signed by the licensee in the presence of two witnesses, who must sign the statement in the presence of the donor. Delivery of the license during the donor's lifetime is not necessary to make the gift valid. The gift shall become invalidated upon expiration, cancellation, revocation, or suspension of the license, and the gift must be renewed upon renewal of each license: Provided, That the statement of gift herein provided for shall contain a provision, including a clear instruction to the donor, providing for a means by which the donor may at his will revoke such gift: Provided further, That nothing in this chapter shall be construed to invalidate a donor card located elsewhere.

(4) The gift may be made to a specified donee or without specifying a donee. If the latter, the gift may be accepted by the attending physician as donee upon or following death. If the gift is made to a specified donee who is not available at the time and place of death, the attending physician upon or following death, in the absence of any expressed indication that the donor desired otherwise, may accept the gift as donee. The physician who becomes a donee under this subsection shall not participate in the procedures for removing or transplanting a part.

(5) Notwithstanding RCW 68.50.400(2), the donor may designate in his will, card, or other document of gift the surgeon or physician to carry out the appropriate procedures. In the absence of a designation or if the designee is not available, the donee or other person authorized to accept the gift may employ or authorize any surgeon or physician for the purpose.

(6) Any gift by a person designated in RCW 68.50.350(2), shall be made by a document signed by him or made by his telegraphic, recorded telephonic, or other recorded message.

§ 68.50.380. Delivery of will, card or other document to specified donee.

If the gift is made by the donor to a specified donee, the will, card, or other document, or an executed copy thereof, may be delivered to the donee to expedite the appropriate procedures immediately after death. Delivery is not necessary to the validity of the gift. The will, card, or other document, or an executed copy thereof, may be deposited in any hospital, bank or storage facility or registry office that accepts it for safekeeping or for facilitation of procedures after death. On request of any interested party upon or after the donor's death, the person in possession shall produce the document for examination.

§ 68.50.390. Amendment or revocation of gift.

(1) If the will, card, or other document or executed copy thereof, has been delivered to a specified donee, the donor may amend or revoke the gift by:

(a) the execution and delivery to the donee of a signed statement;

(b) an oral statement made in the presence of two persons and communicated to the donee;

(c) a statement during a terminal illness or injury addressed to an attending physician and communicated to the donee;

(d) a signed card or document found on his person or in his effects.

(2) Any document of gift which has not been delivered to the donee may be revoked by the donor in the manner set out in subsection (1) above, or by destruction, cancellation, or mutilation of the document and all executed copies thereof.

(3) Any gift made by a will may also be amended or revoked in the manner provided for amendment or revocation of wills, or as provided in subsection (1) above.

§ 68.50.400. Acceptance or rejection of gift — Time of death — Liability for damages.

(1) The donee may accept or reject the gift. If the donee accepts a gift of the entire body, he may, subject to the terms of the gift, authorize embalming and the use of the body in funeral services. If the gift is of a part of the body, the donee, upon the death of the donor and prior to embalming, shall cause the part to be removed without unnecessary mutilation. After removal of the part, custody of the remainder of the body vests in the surviving spouse, next of kin, or other persons under obligation to dispose of the body.

(2) The time of death shall be determined by a physician who tends the donor at his death, or, if none, the physician who certifies the death. The physician shall not participate in the procedures for removing or transplanting a part.

(3) A person who acts in good faith in accord with the terms of RCW 68.50.340 through 68.50.420 or with the anatomical gift laws of another state (or a foreign country) is not liable for damages in any civil action or subject to prosecution in any criminal proceeding for his act.

(4) The provisions of RCW 68.50.340 through 68.50.420 are subject to the laws of this state prescribing powers and duties with respect to autopsies.

§ 68.50.410. Uniformity.

RCW 68.50.340 through 68.50.420 shall be so construed as to effectuate its general purpose to make uniform the law of those states which enact it.

§ 68.50.420. Short title.

RCW 68.50.340 through 68.50.420 may be cited as the "Uniform Anatomical Gift Act".

§ 68.50.500. Identification of potential donors — Hospital procedures.

Each hospital shall develop procedures for identifying potential organ and tissue donors. The procedures shall require that any deceased individual's next of kin or other individual, as set forth in RCW 68.50.350, at or near the time of notification of death be asked whether the deceased was an organ donor. If not, the family shall be informed of the option to donate organs and tissues pursuant to the uniform anatomical gift act. With the approval of the designated next of kin or other individual, as set forth in RCW 68.50.350, the hospital shall then notify an established eye bank, tissue bank, or organ procurement agency including those organ procurement agencies associated with a national organ procurement transportation network or other eligible donee, as specified in RCW 68.50.360, and cooperate in the procurement of the anatomical gift or gifts. The procedures shall encourage reasonable discretion and sensitivity to the family circumstances in all discussions regarding donations of tissue or organs. The procedures may take into account the deceased individual's religious beliefs or obvious nonsuitability for organ and tissue donation. Laws pertaining to the jurisdiction of the coroner shall be complied with in all cases of reportable deaths pursuant to RCW 68.50.010.

§ 68.50.510. Good faith compliance with RCW 68.50.500 — Hospital liability.

No act or omission of a hospital in developing or implementing the provisions of RCW 68.50.500, when performed in good faith, shall be a basis for the imposition of any liability upon the hospital.

This section shall not apply to any act or omission of the hospital that constitutes gross negligence or wilful and wanton conduct.

§ 68.50.900. Effective date — 1987 c. 331.

See RCW 68.05.900.

WEST VIRGINIA

UNIFORM ANATOMICAL GIFT ACT

§ 16-19-1. Definitions.

(a) "Bank or storage facility" means a facility licensed, accredited, or approved under the laws of any state for storage or distribution of human bodies or parts thereof.

(b) "Certification of death" means a written pronouncement of death by the attending physician. Such certification shall be required before the attending physician shall allow removal of any bodily organs of the decedent for transplant purposes.

(c) "Death" means that a person will be considered dead if in the announced opinion of the attending physician, made in accordance with reasonable medical standards, the patient has sustained irreversible cessation of all functioning of the brain.

(d) "Decedent" means a deceased individual and includes a stillborn infant or fetus.

(e) "Donor" means an individual who makes a gift of all or part of his body.

(f) "Hospital" means a hospital licensed, accredited, or approved under the laws of any state; includes a hospital operated by the United States government, a state, or a subdivision thereof, although not required to be licensed under state laws.

(g) "Part" means organs, tissues, eyes, bones, arteries, blood, other fluids and any other portions of a human body.

(h) "Person" means an individual, corporation, government or governmental subdivision or agency, business trust, estate trust, partnership or association, or any other legal entity.

(i) "Physician" or "surgeon" means a physician or surgeon licensed or authorized to practice under the laws of any state.

(j) "State" includes any state, district, commonwealth, territory, insular possession, and any other area subject to the legislative authority of the United States of America.

§ 16-19-2. Persons who may execute an anatomical gift.

(a) Any individual of sound mind and eighteen years of age or more may give all or any part of his body for any purpose specified in section three [§ 16-19-3] of this article, the gift to take effect upon certification of death.

(b) Any of the following persons, in order of priority stated, when persons in prior classes are not available at the time of certification of death, and in the absence of actual notice of contrary indications by the decedent or actual notice of opposition by a member of the same or a prior class, may give all or any part of the decedent's body for any purpose specified in section three [§ 16-19-3] of this article:

(1) The spouse;

(2) An adult son or daughter;

(3) Either parent;

(4) An adult brother or sister;

(5) A guardian of the person of the decedent at the time of the certification of his death;

(6) Any other person authorized or under obligation to dispose of the body.

(c) If the donee has actual notice of contrary indications by the decedent or that a gift by a member of a class is opposed by a member of the same or a prior class, the donee shall not accept the gift. The persons authorized by subsection (b) of this section may make the gift after or immediately before certification of death.

(d) A gift of all or part of a body authorizes any examination necessary to assure medical acceptability of the gift for the purposes intended.

(e) The rights of the donee created by the gift are paramount to the rights of others except as provided by section seven [§ 16-19-7], subsection (d) of this article.

§ 16-19-3. Persons who may become donees; purposes for which anatomical gifts may be made; compliance with rules and regulations of board.

The following persons may become donees of gifts of bodies or parts thereof for the purposes stated:

(1) The West Virginia board of regents for the scientific purposes of educational institutions for which it may receive or requisition dead bodies; or

(2) Any hospital, surgeon or physician, for medical or dental education, research, advancement of medical or dental science, therapy or transplantation; or

(3) Any accredited medical or dental school, college or university for education, research, advancement of medical or dental science or therapy; or

(4) Any person operating a bank or storage facility for blood, arteries, eyes, pituitaries, or other human parts, for use in medical or dental education, advancement of medical or dental science, research, therapy or transplantation to individuals; or

(5) Any specified individual for therapy or transplantation needed by him.

The use, disposition and control of any such donated bodies or parts thereof by any such donee shall be in accordance with rules and regulations prescribed by the West Virginia board of regents.

§ 16-19-3a. Recovery of corneas; conditions; liability of medical examiner.

(a) In any case where a patient is in need of corneal tissue for a transplant, the chief medical examiner, assistance medical examiner, regional pathologist or any other person designated to perform an autopsy in accordance with article twelve [§ 61-12-1 et seq.], chapter sixty-one of this Code, may provide a cornea for transplant, under rules, regulations and procedures established by the chief medical examiner, upon the request of the medical eye bank of West Virginia, incorporated, under the following conditions:

(1) The body of the decedent having a suitable cornea for the transplant is under the jurisdiction of the chief medical examiner and an autopsy is required, in accordance with article twelve [§ 61-12-1 et seq.], chapter sixty-one of this Code;

(2) The decedent's next of kin makes no objections; and

(3) Transplanting of the cornea will not interfere with the course of any subsequent investigation or autopsy or alter the postmortem facial appearance.

(b) Neither the chief medical examiner, any assistant medical examiner, regional pathologist nor any other person designated to perform an autopsy in accordance with section ten [§ 61-12-10], article twelve, chapter sixty-one of this Code and who provides a cornea in accordance with the provisions of this section, nor the medical eye bank of West Virginia, incorporated, shall be liable for any civil damages if the decedent's next of kin subsequently contends that his authorization was required.

§ 16-19-4. Manner of executing anatomical gifts.

(a) A gift of all or part of the body under subsection (a), section two [§ 16-19-2(a)] of this article may be made by will. The gift becomes effective upon certification of death of the testator without waiting for probate. If the will is not probated, or if it is declared invalid for testamentary purposes, the gift, to the extent that it has been acted upon in good faith, is nevertheless valid and effective.

(b) A gift of all or part of the body under subsection (a), section two [§ 16-19-2(a)] of this article may also be made by document other than a will. The gift becomes effective upon certification of death of the donor. The document, which may be a card designed to be carried on the person, must be signed by the donor in the presence of two witnesses who must sign the document in his presence. If the donor cannot sign, the document may be signed for him at his direction and in his presence in the presence of two witnesses who must sign the document in his presence. Delivery of the document of gift during the donor's lifetime is not necessary to make the gift valid.

(c) The gift may be made to a specified donee or without specifying a donee. If the latter, the West Virginia board of regents will be considered to be the donee unless it declines to accept the gift, or unless there is urgent immediate need for a part of the body for transplant or other purposes in which case the gift may be accepted by the attending physician as donee upon or following certification of death. In case the board of regents is considered the donee it shall be the duty of the person who has charge or control of the body, if he or she has knowledge of the gift, to give notice thereof to the board of regents within twenty-four hours after such body comes under his or her control. Thereafter, he or she shall hold the body subject to the order of the board of regents for at least twenty-four hours after the sending of such notice. If the board of regents makes a requisition for the body within the twenty-four-hour period, it shall be delivered, pursuant to the order of the board, to the board or its authorized agent for transportation to an educational institution which the board deems to be in bona fide need thereof and able to adequately control, use and dispose of the body. If the board of regents shall not so act within the twenty-four-hour period, the gift may be accepted by the attending physician as donee upon or following certification of death. If the gift is made to a specified donee who is not available at the time and place of death, the attending physician upon or following certification of death, in the absence of any expressed indication that the donor desired otherwise, may accept the gift as donee. The physician who becomes a donee under this subsection shall not participate in the procedures for removing or transplanting a part, except that this prohibition shall not apply to the removing or transplanting of an eye or eyes.

(d) Notwithstanding subsection (b), section seven [§ 16-19-7(b)] of this article, the donor may designate in his will, card or other document of gift, the surgeon or physician to carry out the appropriate procedures, or in the case of a gift of an eye or eyes, the surgeon or physician or the technician properly trained in the surgical removal of eyes to carry out the appropriate procedures.

In the event of the nonavailability of such designee, or in the absence of a designation, the donee or other person authorized to accept the gift may employ or authorize for the purpose any surgeon or physician or in the case of a gift of an eye or eyes, any surgeon or physician or technician properly trained in the surgical removal of eyes or also in case of a gift of an eye or eyes, the donee or other person authorized to accept the gift may employ or authorize a licensed funeral director or embalmer licensed pursuant to article six [§§ 30-6-1 et seq.], chapter thirty of this Code who has successfully completed a course in enucleation approved by the medical licensing board of West Virginia to enucleate the eye or eyes for the gift after certification of death by a physician. The qualified funeral director or embalmer shall properly care for the enucleated eye or eyes and promptly deliver the eye or eyes to the donee or other person authorized to accept the gift. A qualified funeral director or embalmer acting in accordance with the terms of this subsection shall not be liable, civilly or criminally for the eye enucleation.

(e) Any gift by a person designated in subsection (b) [§ 16-19-2(b)], section two of this article shall be made by a document signed by him or made by his telegraphic, recorded telephonic or other recorded message.

(f) No particular words shall be necessary for donation of all or part of a body, but the following words, in substance, properly signed and witnessed, shall be legally valid for donations made pursuant to subsection (b) of this section:

"UNIFORM DONOR CARD
of

_____
Print or type name of donor

In the hope that I may help others, I hereby make this anatomical gift, if medically acceptable, to take effect upon certification of my death. The words and marks below indicate my desires.

I give: (a) _____ any needed organs or parts;
            (b) _____ only the following organs or parts _____
_____
                               Specify the organ(s) or part(s)
for the purposes of transplantation, therapy, medical research or education;
            (c) _____ my body for anatomical study if needed.
Limitation or special wishes, if any: _____
Signed by the donor and the following two witnesses in the presence of each other:

_____   _____
Signature of Donor   Date of Birth of Donor

_____   _____
Date Signed   City and State

_____   _____
Witness   Witness

This is a legal document under the Uniform Anatomical Gift Act or similar laws."

§ 16-19-4a. Request for consent to an anatomical gift.

(a) Where, based on accepted medical standards, a patient is a suitable candidate for organ or tissue donation, the person in charge of a hospital, or his or her designated representative other than a person connected with the determination of death, shall at the time of death request persons listed in this section for consent to an anatomical gift. In the order of priority stated and in the absence of actual notice of contrary indications by the decedent or actual notice of opposition by a member of the same or a prior class, any of the following persons may give all or any part of the decedent's body for any purpose specified in this article:

    (1) The spouse;

    (2) An adult son or daughter;

    (3) Either parent;

    (4) An adult brother or sister;

    (5) A guardian of the person of the decedent at the time of his death.

Where the person in charge of a hospital or his or her designee has received actual notice of opposition from any of the persons named in this subsection or where there is otherwise reason to believe that an anatomical gift is contrary to the decedent's religious beliefs, such gift of all or any part of the decedent's body shall not be requested. Where a donation is requested, consent or refusal need only be obtained from the person or persons in the highest priority class available.

(b) Where a donation is requested, the person in charge of a hospital or his designated representative shall complete a certificate of request for an anatomical gift, on a form supplied by the hospital. Said certificate shall include a statement to the effect that a request for consent to an anatomical gift has been made, and shall further indicate thereupon whether or not consent was granted, the name of the person granting or refusing the consent, and his or her relationship to the decedent. Upon completion of the certificate, said person shall attach the certificate of request for an anatomical gift to the death certificate.

(c) A gift made pursuant to the request required by this section shall be executed pursuant to applicable provisions of article nineteen [§ 16-19-1 et seq.] of this chapter.

(d) The director of health shall establish regulations concerning the training of hospital employees who may be designated to perform the request, and the procedures to be employed in making it.

(e) The director of health shall establish such additional regulations as are necessary for the implementation of this section.

(f) No hospital or person in charge of a hospital or his or her designated representatives shall be liable for damages for any action taken in good faith in the administering of the provisions of the article.

§ 16-19-5. Delivery of document of gift.

If the gift is made by the donor to a specified donee, the will, card, or other document, or an executed copy thereof, may be delivered to the donee to expedite the appropriate procedures immediately after death. Delivery is not necessary to the validity of the gift. The will, card, or other document, or an executed copy thereof, may be deposited in any hospital, bank or storage facility or registry office that accepts it for safekeeping or for facilitation of procedures after death. On request of any interested party upon or after the donor's death, the person in possession shall produce the document for examination.

§ 16-19-6. Amendment or revocation of the gift.

(a) If the will, card, or other document or executed copy thereof, has been delivered to a specified donee, the donor may amend or revoke the gift by:

(1) The execution and delivery to the donee of a signed statement; or

(2) An oral statement made in the presence of two persons and communicated to the donee; or

(3) A statement during a terminal illness or injury addressed to an attending physician and communicated to the donee; or

(4) A signed card or document found on his person or in his effects.

(b) Any document of gift which has not been delivered to the donee may be revoked by the donor in the manner set out in subsection (a) of this section or by destruction, cancellation, or mutilation of the document and all executed copies thereof.

(c) Any gift made by a will may also be amended or revoked in the manner provided for amendment or revocation of wills, or as provided in subsection (a) of this section.

§ 16-19-7. Rights and duties at death.

(a) The donee may accept or reject the gift. If the donee accepts a gift of the entire body, he may, subject to the terms of the gift, authorize embalming and the use of the body in funeral services. If the gift is of a part of the body, the donee, upon the death of the donor and prior to embalming, shall cause the part to be removed without unnecessary mutilation. After removal of the part, custody of the remainder of the body vests in the surviving spouse, next of kin, or other persons under obligation to dispose of the body.

(b) The time of death shall be determined by a physician who tends the donor at his death, or, if none, the physician who certifies the death. Such physician shall not participate in the procedures for removing or transplanting a part.

(c) A person who acts in good faith in accord with the terms of this article or with the anatomical gift laws of another state or a foreign country is not liable for damages in any civil action nor subject to prosecution in any criminal proceeding for his act.

(d) The provisions of this article are subject to the laws of this State prescribing powers and duties with respect to autopsies.

§ 16-19-7a. Prohibition of sales and purchases of human organs; penalties.

It shall be unlawful for any person to knowingly acquire, receive, or otherwise transfer for valuable consideration any human organ for use in human transplantation. The term human organ means the human kidney, liver, heart, lung, bone marrow, and any other human organ or tissue as may be designated by the director of health but shall exclude blood. The term "valuable consideration" does not include the reasonable payments associated with the removal, transportation, implantation, processing, preservation, quality control, and storage of a human organ or the expenses of travel, housing, lost wages incurred by the donor of a human organ in connection with the donation of the organ, or expenses incurred by nonprofit agencies or corporations to recover expenses incurred while offering services related to the location, maintenance and distribution of said human organs. Any person who violates this section is guilty of a misdemeanor, and, upon conviction thereof, shall be fined not less than five hundred nor more than one thousand dollars.

§ 16-19-8. Uniformity of interpretation.

This article shall be so construed as to effectuate its general purpose to make uniform the law of those states which enact it.

§ 16-19-9. Short title.

This article may be cited as the "Uniform Anatomical Gift Act."

WISCONSIN

UNIFORM ANATOMICAL GIFT ACT

§ 157.06. Uniform anatomical gift act.

(1) Definitions. (a) "Anatomical research" means a gift of the entire body to a medical or dental school anatomy department for purposes of dissection or other like purpose.

(am) "Bank or storage facility" means a facility licensed, accredited or approved under the laws of any state for storage of human bodies or parts thereof.

(b) "Decedent" means a deceased individual and includes a stillborn infant or fetus.

(c) "Donor" means an individual who makes a gift of all or part of his body.

(d) "Hospital" means a hospital licensed, accredited or approved under the laws of any state and includes a hospital operated by the U.S. government, a state, or a subdivision thereof, although not required to be licensed under state laws.

(e) "Part" means organs, tissues, eyes, bones, arteries, blood, other fluids and any other portions of a human body.

(f) "Physician" or "surgeon" means a physician or surgeon licensed or authorized to practice under the laws of any state.

(2) Persons who may execute an anatomical gift. (a) Except as provided in this paragraph, any individual of sound mind may give all or any part of his or her body for any purpose specified in sub. (3), the gift to take effect upon death. If a decedent has given his or her entire body to any donee for the purpose of anatomical research, a parent of an unmarried decedent under 18 years of age may revoke the gift. If a decedent has given his or her entire body to any donee for the purpose of anatomical research, unless the surviving spouse gave consent to the donation in writing prior to the donor's death, the surviving spouse of the decedent may revoke the gift.

(b) Any of the following persons, in order of priority stated, when persons in prior classes are not available at the time of death, and in the absence of actual notice of contrary indications by the decedent or actual notice of opposition by a member of the same or a prior class, may give all or any part of the decedent's body for any purpose specified in sub. (3):

1. The spouse.
2. An adult son or daughter.
3. Either parent.
4. An adult brother or sister.
5. A guardian of the person of the decedent at the time of his death.
6. Any other person authorized or under obligation to dispose of the body.

(c) If the donee has actual notice of contrary indications by the decedent or that a gift by a member of a class is opposed by a member of the same or a prior class, the donee shall not accept the gift. The persons authorized by par. (b) may make the gift after or immediately before death.

(d) A gift of all or part of a body authorizes any examination necessary to assure medical acceptability of the gift for the purposes intended.

(e) The rights of the donee created by the gift are paramount to the rights of others except as provided by subs. (2)(a) and (7)(d).

(2m) Hospital policy. (a) Each hospital shall have a policy based on accepted medical standards that requires, except as provided in par. (b), when a patient who is a suitable candidate for the gift of all or part of his or her body dies in the hospital, that the persons specified in sub. (2)(b) in the order and according to the procedure stated in sub. (2)(b) be requested to consider consenting to the gift of all or any part of the decedent's body, which has not already been given under sub. (2), for the purposes specified in sub. (3).

(b) The policy required under par. (a) does not have to require a request to consider consenting to a gift if the hospital has actual notice of contrary indications by the decedent or actual notice that a gift by a member of a class is opposed by a member of the same or a prior class under sub. (2)(b).

(c) If a gift is requested under par. (a), the hospital shall include in the decedent's medical records a statement that a request to consider consent to an anatomical gift has been made and the name of the person of whom the request is made, the person's relationship to the decedent and whether the person consented to or refused the request.

(3) Persons who may become donees; purposes for which anatomical gifts may be made. The following persons may become donees of gifts of bodies or parts thereof for the purposes stated:

(a) Any hospital, surgeon or physician, for medical or dental education, research, advancement of medical or dental science, therapy or transplantation; or

(b) Any accredited medical or dental school, college or university, for education, research, advancement of medical or dental science or therapy; or

(c) Any bank or storage facility, for medical or dental education, research, advancement of medical or dental science, therapy or transplantation; or

(d) Any specified individual for therapy or transplantation needed by him.

(4) Manner of executing anatomical gifts. (a) A gift of all or part of the body under sub. (2)(a) may be made by will. The gift becomes effective upon the death of the testator without waiting for probate. If the will is not probated, or if it is declared invalid for testamentary purposes, the gift, to the extent that it has been acted upon in good faith, is nevertheless valid and effective.

(b) A gift of all or part of the body under sub. (2)(a) may also be made by document other than a will. The gift becomes effective upon the death of the donor. The document, which may be a card designed to be carried on the person, must be signed by the donor in the presence of 2 witnesses who must sign the document in his presence. If the donor cannot sign, the document may be signed for him at his direction and in his presence in the presence of 2 witnesses who must sign the document in his presence. Delivery of the document of gift during the donor's lifetime is not necessary to make the gift valid.

(c) The gift may be made to a specified donee or without specifying a donee. If the latter, the gift may be accepted by the attending physician as donee upon or following death. If the gift is made to a specified donee who is not available at the time and place of death, the attending physician upon or following death, in the absence of any expressed indication that the donor desired otherwise, may accept the gift as donee. The physician who becomes a donee under this subsection shall not participate in the procedures for removing or transplanting a part.

(d) Notwithstanding sub. (7)(b), the donor may designate in his will, card or other document of gift the surgeon or physician to carry out the appropriate procedures. In the absence of a designation or if the designee is not available, the donee or other person authorized to accept the gift may employ or authorize any surgeon or physician for the purpose.

(e) Any gift by a person designated in sub. (2)(b) shall be made by a document signed by him or made by his telegraphic, recorded telephonic or other recorded message.

(5) Delivery of document of gift. If the gift is made by the donor to a specified donee, the will, card or other document, or an executed copy thereof, may be delivered to the donee to expedite the appropriate procedures immediately after death. Delivery is not necessary to the validity of the gift. The will, card or other document, or an executed copy thereof, may be deposited in any hospital, bank or storage facility or registry office that accepts it for safekeeping or for facilitation of procedures after death. On request of any interested party upon or after the donor's death, the person in possession shall produce the document for examination.

(6) Amendment or revocation of the gift. (a) If the will, card or other document, or executed copy thereof, has been delivered to a specified donee, the donor may amend or revoke the gift by:

1. The execution and delivery to the donee of a signed statement; or

2. An oral statement made in the presence of 2 persons and communicated to the donee; or

3. A statement during a terminal illness or injury addressed to an attending physician and communicated to the donee; or

4. A signed card or document found on his or her person or in his or her effects; or

5. Crossing out the donor authorization in the space provided on the driver's license as prescribed in s. 343.17(1)(c).

(b) Any document of gift which has not been delivered to the donee may be revoked by the donor in the manner set out in par. (a), or by destruction, cancellation or mutilation of the document and all executed copies of the document or by crossing out the authorization in the space provided on the license as prescribed in s. 343.17(1)(c).

(c) Any gift made by a will may also be amended or revoked in the manner provided for amendment or revocation of wills, or as provided in par. (a).

(7) Rights and duties at death. (a) The donee may accept or reject the gift. If the entire body is given for the purpose of anatomical research, it shall not be delivered to the donee or his agent if the surviving spouse or other person who assumes custody of the body requests a funeral service or other last rites for the deceased. If such a request is made, the body shall not be delivered until after the rites have been conducted. If the entire body is given for any purpose other than anatomical research or if the gift is of a part of the body, the donee, upon the death of the donor and prior to embalming, shall cause any parts given which it intends to remove to be removed without unnecessary mutilation. After removal of any such parts, custody of the remainder of the body vests in the surviving spouse, next of kin or other persons under obligation to dispose of the body.

(b) The medical certification of death under s. 69.18(2) shall be determined by a physician who tends the donor at his or her death or, if none, the physician who certifies the death. The physician shall not participate in the procedures for removing or transplanting a part.

(c) A person who acts in good faith in accord with the terms of this section or with the anatomical gift laws of another state (or a foreign country) is not liable for damages in any civil action or subject to prosecution in any criminal proceeding for his act.

(d) This section is subject to the laws of this state prescribing powers and duties of the coroner, medical examiner and other physicians licensed to perform autopsies with respect to autopsies and the reporting of certain deaths under ch. 979.

(e) Except as expressly provided in this section, nothing in this section affects rights or obligations of next of kin of a decedent.

(7m) Removal of eyes by funeral directors and persons acting under direction of physician.

In addition to any physician licensed to practice medicine and surgery under ch. 448, any person acting under the direction of a physician or any funeral director licensed under ch. 445, who has completed a course in eye enucleation and holds a valid certificate of competence from a medical college approved by the medical examining board under s. 448.05(2), may enucleate the eyes of a deceased donor under this section. A certificate of competence shall be valid for 3 years. No licensed funeral director so certified and no funeral establishment with which such a funeral director is affiliated shall be liable for damages resulting from such enucleation.

(8) Uniformity of interpretation. This section shall be so construed as to effectuate its general purpose to make uniform the law of those states which enact it.

(9) Short title. This act may be cited as the uniform anatomical gift act.

WYOMING

ANATOMICAL GIFTS

§ 35-5-101. Definitions.

(a) "Bank or storage facility" means a facility licensed, accredited, or approved under the laws of any state for storage of human bodies or parts thereof.

(b) "Decedent" means a deceased individual and includes a stillborn infant or fetus.

(c) "Donor" means an individual who makes a gift of all or part of his body.

(d) "Hospital" means a hospital licensed, accredited, or approved under the laws of any state; includes a hospital operated by the United States government, a state, or a subdivision thereof although not required to be licensed under state laws.

(e) "Part" means organs, tissues, eyes, bones, arteries, blood, other fluids and any other portions of a human body.

(f) "Person" means an individual, corporation, government or governmental subdivision or agency, business trust, estate, trust, partnership or association, or any other legal entity.

(g) "Physician" or "surgeon" means a physician or surgeon licensed or authorized to practice under the laws of any state.

(h) "State" includes any state, district, commonwealth, territory, insular possession, and any other area subject to the legislative authority of the United States of America.

§ 35-5-102. Donors generally; when donee not to accept gift; when gift to be made; examination of body; rights of donee.

(a) Any individual of sound mind and eighteen (18) years of age or more may give all or any part of his body for any purpose specified in W.S. 35-5-103, the gift to take effect upon death.

(b) Any of the following persons, in order of priority stated, when persons in prior classes are not available at the time of death, and in the absence of actual notice of contrary indications by the decedent or actual notice of opposition by a member of the same or a prior class, may give all or part of the decedent's body for any purpose specified in W.S. 35-5-103:

(i) The spouse;

(ii) An adult son or daughter;

(iii) Either parent;

(iv) An adult brother or sister;

(v) A guardian of the person of the decedent at the time of his death;

(vi) Any other person authorized or under obligation to dispose of the body.

(c) If the donee has actual notice of contrary indications by the decedent or that a gift by a member of a class is opposed by a member of the same or a prior class, the donee shall not accept the gift. The persons authorized by subsection (b) may make the gift after or immediately before death.

(d) A gift of all or part of a body authorizes any examination necessary to assure medical acceptability of the gift for the purposes intended.

(e) The rights of the donee created by the gift are paramount to the rights of others except as provided by W.S. 35-5-107(d).

§35-5-103. Donees generally.

(a) The following persons may become donees of gifts of bodies or parts thereof for the purposes stated:

(i) Any hospital, surgeon, or physician, for medical or dental education, research, advancement of medical or dental science, therapy, or transplantation; or

(ii) Any accredited medical or dental school, college or university for education, research, advancement of medical or dental science, or therapy; or

(iii) Any bank or storage facility, for medical or dental education, research, advancement of medical or dental science, therapy, or transplantation; or

(iv) Any specified individual for therapy or transplantation needed by him.

§ 35-5-104. Gift may be made by will or document; when gift effective; attending physician as donee; designation of surgeon or physician to carry out appropriate procedures.

(a) A gift of all or part of the body under W.S. 35-5-102(a) may be made by will. The gift becomes effective upon the death of the testator without waiting for probate. If the will is not probated, or if it is declared invalid for testamentary purposes, the gift, to the extent that it has been acted upon in good faith, is nevertheless valid and effective.

(b) A gift of all or part of the body under W.S. 35-5-102(a) may also be made by document other than a will. The gift becomes effective upon the death of the donor. The document, which may be a card designed to be carried on the person, must be signed by the donor in the presence of two (2) witnesses who must sign the document in his presence. If the donor cannot sign, the document may be signed for him at his direction and in his presence in the presence of two (2) witnesses who must sign the document in his presence. Delivery of the document of gift during the donor's lifetime is not necessary to make the gift valid.

(c) The gift may be made to a specified donee or without specifying a donee. If the latter, the gift may be accepted by the attending physician as donee upon or following. If the gift is made to a specified donee who is not available at the time and place of death, the attending physician upon or following death, in the absence of any expressed indication that the donor desired otherwise, may accept the gift as donee. The physician who becomes a donee under this subsection shall not participate in the procedures for removing or transplanting a part.

(d) Notwithstanding W.S. 35-5-107(b), the donor may designate in his will, card, or other document of gift the surgeon or physician to carry out the appropriate procedures. In the absence of a designation or if the designee is not available, the donee or other person authorized to accept the gift may employ or authorize any surgeon or physician for the purpose.

(e) Any gift by a person designated in W.S. 35-5-102(b) shall be made by a document signed by him or made by his telegraphic recorded telephonic, or other recorded message.

§ 35-5-105. Delivery of will or other document to specified donee; deposit for safekeeping; examination of document by interested party.

If the gift is made by the donor to a specified donee, the will, card, or other document, or an executed copy thereof, may be delivered to the donee to expedite the appropriate procedures immediately after death. Delivery is not necessary to the validity of the gift. The will, card, or other document, or an executed copy thereof, may be deposited in any hospital, bank or storage facility or registry office that accepts it for safekeeping or for facilitation of procedures after death. On request of any interested party upon or after the donor's death, the person in possession shall produce the document for examination.

§ 35-5-106. Amendment or revocation of gift.

(a) If the will, card, or other document or executed copy thereof, has been delivered to a specified donee, the donor may amend or revoke the gift by:

(i) The execution and delivery to the donee of a signed statement; or

(ii) An oral statement made in the presence of two (2) persons and communicated to the donee; or

(iii) A statement during a terminal illness or injury addressed to an attending physician and communicated to the donee; or

(iv) A signed card or document found on his person or in his effects.

(b) Any document of gift which has not been delivered to the donee may be revoked by the donor in the manner set out in subsection (a) of this section, or by destruction, cancellation, or mutilation of the document and all executed copies thereof.

(c) Any gift made by a will may also be amended or revoked in the manner provided for amendment or revocation of wills, or as provided in subsection (a) of this section.

§ 35-5-107. Acceptance or rejection of gift; embalming and use of body in funeral services; removal of part of body; custody or remains; by whom time of death determined; liability; provisions subject to state autopsy laws.

(a) The donee may accept or reject the gift. If the donee accepts a gift of the entire body, he may, subject to the terms of the gift, authorize embalming and the use of the body in funeral services. If the gift is of a part of the body, the donee, upon the death of the donor and prior to embalming, shall cause the part to be removed without unnecessary mutilation. After removal of the part, custody of the remainder of the body vests in the surviving spouse, next of kin, or other person under obligation to dispose of the body.

(b) The time of death shall be determined by a physician who tends the donor at his death, or, if none, the physician who certifies the death.

(c) A person who acts in good faith in accord with the terms of this act [§§ 35-5-101 through 35-5-109] or with the anatomical gift laws of another state is not liable for damages in any civil action or subject to prosecution in any criminal proceeding for his act.

(d) The provisions of this act are subject to the laws of this state prescribing powers and duties with respect to autopsies.

§ 35-5-108. Construction.

This act [§§ 35-5-101 through 35-5-109] shall be so construed as to effectuate its general purpose to make uniform the law of those states which enact it.

§ 35-5-109. Short title.

This act [§§ 35-5-101 through 35-5-109] may be cited as the Uniform Anatomical Gift Act.

§ 35-5-110. Transplantation of tissues, organs or components; exemption from liability; exceptions.

A physician, surgeon, hospital, blood bank, tissue bank, or other person or entity who donates, obtains, prepares, transplants, injects, transfuses or otherwise transfers, or who assists or participates in obtaining, preparing, transplanting, injecting, transfusing or transferring any tissue, organ, blood or component thereof from one (1) or more human beings, living or dead, to another human being, is not liable as the result of any such activity except for his or its own negligence or misconduct.

§ 35-5-111. Eye enucleation; person eligible to perform enucleation; certification requirements.

(a) A licensed funeral director or undertaker as defined in W.S. 33-16-301, a registered nurse licensed to practice in this state, a physician's assistant certified in Wyoming or an ophthalmic technician certified by the American Board of Ophthalmology may upon certification of competence under subsection (b) of this section, enucleate eyes for a gift in accordance with W.S. 35-5-101 through 35-5-109 after proper determination of death by a physician. For purposes of this subsection, proper determination of death does not mean the execution and registration of a formal death certificate.

(b) To perform eye enucleation under subsection (a) of this section, a qualified funeral director, undertaker, registered nurse, physician's assistant or ophthalmic technician shall first successfully complete a course in eye enucleation and receive certification of competence from a medical school in the United States and certified by the American Board of Ophthalmology. The certificate shall provide:

(i) The date of satisfactory completion of required course work; and

(ii) The name, address and qualifications of the person or institution providing certification and the notarized signature of that person or authorized representative of the institution.

§ 35-5-112. Driver's license indication of anatomical organ donors; procedure.

(a) The motor vehicle division of the department of revenue and taxation shall adopt and implement a program whereby anatomical organ donors may be so identified by an appropriate decal, sticker or other marking to be affixed to the driver's license or identification card of the person.

(b) The division shall provide space on every application for a driver's license or renewal thereof in which the applicant may indicate his desire to have the marking provided in subsection (a) of this section on his driver's license. In addition, any person whose license has not expired or who has already obtained a license may have the marking affixed by the division upon request.

(c) The division shall publish the existence of the program along with information regarding the procedures for having the marking affixed by the division upon request.

(d) The division shall notify its counterparts in each of the other states as to the existence of the program and the significance of the marking.

(e) No provision of this section shall be construed to modify or repeal any provisions of the Uniform Anatomical Gift Act [§§ 35-5-101 through 35-5-109], and the actual donation of an anatomical organ shall be in conformity with and subject to all provisions of the Uniform Anatomical Gift Act.

ASSOCIATIONS

American Association of Blood Banks
1117 N. 19th Street, Suite 600
Arlington, VA 22209
703-528-8200

American Association of Kidney Patients
211 East 43rd Street, Suite 301
New York, NY 10017
212-867-4486

American Association of Tissue Banks
1350 Beverly Road, Suite 220-A
McLean, VA 22101
703-827-9582

American Council on Transplantation
700 North Fairfax, Suite 505
Alexandria, VA 22314
703-836-4301

American Kidney Fund
6110 Executive Boulevard, Suite 1010
Rockville, MD 20852
800-638-8299

American Liver Foundation
998 Pompton Avenue
Cedar Grove, NJ 07009
201-857-2626

Association of Blood Donor Recruiters
1255 N. Milwaukee Avenue
Glenview, IL 60025
312-657-7342

Consortium of Registered Nurses for Eye Acquisition
1511 K Street, N.W., Suite 830
Washington, DC 20005
202-628-4280

Council of Community Blood Centers
725 15th Street, N.W., Suite 700
Washington, DC 20005
202-393-5725

Eye Bank Association of America
1511 K Street, N.W., Suite 830
Washington, DC 20005
202-628-4280

Eye-Bank for Sight Restoration
210 E. 64th Street
New York, NY 10021
212-980-6700

International Society for Heart Transplantation
435 North Michigan Avenue, Suite 1717
Chicago, IL 60611
312-644-0828

Lifebanc
1909 East 101st Street
Cleveland, OH 44106
216-791-5433

Living Bank
P.O. Box 6725
Houston, TX 77265
713-528-2971

Medic Alert Organ Donor Program
P.O. Box 1009
Turlock, CA 95381
209-668-3333

National Kidney Foundation
Two Park Avenue
New York, NY 10003
212-889-2210

National Organ Transplant Education Foundation
1275 K Street, N.W., Suite 900
Washington, DC 20005
202-371-0393

National Temporal Bone Banks Program of the DRF
Massachusetts Eye and Ear Infirmary
243 Charles Street
Boston, MA 02114
617-523-7900

North American Transplant Coordinators Organization
5000 Van Nuys Boulevard, Suite 400
Sherman Oaks, CA 90405
818-995-7338

Pittsburgh Transplant Foundation
5743 Center Avenue
Pittsburgh, PA 15206
412-366-6771

United Network for Organ Sharing
3001 Hungary Spring Road
P.O. Box 28010
Richmond, VA 23228
804-755-1600

GLOSSARY

Anatomical gift: a donation of all or part of a human body to take effect upon or after death.

Bank or storage facility: a facility licensed, accredited, or approved under the laws of any state for storage of human bodies or parts thereof.

Decedent: a deceased individual and includes a stillborn infant or fetus.

Document of a gift: a card, a statement attached to or imprinted on a motor vehicle operator's or chauffeur's license, a will, or other writing used to make an anatomical gift.

Donor: an individual who makes a gift of all or part of his body.

Enucleator: an individual who is certified by the Department of Ophthalmology to remove or process eyes or parts of eyes.

Eye bank: a nonprofit corporation chartered under the laws of the state to obtain, store, and distribute donor eyes to be used by ophthalmologists for corneal transplants, research, or other medical purposes.

Hospital: a hospital licensed, accredited, or approved under the laws of any state and includes a hospital operated by the United States government, a state, or a subdivision thereof, although not required to be licensed under state laws.

Part: organs, tissues, eyes, bones, arteries, blood, other fluids and any other portions of a human body.

Person: an individual, corporation, government or governmental subdivision or agency, business trust, estate, trust, partnership or association, or any other legal entity.

Physician or surgeon: a physician or surgeon licensed or authorized to practice under the laws of any state.

Procurement agency: any agency that has been certified or recertified by the secretary of the United States department of health and human services or any agency certified by the State Department of Health as a qualified organ or tissue agency.

State: any state, district, commonwealth, territory, insular possession, and any other area subject to the legislative authority of the United States of America.

Technician: any person, who is not a physician or surgeon, who is acting under the direction or supervision of a physician, surgeon, or hospital to remove or process a part.